Advanced Pain Management in Interventional Radiology

Case-Based Approach

J. David Prologo, MD, FSIR
Division Director, Interventional Radiology and Image Guided Medicine
Department of Radiology and Imaging Sciences
Emory University School of Medicine
Atlanta, Georgia, USA

Charles E. Ray Jr., MD, PhD, MHA
Professor and Head, Department of Radiology
University of Illinois College of Medicine;
Associate Chief Executive Officer, Strategic Alignment
University of Illinois Health
Chicago, Illinois, USA

476 illustrations

Thieme
New York • Stuttgart • Delhi • Rio de Janeiro

Library of Congress Cataloging-in-Publication Data is available from the publisher.

Important note: Medicine is an ever-changing science undergoing continual development. Research and clinical experience are continually expanding our knowledge, in particular our knowledge of proper treatment and drug therapy. Insofar as this book mentions any dosage or application, readersmay rest assured that the authors, editors, and publishers have made every effort to ensure that such references are in accordance with **the state of knowledge at the time of production of the book.**

Nevertheless, this does not involve, imply, or express any guarantee or responsibility on the part of the publishers in respect to any dosage instructions and forms of applications stated in the book. **Every user is requested to examine carefully** the manufacturers' leaflets accompanying each drug and to check, if necessary in consultation with a physician or specialist, whether the dosage schedules mentioned therein or the contraindications stated by the manufacturers differ from the statements made in the present book. Such examination is particularly important with drugs that are either rarely used or have been newly released on the market. Every dosage schedule or every form of application used is entirely at the user's own risk and responsibility. The authors and publishers request every user to report to the publishers any discrepancies or inaccuracies noticed. If errors in this work are found after publication, errata will be posted at www.thieme.com on the product description page.

Some of the product names, patents, and registered designs referred to in this book are in fact registered trademarks or proprietary names even though specific reference to this fact is not always made in the text. Therefore, the appearance of a name without designation as proprietary is not to be construed as a representation by the publisher that it is in the public domain.

Thieme addresses people of all gender identities equally. We encourage our authors to use gender-neutral or gender-equal expressions wherever the context allows.

Thieme Publishers New York
333 Seventh Avenue, 18th Floor
New York, NY 10001, USA
www.thieme.com
+1 800 782 3488, customerservice@thieme.com

Cover design: © Thieme
Cover image source: © Thieme
Typesetting by TNQ Technologies, India

Printed in India by Replika Press Pvt. Ltd.   5 4 3 2 1

DOI: 10.1055/b000000387

ISBN: 978-1-68420-140-2

Also available as an e-book:
eISBN (PDF): 978-1-68420-141-9
eISBN (epub): 978-1-63853-672-7

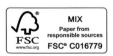

To Dana, for her unconditional support across a wildly expansive barrage of projects and interests—through which she has shown nothing but enthusiasm, encouragement, and love.

J. David Prologo, MD, FSIR

To Laura, for her support and understanding during the writing and editing of this book; and Carly, Erich, Ender, and Finley for reminding me of what matters most.

Charles E. Ray, Jr., MD, PhD, MHA

Contents

Videos

Preface

Pain is ubiquitous. Unfortunately, we all suffer some degree of pain at some point in our lives. As children, young adults, during middle age, and at the end of life, we will all experience ache, hurt, and smart. Most of our pain is self-limiting, and thankfully a majority of us will not suffer from unremitting, debilitating pain. However, this book is intended to help those individuals who do experience severe and life-limiting pain. Minimally invasive techniques are constantly being developed to aid these patients who trust the medical establishment to provide the best opportunity for relief with the fewest potential complications. Advancements have been spectacular, and development continues at a rapid pace, but discoveries cannot end now. It is not just the further advancement of techniques but also the adoption by individuals unfamiliar with the techniques that are already established which will further promote the field of advanced image-guided interventional techniques in the treatment of unrelenting pain. This book is for those practitioners who are interested in taking their practice to the next level.

J. David Prologo, MD, FSIR
Charles E. Ray, Jr., MD, PhD, MHA

Acknowledgements

We wish to acknowledge the tireless and creative efforts of Dr. Maxwell Edison Cooper in the creation of the videos for this book.

We would also like to express our sincere gratitude to Ms. Sumbul Jafri, project manager, and all the staff at Thieme for their professionalism and persistence in bringing this book through the production process.

J. David Prologo, MD, FSIR
Charles E. Ray, Jr., MD, PhD, MHA

Contributors

Sunil Agarwal, MD
Pain Medicine Physician
Department of Anesthesiology
Emory University School of Medicine
Atlanta, Georgia, United States

Osman Ahmed, MD
Associate Professor
Vascular and Interventional Radiology
University of Chicago
Chicago, Illinois, USA

Nicolas Amoretti, MD, HDR
Interventional Radiologist
Department of Radiology
Centre Hospitalier Universitaire de Nice
Hôspital Pasteur 2
Nice, France

Alexandra K. Banathy, MD
Resident Physician
Division of Vascular and Interventional Radiology
Department of Radiology & Medical Imaging
University of Virginia Health System
Charlottesville, Virginia, USA

Ross Bittman, MD
Resident Physician
Department of Radiology and Imaging Sciences
Emory University School of Medicine
Atlanta, Georgia, USA

Robert L. Bowers, DO, PhD
Assistant Professor, Orthopaedics
Assistant Professor, Physical Medicine and Rehab
Emory University School of Medicine
Emory Sports Medicine Centre;
Director, Baseball Medicine Program;
Team Physician
Atlanta Braves, Georgia Tech Baseball, College Park
    Skyhawks, Woodward Academy
Atlanta, Georgia, USA

Samuel E. Broida, BS, MD
Resident
Department of Orthopedic Surgery
Emory University School of Medicine
Atlanta, Georgia, USA

Anthony Brown, MD
Interventional Radiologist
Radiology Imaging Associates Endovascular
Denver, Colorado, USA

Juan C. Camacho, MD
Clinical Associate Professor
Department of Clinical Sciences
Florida State University;
Vascular & Interventional Radiologist
Radiology Associates of Florida
Sarasota, Florida, USA

Jordan Castle, MD
Interventional Radiologist
Inland Imaging
Spokane, Washington, USA

Aron Chary, MD
Assistant Professor of Radiology
Department of Radiology and Imaging Sciences
Emory University School of Medicine
Atlanta, Georgia, USA

Avneesh Chhabra, MD, MBA
Division Chief and Professor
Musculoskeletal Radiology
UT Southwestern Medical Center;
Professor
Department of Orthopaedic Surgery
UT Southwestern Medical Center;
Adjunct Faculty
University of Dallas
Dallas, Texas, USA;
Adjunct Faculty
John Hopkins University
London, United Kingdom;

Adjunct Faculty
Walton Centre for Neuroscience
Liverpool, United Kingdom

Daniel E. Dalili, MBBS, BSc
Interventional Radiologist
Department of Radiology, Southend University Hospital
Mid and South Essex NHS Trust
Essex, United Kingdom

Danoob Dalili, MBBS, FRCR, EDiMSK
Director of Interventional Spine
Academic Surgical Unit, South West London Elective
    Orthopaedic Centre
Epsom, Surrey, United Kingdom;
Department of Radiology
Epsom & St Helier University Hospitals NHS Trust
London, United Kingdom

A. Michael Devane, MD FSIR
Vice Chair Academic Affairs
Department of Radiology
Prisma Health Upstate;
Associate Professor
University of South Carolina School of Medicine
Greenville, South Carolina, USA

Faramarz Edalat, MD
Assistant Professor of Radiology
Department of Radiology and Imaging Sciences
Emory University School of Medicine
Atlanta, Georgia, USA

Nicholas Feinberg, MD
Instructor of Radiology
Department of Radiology
University of Chicago
Billings Hospital
Chicago, Illinois, USA

Dimitrios Filippiadis, MD, PhD, MSc, EBIR
Associate Professor of Diagnostic and
    Interventional Radiology
2nd Department of Radiology
University General Hospital "ATTIKON"
Medical School, National and Kapodistrian
    University of Athens
Chaidari, Athens, Greece

Christopher Florido, MD
Department of Radiology
University of Illinois
Chicago, Illinois, USA

Jan Fritz, MD, PD, RMSK
Associate Professor
Division Chief of Musculoskeletal Radiology
Department of Radiology
New York University Grossman School of Medicine
New York, New York, USA

Anne Gill, MD
Associate Professor
Department of Radiology & Imaging Sciences
Division of Interventional Radiology and
    Image-Guided Medicine
Emory University School of Medicine
Atlanta, Georgia, USA

Felix M. Gonzalez, MD
Senior MSK Interventional Radiologist
AdventHealth Radiology
Orlando, Florida, USA

Shenise Gilyard, MD
Assistant Professor
Division of Interventional Radiology
Department of Radiology
University of California School of Medicine
Los Angeles, California, USA

Andrew J. Gunn, MD
Associate Professor
Division of Vascular and Interventional Radiology
Department of Radiology
University of Alabama at Birmingham
Birmingham, Alabama, USA

John R. Hermansen, MD
Staff Physician
Co-director, Amputee and Musculoskeletal
    Medicine Fellowship
Department of Physical Medicine and
    Rehabilitation (PM&R)
Central Virginia Veterans Healthcare System
Department of PM&R
Virginia Commonwealth University
Richmond, Virginia, USA

Joshua A. Hirsch, MD
Professor
Department of Radiology
Massachusetts General Hospital
Boston, Massachusetts, USA

Junjian Huang, MD
Assistant Professor
Department of Radiology
Massachusetts General Hospital
Boston, Massachusetts, USA;
Department of Radiology
University of Alabama at Birmingham
Birmingham, Alabama, USA

Amanda Isaac, MBChB, MRCS, FRCR
Associate Professor
School of Biomedical Engineering & Imaging Sciences
Kings College London;
Department of Radiology
Guy's and St Thomas' NHS Foundation Trust
London, United Kingdom

Jack W. Jennings
Professor of Radiology and Orthopaedic Surgery
Mallinckrodt Institute of Radiology
Washington University in Saint Louis
Saint Louis, Montana, USA

Jerry P. Kalangara, MD
Associate Professor
Department of Anesthesiology
Division of Pain Medicine
Emory University School of Medicine
Atlanta, Georgia, USA

Amit Anand Karandikar, MBBS, FRCR, FAMS
Senior Consultant
Department of Diagnostic Radiology
Tan Tock Seng Hospital
Singapore

Alexis Kelekis, MD, PhD, MSc, EBIR
Professor of Diagnostic and Interventional Radiology
2nd Department of Radiology
University General Hospital "ATTIKON"
Medical School, National and Kapodistrian
    University of Athens
Chaidari, Athens, Greece

Kody Kleinrichert, MD
Lieutenant
Medical Corps US Navy;
Flight Surgeon
Marine Fighter Attack Training Squadron 501
Beaufort, South Carolina, USA

Nima Kokabi, MD
Associate Professor
Department of Radiology and Imaging Sciences
Emory University School of Medicine
Atlanta, Georgia, USA;
Division of Vascular and Interventional Radiology
Department of Radiology, University of North Carolina
Chapel Hill, North Carolina, USA

Jason Levy, MD, FSIR
Interventional Radiologist
Department of Interventional Radiology
Northside Hospital
Atlanta, Georgia, USA

Ming-Yann Lim, MBBS, DOHNS, MMed, FRCS, FAMS
Senior Consultant and Head
Department of Otorhinolaryngology and Head and
    Neck Surgery
Tan Tock Seng Hospital
Singapore

Will S. Lindquester, MD
Independent Interventional Radiology Resident
Department of Radiology
Emory University School of Medicine
Atlanta, Georgia, USA

Siu Cheng Loke, MBChB, MMED, FRCR
Senior Consultant
Department of Diagnostic Radiology
Tan Tock Seng Hospital
Singapore

Venkata Macha, BS
Medical Student (M4)
University of Alabama at Birmingham School of Medicine
Birmingham, Alabama, USA

Aneesa Majid, MD, MBA, FSIR
Interventional Radiologist
No Limits Radiology
Dallas, Texas, USA

Jon Marshall, DO
Interventional Radiologist
The Core Institute
North Phoenix Clinic
Phoenix, Arizona, USA

R. Amadeus Mason, MD
Assistant Professor
Department of Orthopaedics and Family Medicine
Emory University School of Medicine
Atlanta, Georgia, USA

Kenneth Mautner, MD
Associate Professor
Department of Orthopaedics and
    Rehabilitation Medicine
Emory University School of Medicine
Atlanta, Georgia, USA

J. Kevin McGraw, MD, FSIR
Medical Director, Interventional Radiology
Riverside Radiology and Interventional Associates, Inc.
Columbus, Ohio, USA

J. Reed McGraw, BS
Clinical Research Fellow
Hospital of the University of Pennsylvania
Philadelphia, Pennsylvania, USA

Jason W. Mitchell, MD, MPH, MBA, FSIR
Tallahassee, Florida, USA

James Morrison, MD
Interventional Radiologist
Department of Radiology
Michigan State University
Corewell Health
Grand Rapids, Michigan, USA

Amgad M. Moussa, MD
Assistant Professor
Interventional Radiology Service
Department of Radiology
Memorial Sloan Kettering Cancer Center;
Assistant Professor of Radiology
Weill Cornell University
Manhattan, New York, USA

Thomas Murphy, MD
Interventional Radiologist
Quantum Interventional Radiology
Atlanta, Georgia, USA

Nariman Nezami, MD
Associate Professor
Department of Diagnostic Radiology and
    Nuclear Medicine
University of Maryland School of Medicine
Baltimore, Maryland, USA;
Experimental Therapeutics Program
University of Maryland Marlene & Stewart
    Greenebaum Comprehensive Cancer Center
Baltimore, Maryland, USA;
Fischell Department of Bioengineering
University of Maryland
College Park, Maryland, USA

Ashley M. L. Nguyen, MD
Pre-Medical Student
Neuroradiology and Pain Solutions of Oklahoma
Oklahoma, Oklahoma, USA

Dan T. D. Nguyen, MD
Medical Director
Neuroradiology and Pain Solutions of Oklahoma
Oklahoma, Oklahoma, USA

William G. O'Connell, MD
Assistant Professor
Department of Radiology and Imaging Sciences
Emory University School of Medicine
Atlanta, Georgia, USA

Oluseun A. Olufade, MD
Assistant Professor
Department of Orthopaedics
Emory University School of Medicine
Atlanta, Georgia, USA

David J. Park, MD
Former Chief Resident
Department of Orthopaedics and Rehabilitation Medicine
Tufts Medical Center
Boston, Massachusetts, USA

Parham Pezeshk, MD
Associate Professor
Division of Musculoskeletal Radiology
Department of Radiology
UT Southwestern Medical Center
Dallas, Texas, USA

Sudheer Potru
Assistant Professor
Anesthesiology Service Line
Health Care System
Atlanta, Virginia, USA;
Department of Anesthesiology
Division of Pain Medicine
Emory University School of Medicine
Atlanta, Georgia, USA

J. David Prologo, MD, FSIR
Associate Professor
Division of Interventional Radiology
Department of Radiology and Imaging Sciences
Emory University School of Medicine
Atlanta, Georgia, USA

Uei Pua, MBBS, FRCR (UK), MMed, FAMS, FCIRSE, FSIR
Professor
Department of Diagnostic Radiology
Tan Tock Seng Hospital;
Yong Loo Lin School of Medicine
National University of Singapore
Singapore

Charles E. Ray Jr., MD, PhD, MHA
Professor and Head, Department of Radiology
University of Illinois College of Medicine;
Associate Chief Executive Officer, Strategic Alignment
University of Illinois Health
Chicago, Illinois, USA

Ernesto Santos
Attending Radiologist
Division of Interventional Radiology
Memorial Sloan Kettering Cancer Center
New York, New York, USA

Daniel P. Sheeran, MD
Assistant Professor
Division of Vascular and Interventional Radiology
Department of Radiology & Medical Imaging
University of Virginia Health System
Charlottesville, Virginia, USA

Vinita Singh, MD
Associate Professor
Department of Anesthesiology
Division of Pain Medicine
Emory University School of Medicine
Atlanta, Georgia, USA

Kyle Sonnabend, DO, MD
Chief Resident
Department of Radiology
University of Illinois
Chicago, Illinois, USA

Walter I. Sussman, DO
Assistant Clinical Professor
Department of Orthopaedics and Rehabilitation
Tufts University
Boston, Massachusetts, USA;
Managing partner
Boston Sports & Biologics
Wellesley, Massachusetts, USA

Uma Thakur, MD
Assistant Professor
Division of Musculoskeletal Radiology
Department of Radiology
UT Southwestern Medical Center
Dallas, Texas, USA

Nicolas Theumann, MD
Professor
Department of Radiology
Bois-Cerf Clinic
Lausanne, Switzerland

Anderanik Tomasian, MD
Associate Professor
Department of Radiological Sciences
University of California Irvine
Orange, California, USA

Vibhor Wadhwa, MD
Interventional Radiology Fellow
Division of Interventional Radiology
Department of Radiology
Weill Cornell Medical Center
New York, New York, USA

Luke R. Wilkins, MD, FSIR
Associate Professor
Division of Vascular and Interventional Radiology
Department of Radiology & Medical Imaging
University of Virginia Health System
Charlottesville, Virginia, USA

Roger Williams, DO
Interventional Radiologist
Quantum Interventional Radiology
Atlanta, Georgia, USA

Nan Xiang, MD
Assistant Professor
Department of Anesthesiology
Division of Pain Medicine
Emory University School of Medicine
Atlanta, Georgia, USA

Zohyra E. Zabala, MD
Post Doctoral Research Fellow
Department of Endocrinology
Division of Endocrinology, Metabolism & Lipids
Emory University School of Medicine
Atlanta, Georgia, USA

1 The Opioid Crisis: A Brief History

Christopher Florido, Kyle Sonnabend and Charles E. Ray Jr.

1.1 History

The opium poppy (*Papaver somniferum*) is a domesticated annual plant and today it is found only in association with human activity, seen either in planted fields or incidentally in environments near these cultivated areas.[1] The exact origins of the plant have not been identified, and no wild progenitor is known.[1] Throughout history the opium poppy has been used for a variety of purposes including as food and for oil from its seeds, as well as animal fodder and heating fuel from its stalks. Most notoriously, it has been used for its analgesic and euphoric properties. The poppy capsule contains more than 50 alkaloids including morphine, codeine, thebaine, and papaverine, among others.[1] These compounds can be obtained by slicing the capsule and extracting the opium latex and, in more recent history, have been isolated and concentrated for both medicinal and recreational use.

It is difficult to pinpoint the first recorded cultivation and use of the opium poppy because descriptions of drugs and medications by ancient authors tend to be ambiguous. That said, many sources seem to agree that the Sumerians of ancient Mesopotamia (a region of Western Asia roughly corresponding to modern-day Iraq, Kuwait, Eastern Syria, and Southeastern Turkey) cultivated poppies and isolated opium from poppy seeds in the third millennium BC.[2] They referred to the poppy as "hul gil" or "the plant of joy." Early descriptions of opium poppy use suggest it was taken orally or inhaled from heated vessels as part of religious rituals. It would eventually become widely used for both medicinal and recreational purposes. Wherever it originated, opium cultivation spread to ancient Greek, Persian, and Egyptian societies.

Egyptians obtained knowledge of the opium poppy from the ancient Sumerians and began cultivation of opium around 1300 BC.[3] The opium trade flourished during the reign of Thutmose IV, Akhenaton, and King Tutankhamen. The trade route extended to the Phoenicians and Minoans who would move the opium poppy into Greece, Carthage, and Europe.[3]

There are many references to the opium poppy in the ancient Greek culture. The divinities Hypnos (Sleep), Nxy (Night), and Thanatos (Death) were portrayed wearing wreaths containing poppies or with poppies in their hands.[4] In *The Odyssey*, the Greek author Homer refers to a preparation given to Telemachus and his friends by Helen, the daughter of Zeus, to forget their grief over Odysseus' absence. Some modern pharmacologists believe that this preparation contained opium.[2] Hippocrates, the "father of modern medicine," mentions the inclusion of the opium poppy in medicinal preparations for use as a hypnotic, narcotic, and cathartic.[4]

Starting around the 8th century AD, Arab traders brought the opium poppy to India and China. Between the 10th and 13th centuries trade extended from Asia to all parts of Europe.[2] Manuscripts from the 16th century describe opioid abuse and tolerance in Turkey, Egypt, Germany, and England. The problem of addiction was perhaps most rampant in China where the practice of smoking opium became commonplace in the mid-17th century when tobacco smoking was banned.[2] Although suppression of the sale and use of opium in China was attempted, these efforts ultimately failed because the British and French forced the Chinese to permit opium trade through various means.[2]

German pharmacist Friedrich Wilhelm Adam Sertürner isolated the active ingredient in opium between 1803 and 1806.[2] He named this alkaloid "morphine" after Morpheus, the "god of dreams."[2] It was first marketed commercially by Merck pharmaceuticals in 1827.[5] Its use became more widespread after the invention of the hypodermic syringe and hollow needle in the 1850s. It was at this time that morphine began to be used for minor surgical procedures, postoperative pain, chronic pain, and as an adjunct to general anesthetics.[2] Although the problem of opium addiction was well known at this time both in the United States and abroad, it was assumed that because injected morphine could control pain at much lower doses, it would be less likely to cause addiction.[6] When heroin was first synthesized in 1898, it was similarly pronounced to be more potent and therefore have less potential for addiction.[2] These examples are the first instances when such unfounded (and ultimately untrue) claims have been made about an opioid drug, but not the last.

The discovery of morphine and heroin would lead to the first wave of opioid addiction in the United States. This first epidemic had diverse origins stemming from a poor understanding of the etiology of painful conditions to the lack of alternative therapies. These drugs saw uses including (but not limited to) treatment of the common cold, diarrhea, hangovers, and painful injuries.[7]

In the first half of the 20th century, the addictive potential of morphine and heroin became the subject of much political debate in the United States. Initially, individual states were allowed to regulate the manufacture and sale of these substances. Then, the "Harrison Act" was passed in 1914 which imposed taxes on all aspects of opioid import, production, and sale, and also (more or less) restricted the legal use of opioids to patients with a medical prescription. Interestingly, the Supreme Court's interpretation of the act ultimately decided that opioids could be prescribed for symptomatic treatment of pain but not for maintenance of addiction.[6] Following the "Harrison Act," increasingly severe laws regarding the sale and possession of opiates were passed at the federal level. This ultimately led toward mandatory minimum prison sentences of 10 years by 1956.

In addition to increasingly strict laws and policies, additional social strategies were employed in the first half of the 20th century. The primary tactics of these campaigns were silence and exaggeration.[6] Silence took the form of suppression of exposure to opioids, such as banning films that depicted narcotic use. Exaggeration took the form of a national campaign launched in 1924 which made false claims, for example, the claim that one ounce of heroin could addict 2000 people.[6] The goal of these strategies was to discourage experimentation and abuse, but ultimately these tactics led to widespread ignorance and ultimately a loss of credibility regarding government statements on narcotics. This paved the way for a renewed enthusiasm for narcotic use starting in the 1960s. For the remainder of the

20th century, opioid addiction epidemics in the United States primarily resulted from transient increases in illicit heroin use in urban areas.[7] Starting in the 1990s that would change.

The opioid crisis in the United States was declared a national public health emergency in 2017.[8] Although continued illicit production and sale of opioids are factors in this epidemic, sanctioned medical use also plays a significant role. In the 1990s, the American Pain Society pronounced pain as a "fifth vital sign" in an effort to improve patient care. The American Pain Society, in partnership with the American Academy of Pain Medicine, also released a consensus statement endorsing the use of opioids to treat chronic pain in noncancer patients. Concurrently, the pharmaceutical industry initiated aggressive marketing campaigns that advocated long-term use of opioids to treat chronic pain and simultaneously minimize the risks of addiction. In tandem with the efforts of the American Pain Society to improve patient care with regard to pain, state medical boards loosened restrictions on opioid prescription. As a result, retail sales of the drugs oxycodone and hydrocodone increased by 866 and 280%, respectively, from 1997 to 2007.[9] Aggressive marketing campaigns and concordant high-volume prescriptions are believed to be major contributors to increasing opioid abuse and opioid-related deaths. In fact, an estimated 80% of Americans who become addicted to heroin start with prescription opioids.[9]

The modern opioid epidemic is a challenging problem with a complex history. Chronic opioid addiction is a life-threatening disease, and efforts to combat the epidemic must contend with all facets of the problem, including illicit production, as well as medical use under prescriptive authority.

1.2 Epidemiology

The World Health Organization (WHO) and Centers for Disease Control and Prevention (CDC) track cases of illicit drug use, nonfatal overdose, and drug-related deaths. According to the WHO, an estimated 275 million people (worldwide) used an illicit drug at least once in 2016.[10] Out of those, an estimated 34 million people used opioids and an estimated 27 million people suffered from opioid use disorders.[10] The majority of people with opioid dependence are reported to use illicit substances such as heroin but there are an increasing proportion of people using prescription opioids.[10]

The WHO data show that approximately 450,000 people (globally) died as a result of drug overdose in 2015, with approximately 118,000 of those deaths associated with opioid use disorders.[10] The WHO also notes that overdose is implicated in one-third to one-half of all drug-related deaths, and that most cases are attributable to opioids.[10] Of these data, perhaps most disconcerting is the fact that the lifetime prevalence of witnessed overdose in drug users is around 70% but yet less than 10% of people receive effective treatment for opioid dependence.[10]

Opioid overdose can be identified by a triad of signs and symptoms which include pinpoint pupils, loss of consciousness, and respiratory depression. Respiratory depression in particular is typically the cause of death in cases of opioid overdose.[10] Because of this, combining opioids with other sedative medications or alcohol can result in an increased risk of death.[10] Furthermore, people with opioid dependence are the most likely to suffer from an overdose. This likely relates to drug tolerance experienced by these individuals, which in turn leads to increasing doses and the potential for more profound respiratory depression.[10]

The WHO information sheet on opioid overdose released in August 2018 reveals that in the United States there were an estimated 63,632 deaths related to drug overdose in 2016. This number reflects a 21% increase from previous years and is thought to be largely related to an increase in deaths associated with opioids, more specifically prescription opioids.[10] In fact, prescription opioids (with the exception of methadone, which is used to treat opioid dependence) were associated with 19,413 deaths in the United States in 2016 alone.[10]

The CDC released a National Center for Health Statistics (NCHS) data brief on drug overdose deaths in the United States (1999–2018) in January 2020. The data revealed 67,367 drug overdose deaths in the United States in 2018, with opioids implicated in 46,802 of those deaths (approximately 70% of all drug overdose deaths).[11] Of the opioid overdose deaths, two out of three involved synthetic opioids (excluding methadone).

Overall, the NCHS data demonstrate a significant increasing trend in drug overdose deaths (for all drugs combined) from 1999 to 2018. The age-adjusted rate of drug overdose deaths increased from 6.1 per 100,000 standard population in 1999 to 21.7 per 100,000 standard population in 2017. Interestingly, there was a statistically significant decrease in drug overdose deaths (for all drugs combined) of 4.6% from 2017 to 2018. Despite this, the rate of drug overdose deaths involving synthetic opioids (excluding methadone) increased by 10% in the same 1-year period.[11]

Opioids were implicated in 446,032 deaths in the United States from 1999 to 2018. As previously mentioned, rates of overdose deaths for all drugs decreased from 2017 to 2018. This includes decreased deaths from all opioids (down 2%), prescription opioids (down 13.5%), and heroin (down 4.1%); an increase in death rates was seen only with synthetic opioids (up 10%).[12] This recent downward trend in prescription opioid-related deaths is encouraging, and may at least in part reflect efforts to reduce high dose opioid prescribing. The smaller decrease in heroin-related deaths could be explained by at least two factors: decreased use of heroin in favor of synthetic opioids such as fentanyl and expansion of naloxone access for heroin users.[12]

The CDC also publishes data on opioid prescribing rates in the United States. These data show an increasing rate of prescriptions from 2006 to 2012 (215,917,663 to 255,207,954) with a decreasing rate from 2012 to 2018 (down to 168,158,611 in 2018).[13] This favorable change in prescribing patterns seems to be producing results, and mirrors the recent 13.5% decrease in deaths related to prescription opioids. Although encouraging, the reduced availability of prescription opioids could be a driving force behind the increasing death rate related to synthetic opioids. In fact, not only is the death rate related to synthetic opioids increasing, but individuals with reported law-enforcement encounters testing positive for synthetic opioids such as fentanyl are on the rise since 2013. Most of the recent deaths related to synthetic opioids do not involve prescription opioids but rather are related to illicitly produced fentanyl, which is mixed with or sold as heroin, sometimes without the user's knowledge.[14] Continued investigation into these trends is paramount in the ongoing efforts to combat the opioid epidemic.

The epidemiologic data discussed above show that the opioid epidemic is complex and multifactorial. Strategies aimed at solving this problem must therefore take into account these myriad facets of the problem. Strategies that target illicit production, sale, and use of heroin as well as synthetic opioids may differ from those that target dependence and abuse related to prescription opioids.[15] Although the aforementioned recent data regarding prescription opioids are promising, there remains much work to be done. This is perhaps most poignantly illustrated by a CDC study of opioid-related hospitalizations published in November of 2019, which shows that 90% of opioid-related hospitalizations in the United States in all years from 2011 to 2015 involved patients with two or more chronic conditions. The highest prevalence was noted in patients aged 35 to 54 years suffering from conditions including cancer, stroke, obesity, asthma, liver disease, and arthritis.[15] These findings suggest that alternative approaches (those that seek to decrease or eliminate the role of opioids) to chronic pain management are essential in order to truly curb the worsening of the opioid epidemic.

1.3 Drugs

Following the discovery of morphine in 1827, many new synthetic and semi-synthetic opioids have been produced, some of which are commonly used for the treatment of pain. Each drug is different, each with unique properties including different side effects. In order to most safely and effectively prescribe these drugs, knowledge of these differences is essential. The following section contains pertinent facts regarding commonly used opioid medications; ▶ Table 1.1 provides an overview of many of these drugs.

1.3.1 Opioids

Morphine: Intravenous, epidural, or intrathecal administration of morphine should only be performed if supplemental oxygen and the equipment for emergency airway placement are present, as potentially fatal respiratory depression can occur.[16,17] Morphine is primarily metabolized by the liver and secreted through the urinary system. Care must be taken in elderly patients and in patients with renal insufficiency, as the buildup of morphine metabolites can cause unwanted side effects or increased potency.[16]

Codeine: Compared to the other opioids, codeine is a weak agonist of the opioid receptor with minimal analgesic effect.[16] The analgesic effects of codeine come from its metabolites morphine-6-glucuronide and morphine-3-glucuronide.[16] Intravenous use is not recommended as it is associated with a significant risk of severe hypotension.

Table 1.1 Opioids commonly used to treat chronic pain

Drug	Route/Dose	Duration and Half-Life	Side Effects	Reversal Agent
Natural Opioids				
Morphine	Intravenous: 1–4 mg every 1 to 4 hours as needed Oral: 10 mg every 4 hours as needed	Intravenous onset: 5–10 minutes Duration: 3–4 hours Half-life: 1.5–2 hours Oral onset: 30 minutes Duration: 3–5 hours	Respiratory depression, hypotension, bradycardia, seizures, confusion, itching, rash	Naloxone
Semi-synthetic				
Oxycodone	Oral (immediate release): 5 to 15 mg tablets every 4 to 6 hours as needed	Onset: 10–15 minutes Duration: 3–6 hours Half-life: 4 hours	Respiratory depression, drowsiness, nausea, constipation	Naloxone
Hydrocodone (commonly combined with acetaminophen)	Oral: 5 mg/325 mg tablet (hydrocodone/acetaminophen) One to two tablets every 4–6 hours Maximum adult acetaminophen dose: 4,000 mg per 24 hours	Onset: Within 60 minutes Duration: 12–24 hours Half-life: 7–13 hours	Respiratory depression, drowsiness, nausea, constipation	Naloxone
Hydromorphone	Oral: 2–4 mg tablet every 4–6 hours as needed	Onset: 15–30 minutes Duration: 12–24 hours Half-life: 11 hours	Respiratory depression, drowsiness, nausea, constipation	Naloxone
Oxymorphone	Oral: 2.5–5 mg tablet every 4–6 hours as needed	Onset: 10–15 minutes Duration: 3–6 hours Half-life: 7–9 hours	Respiratory depression, drowsiness, nausea, constipation	Naloxone
Synthetic				
Tramadol	Oral: 25–50 mg tablet every 6 hours as needed	Onset: Within 60 minutes Duration: 6–9 hours Half-life: 5–6 hours	Respiratory depression, drowsiness, nausea, constipation	Diazepam–Naloxone combination
Fentanyl	Transdermal: 12–25 μg patch applied every 72 hours	Onset: 6 hours Duration: 48–72 hours with effects lasting up to 12 hours after patch removal Half-life: 17 hours following patch removal	Respiratory depression, drowsiness, nausea, constipation	Naloxone

Fentanyl: Intravenous fentanyl is not very effective for long-term pain relief because the half-life is relatively short.[16] For this reason, the transdermal formulation of fentanyl plays an important role by increasing the duration of effect. Additionally, transdermal use can also be effective in patients who are not able to swallow or who are noncompliant[16]; transdermal administration, however, is not effective in the treatment of acute pain. Of note, lower rates of constipation, nausea, vomiting, drowsiness, and urinary retention have been reported with transdermal fentanyl compared to oral morphine.[18]

Hydrocodone: Although oral hydrocodone is equipotent to oral morphine,[16] the American Pain Society guidelines recommend a dose reduction of between 25 and 50% when converting between any two opioids.[19,20] There are immediate release and extended release formulations as well as formulations combined with acetaminophen or ibuprofen.

Hydromorphone: Hydromorphone can be administered by oral tablets, liquids, and suppositories, among other routes. Hydromorphone metabolites can cause opioid neurotoxicity with symptoms including myoclonus, hyperalgesia, and seizures, so care must be taken in patients with neurological disorders.[16]

Oxycodone and Oxymorphone: Oxycodone is available in immediate release and extended release formulations, as well as in formulations combined with acetaminophen. The combination with acetaminophen may have additive analgesic effects and permit lower oxycodone doses.[16] Oxymorphone is available in immediate release and extended release formulations, and acts on the mu-opioid receptor.[16]

Methadone: Methadone is a long-acting mu-opioid receptor agonist and is available in oral and intravenous formulations. The half-life is widely variable (from 8 to 59 hours).[16] Given its long half-life, it is useful as a treatment for chronic opioid addiction, but its use should be monitored by an experienced pain or palliative care specialist. Short-acting pain relief medications should also be available, as breakthrough pain can be an issue when first starting the drug. This is most important in the first 4 to 7 days of use, as the steady state of the drug may not be reached for several days (up to 2 weeks).[16]

In patients with dysrhythmias, there is evidence suggesting that higher doses of methadone may lead to QTc prolongation and Torsades de pointes.[16] Thus, it can occur at doses of 120 mg and above. Baseline and follow-up electrocardiograms should be obtained in patients being treated with high doses of methadone. Additional care must be taken in patients taking tricyclic antidepressants as this class of drug is also known to prolong the QTc interval.[21] Routine laboratory monitoring of the patient's potassium, magnesium, and calcium levels should be performed.[16]

Tramadol: Tramadol is used for treating moderate to severe pain and is available in immediate and extended release formulations. Tramadol is about one-tenth as potent as morphine.[16] Tramadol is a weak mu opioid agonist with some norepinephrine and serotonin reuptake inhibition.[16] Tramadol should be used with caution in patients who are also taking serotonergic and monoamine oxidase inhibitors due to the risk of serotonin syndrome.[22]

1.3.2 Nonopioid Analgesics

Acetaminophen: Acetaminophen has analgesic and antipyretic properties, but lacks anti-inflammatory properties.[23] Care must be taken when using acetaminophen since hepatotoxicity and renal impairment can occur.[24,25] The Food and Drug Administration (FDA) recommends that no more than 4,000 mg of acetaminophen be taken at any one time in order to reduce the risk of liver failure. Acetaminophen was the leading cause of acute liver failure from 1998 to 2003.[26,27]

1.3.3 Nonsteroidal Anti-inflammatory Drugs (NSAIDs)

NSAIDs work by blocking the biosynthesis of prostaglandins, which are inflammatory mediators that initiate, cause, intensify, or maintain pain.[16] Certain NSAIDs are contraindicated in patients with a history of peptic ulcer disease, gastrointestinal bleeding, or perforation.[16] Renal insufficiency is also a concern in patients with compromised fluid status, concomitant use of other nephrotoxic drugs, and renally excreted chemotherapy agents.[16] In 2005, the FDA issued a warning that NSAIDs may increase the risk of heart attack or stroke, even in patients with short-term NSAID use. Increased risk for these severe events is reported with higher dose exposures.[28] Of note, topical NSAIDs such as diclofenac gel or patch may be useful in patients taking prophylactic or therapeutic anticoagulation.[16]

1.4 Interventional Radiology (IR) Procedures in Pain Management

The use of interventional radiologic procedures for the primary treatment of pain has benefited many patients and improved their quality of life. These procedures often help patients to reduce or stop taking chronic pain medications. This is advantageous in reducing health care costs and side effects from chronic medication administration. Many of these procedures are safe and effective, and can be performed as same-day outpatient procedures. IR pain management procedures are described in depth later in this book and are beyond the scope of this chapter. An introduction to these procedures dedicated to pain relief in lieu of opioid administration is included here.

1.4.1 Spinal Procedures

It has been suggested that the approach to a patient with pain can be simplified into four categories: spinal pain secondary to neoplasm, spine pain that is nonneoplastic, nonspinal pain secondary to neoplasm, and nonspinal pain that is nonneoplastic in origin.[29]

Spinal metastatic disease often results in pathologic vertebral body fractures. A stepwise approach is useful in the evaluation of the patient with pain secondary to a neoplastic spine lesion. First, is the pain referable to the lesion? If not, other etiologies should be considered. If yes, is there an associated fracture? If not, cryoablation should be considered. If there is an associated fracture, is the lesion lytic? If not, alternative therapies (such as external beam radiotherapy) should be considered first. If the lesion is lytic, is there epidural involvement? If not, then radiofrequency ablation (RFA) should be considered. Percutaneous coaxial RFA and cementoplasty can also be useful in many of these patients.[30,31,32,33,34]

The evaluation of the patient with nonspinal pain secondary to neoplasm is similar to the workup of a patient with spinal pain related to a neoplasm. If the pain is referable to a lesion, is it accessible to a percutaneous approach under image guidance? If yes, are there adjacent structures that could be damaged by ablation? If yes, adjunctive maneuvers (such as hydrodissection) should be considered. The next step is to determine if the lesion is blastic. If not, cryoablation can be performed. If it is blastic, then coaxial or juxtacortical cryoablation should be considered. The use of cryoablation allows for visualization of the ablation zone and has improved analgesia compared with heat-mediated systems.[35,36,37,38] Additionally, various ablation configurations and sizes can be obtained using different cryoablation probes. Polymethylmethacrylate (PMMA) can be used after ablation, but its use could lead to slower recovery and may act as a fulcrum for future fracture[29] (although this point is debatable).

Spine pain that is unrelated to cancer can be divided into two broad categories: axial and radicular. The area of greatest concern can be identified by asking the patient, "If treatment was only possible at one site, would it be the back or the extremity?" Axial pain can be further subdivided into facet, diskogenic, and sacroiliac pain, or pain secondary to a compression fracture. Facet pain can be treated with a medial branch block, facet block, or rhizotomy using a percutaneous approach with image guidance.[39] The treatment of diskogenic pain is currently limited to epidural injections. However, many potential procedures could provide pain relief such as stem cell therapy, platelet-rich plasma, ozone therapy, chemonucleolysis, decompression, laser therapy, and drug delivery.[40,41,42]

1.4.2 Kyphoplasty/Vertebroplasty/Sacroplasty

Vertebral compression fractures (VCFs) are common in the osteoporotic population, with over 700,000 new compression fractures a year in the United States.[43] VCFs have a negative impact on patient's quality of life comparable to chronic diseases such as diabetes and heart disease.[44] In addition to this, the morbidity of symptomatic fractures is greater than hip fractures. From a financial perspective, the total expenditures for a patient with VCF is now greater than $5 billion from inpatient admission and emergency room visits only.

About 84% of patients with symptomatic VCFs present with midline back pain. In severe cases, bony retropulsion into the central canal can occur with resultant neural foramen compression that can cause decreased functional status, decreased mobility, and increased dependence on analgesics and narcotics. In addition to significant morbidity these factors can also lead to increased mortality.[45]

Percutaneous vertebroplasty has been used since 1984 to treat spinal hemangiomas. The first vertebroplasty for treatment of osteoporotic VCFs was performed in the 1990s.[46,47] Vertebroplasty can also be used to treat pathologic and traumatic fractures as well as painful neoplastic lesions.[45]

Vertebroplasty can be performed under fluoroscopy or computed tomography (CT) guidance. After the administration of subcutaneous and periosteal anesthesia, a coaxial needle introducer is advanced to the periosteum. A transpedicular or peripedicular approach can be used; however, the vast majority of operators will choose the former approach. It is important to traverse the middle of the pedicle's trabecular bone while avoiding the bony cortex of the neural foramen and the spinal canal. The needle tip should reside in the center of the vertebral body, and the cannula should cross the midline if a unipedicular approach is used. Advances in commercially available cannulas aid in accomplishing this. PMMA is activated with a catalyst and mixed into a toothpaste-like consistency, and slowly injected into the vertebral body. A volume of 2 to 6 mL is injected under continual image guidance to monitor for extravasation. Cement placement into the trabeculated spine, seen as interdigitation, is crucial. Complete filling of the vertebral body is rarely achieved, but is unnecessary; the goal is to stabilize the existing vertebral body height.

Kyphoplasty was introduced clinically in 2001, and varies from vertebroplasty in that a high pressure balloon is inserted into the vertebral body and inflated in order to create a cavity that is subsequently filled with cement. Depending on the source, kyphoplasty is often viewed as interchangeable with vertebroplasty with regard to outcomes.

Sacroplasty is used in the treatment of sacral insufficiency fractures, which are similar to VCFs as they are equally debilitating and a source of low back pain. Sacroplasty was first described in 2003. Detection is usually achieved by magnetic resonance imaging (MRI) or bone scintigraphy, since radiographs are insensitive for detection. As with kyphoplasty and vertebroplasty, sacroplasty is performed with either CT or fluoroscopic guidance using similar technique, equipment, and materials. The benefits of sacroplasty are similar to the benefits of vertebroplasty and kyphoplasty with improvements in pain, mobility, and narcotic use.[48,49]

1.4.3 Celiac Plexus Block

CT-guided celiac plexus block was first described in 1977,[50] and was traditionally performed under fluoroscopic guidance by anesthetists. The indications include persistent and intractable abdominal pain which can be caused by pancreatic, gastric, esophageal, or biliary malignancies, retroperitoneal lymph node metastasis, and metastatic liver cancer.[51] There is an 80% response rate for patients with malignancies such as pancreatic cancer.

Contraindications to celiac plexus neurolysis include severe uncorrectable coagulopathy or thrombocytopenia, abdominal aortic aneurysm, aortic mural thrombosis, or an eccentric origin of the celiac artery.[51] Sepsis as well as intraabdominal infections are also contraindications for celiac plexus neurolysis. Gastrointestinal motility is also increased with celiac plexus block, so patients with bowel obstruction should not undergo this procedure.

The use of CT helps to identify the precise location of the celiac plexus. A celiac plexus block is usually performed by an anterior or posterior approach. A small amount of contrast media or air is administered to outline the aorta and retroperitoneum between the celiac axis and superior mesenteric artery. Once proper positioning is obtained, a mixture of 20 to 40 mL 95% alcohol and long-acting anesthetic is injected.

1.4.4 Osteoid Osteoma Ablation

Osteoid osteoma is relatively common, and treatment with RFA was first described in 1989.[52] The most common presenting symptom is bone pain which will often worsen at night. The pain has been commonly described as a dull ache, but can also be severe, awakening the patient from sleep. Patients will often take NSAIDs to help reduce pain; in some cases, the patient will progress to taking opioids.

Previously, the standard treatment for osteoid osteoma was surgical resection.[53] Following surgery, the average hospital stay for a patient was 3 to 5 days with limited weight-bearing activity for 1 to 6 months. Surgical resection could leave the patient prone to fracture, and sometimes internal fixation with bone grafting was necessary.[54] However, the low rate of complications of percutaneous RFA compared to surgical resection has made RFA a popular choice.

RFA is usually performed with CT guidance in conjunction with general, spinal, or propofol induced anesthesia. The average procedure lasts 90 minutes. Postprocedural monitoring is usually less than 24 hours, and all daily activities can be resumed immediately after the procedure is complete. The use of RFA is contraindicated for lesions located less than 1 cm from vital structures such as nerves in the hand or spine. Additional contraindications include pregnancy, cellulitis, sepsis, and coagulopathy.

1.5 Public Perception of the Opioid Crisis

Americans perceive multiple factors as the cause of the current opioid epidemic. Up to 44% of Americans perceive prescription opioids as a very serious problem or crisis in their region, with 30% of people feeling that drug abuse is a cause of trouble for their family.[55] Approximately 55% of Americans place the blame on pharmaceutical companies for encouraging doctors to use opioids, with 53% of Americans placing the blame on physicians for overprescribing opioids. This could in part be related to prior legal issues with pharmaceutical companies that have allegedly bribed physicians to prescribe certain medications.[56] In addition to this, so-called "pill mills," described as clinics, physicians, or pharmacies that may be facilitating drug-seeking endeavors, have been exposed by law enforcement. In 2016, a physician had his license revoked for only accepting cash for prescribing fentanyl and other analgesic medications to patients in 11 different states.[57] This is particularly concerning because 19% of people thought it would be "extremely easy" to obtain a large amount of prescription opioids without needing them for a medical purpose and another 27% thought that it would be "somewhat easy."[58] In a separate study, around 8% of people felt that opioids are "not safe at all," and an additional 23% felt that opioids are "not very safe."[55] An American Psychiatric Association public opinion poll about opioids reported that only 46% of people completely agreed that people can recover from an opioid addiction.[58] Given the above findings, it is not surprising that 78% of Americans would prefer not to have pain medications be the first step in treatment and would seek alternatives.[55]

A survey conducted in 2018 showed that 8 out of 10 respondents felt that the federal government should be doing more to address the opioid crisis[59]; additionally, up to 43% of Americans believe the country is headed in the wrong direction regarding the opioid epidemic.[60,61] In addition to this, 37% of Americans feel that the nation has lost ground with the opioid epidemic.[62] It is fair to say that the opioid epidemic is a concern among Americans. A majority of Americans would prefer policymakers to increase access to treatment, and public opinion polls demonstrate a preference for treatment over arrests.[63,64] In at least one study a significant minority (one in four) advocated for stricter punishments and enforcement.[61]

1.6 Legislation

On October 24, 2018, the Substance Use-Disorder Prevention that Promotes Opioid Recovery and Treatment (SUPPORT) for Patients and Communities Act was passed into law. The law is focused on addressing the nation's opioid overdose epidemic by increasing support for treatment facilities. This includes numerous provisions that will increase access to treatment programs and expand access to substance use disorder prevention.[65,66] The new law will partially lift for 5 years a restriction that blocked states from using federal Medicaid dollars on medication assisted treatment. This will allow residential addiction treatment centers to provide treatment for up to 30 days in a 12-month period.[66] The CDC will also be authorized to provide grants to state and local governments to improve their prescription drug monitoring programs, collect public health data, implement evidence-based prevention strategies, encourage data sharing between states, and support prevention and research activities related to controlled substances which include awareness and education efforts.[67]

The law also focuses on protecting pregnant women and infants, with an increase in funding for residential treatment programs aimed at combatting neonatal abstinence syndrome (NAS). With the rise in opioid use since the 1970s, the prevalence of NAS has increased fivefold from 2000 to 2012 (with the number of cases rising to 21,732).[68] NAS may affect anywhere from 55 to 94% of women taking opioids during pregnancy.[69] The CDC will also develop educational material for pregnant women on the use of pain management during pregnancy that focuses on shared decision-making between the woman and the health care provider.[66]

In order to increase the number of health care workers dedicated to the treatment of opioid abuse, loan repayment of up to $250,000 will be provided to these workers when working in mental health shortage areas where the drug overdose death rate is higher than the national average. The provider will be required to practice for 6 years in these underserved areas. Up to $25 million are being appropriated for this cause through 2023.[65,66,67] Resources will also be available for pain care training and education with a focus on the dangers of opioid abuse, and early warning signs of opioid use disorders. Alternatives to opioid-based pain treatment will also be emphasized.

There will also be an increase in shipment tracking between the US Postal Service and US Customs and Border Protection regarding international shipments of controlled substances. It is hoped that this may help decrease the amount of illegal opioid distribution. A focus on synthetic fentanyl and its analogs is a concern due to their significant percentage of opioid-related overdose deaths.[66,67]

1.7 Summary

The medical field including the pharmaceutical industry has evolved and changed considerably since the original discovery of morphine in 1827. Many new synthetic and semi-synthetic opioids have since been discovered and are commonly used today for pain management. Despite these new discoveries, the age-old problem of opioid addiction and abuse remains, and now appears to be more profound and extensive than ever before. Procedures performed by interventional radiologists that focus on pain relief play an increasingly important role in decreasing opioid use in select populations. As the fight against the opioid epidemic continues, effective policy-making will be key to enacting real change.

References

[1] Hobbs J. Troubling fields: the opium poppy in Egypt. Geogr Rev. 1998; 88(1): 64–85

[2] Brownstein MJ. A brief history of opiates, opioid peptides, and opioid receptors. Proc Natl Acad Sci U S A. 1993; 90(12):5391–5393

[3] Booth M. Opium: A History. New York, New York: Simon & Schuster; 1996:15–17

[4] Kritikos PG, Papadaki SP. The history of the poppy and of opium and their expansion in antiquity in the eastern Mediterranean area. The United Nations. https://www.unodc.org/unodc/en/data-and-analysis/bulletin/bulletin_1967–01–01_3_page004.html. Published 1967. Accessed June 26, 2020

[5] Courtwright D. Forces of Habit: Drugs and the Making of the Modern World. Harvard University Press; 2009:36

[6] Musto DF. Opium, cocaine and marijuana in American history. Sci Am. 1991; 265(1):40–47

[7] Kolodny A, Courtwright DT, Hwang CS, et al. The prescription opioid and heroin crisis: a public health approach to an epidemic of addiction. Annu Rev Public Health. 2015; 36:559–574

[8] Health and Human Services. HHS acting secretary declares public health emergency to address national opioid crisis. https://www.hhs.gov/about/news/2017/10/26/hhs-acting-secretary-declares-public-health-emergency-address-national-opioid-crisis.html. Published 2017. Accessed June 26, 2020

[9] Chisholm-Burns MA, Spivey CA, Sherwin E, Wheeler J, Hohmeier K. The opioid crisis: origins, trends, policies, and the roles of pharmacists. Am J Health Syst Pharm. 2019; 76(7):424–435

[10] World Health Organization. Information sheet on opioid overdose. https://www.who.int/substance_abuse/information-sheet/en/. Published 2018. Updated August 2018. Accessed

[11] Hedegaard H, Miniño AM, Warner MP. Drug overdose deaths in the United States, 1999–2018. NCHS data brief, No. 356. National Center for Health Statistics. https://www.cdc.gov/nchs/data/databriefs/db356-h.pdf. Published 2020. Accessed June 26, 2020

[12] Wilson N, Kariisa M, Seth P, Smith H IV, Davis N. Morbidity and Mortality weekly report—drug and opioid involved overdose deaths—United States, 2017–2018. CDC. https://www.cdc.gov/mmwr/volumes/69/wr/mm6911a4.htm. Published 2020. Accessed June 26, 2020

[13] Centers for Disease Control. Opioid overdose—U.S. prescribing rate maps. https://www.cdc.gov/drugoverdose/maps/rxrate-maps.html. Published 2020. Updated March 5. Accessed June 26, 2020

[14] Centers for Disease Control. Opioid overdose—fentanyl encounters data. https://www.cdc.gov/drugoverdose/data/fentanyl-le-reports.html. Published 2016. Accessed June 26, 2020

[15] Rajbhandari-Thapa J, Zhang D, Padilla HM, Chung SR. Opioid-related hospitalization and its association with chronic diseases: findings from the National Inpatient Sample, 2011–2015. Prev Chronic Dis. 2019; 16:E157

[16] Swarm RA, Paice JA, Anghelescu DL, et al. BCPS. Adult cancer pain, version 3.2019, NCCN Clinical Practice Guidelines in Oncology. J Natl Compr Canc Netw. 2019; 17(8):977–1007

[17] UpToDate. Morphine: Drug Information. https://www.uptodate.com/contents/morphine-drug-information - F8776705. Accessed August 7, 2020

[18] Wang DD, Ma TT, Zhu HD, Peng CB. Transdermal fentanyl for cancer pain: trial sequential analysis of 3406 patients from 35 randomized controlled trials. J Cancer Res Ther. 2018; 14(8) Suppl:S14–S21

[19] Chou R, Fanciullo GJ, Fine PG, et al. American Pain Society-American Academy of Pain Medicine Opioids Guidelines Panel. Clinical guidelines for the use of chronic opioid therapy in chronic noncancer pain. J Pain. 2009; 10 (2):113–130

[20] Shaheen PE, Walsh D, Lasheen W, Davis MP, Lagman RL. Opioid equianalgesic tables: are they all equally dangerous? J Pain Symptom Manage. 2009; 38(3): 409–417

[21] McPherson ML, Walker KA, Davis MP, et al. Safe and appropriate use of methadone in hospice and palliative care: expert consensus white paper. J Pain Symptom Manage. 2019; 57(3):635–645.e4

[22] Beakley BD, Kaye AM, Kaye AD. Tramadol, pharmacology, side effects, and serotonin syndrome: a review. Pain Physician. 2015; 18(4):395–400

[23] Stockler M, Vardy J, Pillai A, Warr D. Acetaminophen (paracetamol) improves pain and well-being in people with advanced cancer already receiving a strong opioid regimen: a randomized, double-blind, placebo-controlled cross-over trial. J Clin Oncol. 2004; 22(16):3389–3394

[24] American Geriatrics Society Panel on Pharmacological Management of Persistent Pain in Older P. Pharmacological management of persistent pain in older persons. J Am Geriatr Soc. 2009; 57:1331–1346

[25] Israel FJ, Parker G, Charles M, Reymond L. Lack of benefit from paracetamol (acetaminophen) for palliative cancer patients requiring high-dose strong opioids: a randomized, double-blind, placebo-controlled, crossover trial. J Pain Symptom Manage. 2010; 39(3):548–554

[26] Larson AM, Polson J, Fontana RJ, et al. Acute Liver Failure Study Group. Acetaminophen-induced acute liver failure: results of a United States multicenter, prospective study. Hepatology. 2005; 42(6):1364–1372

[27] Tanne J. Paracetamol causes most liver failure in UK and US. BMJ. 2006; 332 (7542):628

[28] Bally M, Dendukuri N, Rich B, et al. Risk of acute myocardial infarction with NSAIDs in real world use: Bayesian meta-analysis of individual patient data. BMJ. 2017; 357:j1909

[29] Bittman RW, Friedberg EB, Fleishon HB, Prologo JD. Global approach to the patient with pain in interventional radiology. Semin Intervent Radiol. 2018; 35(4):342–349

[30] Greenwood TJ, Wallace A, Friedman MV, Hillen TJ, Robinson CG, Jennings JW. Combined ablation and radiation therapy of spinal metastases: a novel multimodality treatment approach. Pain Physician. 2015; 18(6):573–581

[31] Anchala PR, Irving WD, Hillen TJ, et al. Treatment of metastatic spinal lesions with a navigational bipolar radiofrequency ablation device: a multicenter retrospective study. Pain Physician. 2014; 17(4):317–327

[32] Wallace AN, Robinson CG, Meyer J, et al. The metastatic spine disease multidisciplinary working group algorithms. Oncologist. 2015; 20(10): 1205–1215

[33] Lea W, Tutton S. Decision making: osteoplasty, ablation, or combined therapy for spinal metastases. Semin Intervent Radiol. 2017; 34(2):121–131

[34] Kam NM, Maingard J, Kok HK, et al. Combined vertebral augmentation and radiofrequency ablation in the management of spinal metastases: an update. Curr Treat Options Oncol. 2017; 18(12):74

[35] Prologo JD, Patel I, Buethe J, Bohnert N. Ablation zones and weight-bearing bones: points of caution for the palliative interventionalist. J Vasc Interv Radiol. 2014; 25(5):769–775.e2

[36] Callstrom MR, Dupuy DE, Solomon SB, et al. Percutaneous image-guided cryoablation of painful metastases involving bone: multicenter trial. Cancer. 2013; 119(5):1033–1041

[37] Prologo JD, Passalacqua M, Patel I, Bohnert N, Corn DJ. Image-guided cryoablation for the treatment of painful musculoskeletal metastatic disease: a single-center experience. Skeletal Radiol. 2014; 43(11):1551–1559

[38] Thacker PG, Callstrom MR, Curry TB, et al. Palliation of painful metastatic disease involving bone with imaging-guided treatment: comparison of patients' immediate response to radiofrequency ablation and cryoablation. AJR Am J Roentgenol. 2011; 197(2):510–515

[39] Stout A, Dreyfuss P, Swain N, Roberts S, Loh E, Agur A. Proposed optimal fluoroscopic targets for cooled radiofrequency neurotomy of the sacral lateral

branches to improve clinical outcomes: an anatomical study. Pain Med. 2018; 19(10):1916–1923

[40] Knezevic NN, Mandalia S, Raasch J, Knezevic I, Candido KD. Treatment of chronic low back pain—new approaches on the horizon. J Pain Res. 2017; 10: 1111–1123

[41] Pettine KA, Suzuki RK, Sand TT, Murphy MB. Autologous bone marrow concentrate intradiscal injection for the treatment of degenerative disc disease with three-year follow-up. Int Orthop. 2017; 41(10):2097–2103

[42] Centeno C, Markle J, Dodson E, et al. Treatment of lumbar degenerative disc disease-associated radicular pain with culture-expanded autologous mesenchymal stem cells: a pilot study on safety and efficacy. J Transl Med. 2017; 15(1):197

[43] McDonald RJ, Lane JI, Diehn FE, Wald JT. Percutaneous vertebroplasty: overview, clinical applications, and current state. Appl Radiol. 2017; 46(1):24–30

[44] Cummings SR, Melton LJ. Epidemiology and outcomes of osteoporotic fractures. Lancet. 2002; 359(9319):1761–1767

[45] Kallmes DF, Jensen ME. Percutaneous vertebroplasty. Radiology. 2003; 229 (1):27–36

[46] Galibert P, Deramond H, Rosat P, Le Gars D. [Preliminary note on the treatment of vertebral angioma by percutaneous acrylic vertebroplasty] [in French]. Neurochirurgie. 1987; 33(2):166–168

[47] Debussche-Depriester C, Deramond H, Fardellone P, et al. Percutaneous vertebroplasty with acrylic cement in the treatment of osteoporotic vertebral crush fracture syndrome. Paper presented at Proceedings of the XIV Symposium Neuroradiologicum, 1991, Berlin, Heidelberg. pp. 149–152. https://doi.org/10.1007/978-3-642-49329-4_50

[48] Garfin SR, Yuan HA, Reiley MA. New technologies in spine: kyphoplasty and vertebroplasty for the treatment of painful osteoporotic compression fractures. Spine. 2001; 26(14):1511–1515

[49] Hulme PA, Krebs J, Ferguson SJ, Berlemann U. Vertebroplasty and kyphoplasty: a systematic review of 69 clinical studies. Spine. 2006; 31(17):1983–2001

[50] Haaga JR, Reich NE, Havrilla TR, Alfidi RJ. Interventional CT scanning. Radiol Clin North Am. 1977; 15(3):449–456

[51] Kambadakone A, Thabet A, Gervais DA, Mueller PR, Arellano RS. CT-guided celiac plexus neurolysis: a review of anatomy, indications, technique, and tips for successful treatment. Radiographics. 2011; 31(6):1599–1621

[52] Tillotson CL, Rosenberg AE, Rosenthal DI. Controlled thermal injury of bone. Report of a percutaneous technique using radiofrequency electrode and generator. Invest Radiol. 1989; 24(11):888–892

[53] Motamedi D, Learch TJ, Ishimitsu DN, et al. Thermal ablation of osteoid osteoma: overview and step-by-step guide. Radiographics. 2009; 29(7): 2127–2141

[54] Rosenthal DI, Hornicek FJ, Wolfe MW, Jennings LC, Gebhardt MC, Mankin HJ. Percutaneous radiofrequency coagulation of osteoid osteoma compared with operative treatment. J Bone Joint Surg Am. 1998; 80(6):815–821

[55] Gallup. Americans prefer drug-free pain management over opioids. https://news.gallup.com/reports/217676/americans-prefer-drug-free-pain-management-opioids.aspx. Published 2017. Accessed January 8, 2020

[56] Concepcion M. Former Insys sales exec settles with Arizona for $9.5 M in opioid bribe case. https://www.12news.com/article/news/local/arizona/former-insys-sales-exec-settles-with-arizona-for-95m-in-opioid-bribe-case/75-4cc388eb-ed68-4314-be05-779b36c31db5. Published 2019. Updated April 1, 2019. Accessed January 8, 2020

[57] The Associated Press. Regulators: Illinois doctor's pill mill supplied 11 states. https://chicago.cbslocal.com/2016/11/30/regulators-illinois-doctors-pill-mill-supplied-11-states/. Published 2016. Accessed January 8, 2020

[58] Association AP. APA public opinion poll—annual meeting 2018. https://www.psychiatry.org/newsroom/apa-public-opinion-poll-annual-meeting-2018. Published 2018. Accessed January 8, 2020

[59] De Pinto J, Backus F, Khanna K, Salvanto A. Opioid addiction in U.S.: 7 in 10 say it's a very serious problem—CBS news poll. Published 2018. Accessed January 8, 2020

[60] Cook AK, Worcman N. Confronting the opioid epidemic: public opinion toward the expansion of treatment services in Virginia. Health Justice. 2019; 7(1):13

[61] American Psychiatric Association. APA public opinion pol—annual meeting 2017. https://www.psychiatry.org/News-room/News-Releases/New-National-Poll-Finds-Americans-Show-Strong-Supp. Published 2017. Accessed January 8, 2020

[62] Brenan M. More in U.S. say illegal drugs are a more serious problem. Gallup. https://news.gallup.com/poll/221147/say-illegal-drugs-serious-problem.aspx. Published 2017. Accessed January 8, 2020

[63] Cook A, Brownstein H. Public opinion and public policy: heroin and other opioids. Crim Justice Policy Rev. 2017; 30(8):1163–1185

[64] Pew Research Center. America's new drug policy landscape: two-thirds favor treatment, not jail, for use of heroin, cocaine. https://www.people-press.org/2014/04/02/americas-new-drug-policy-landscape/. Published 2014. Accessed January 8, 2020

[65] American Society of Addiction Medicine. The SUPPORT for Patients and Communities Act (H.R. 6). https://www.asam.org/advocacy/the-support-for-patients-and-communities-act-(h.r.-6). Published 2020. Accessed January 8, 2020

[66] Congress.gov. H.R.6—SUPPORT for Patients and Communities Act. 115th Congress (2017–2018). https://www.congress.gov/bill/115th-congress/house-bill/6. Accessed January 8, 2020

[67] O'Reilly K. 10 ways the new opioids law could help address the epidemic. American Medical Association. https://www.ama-assn.org/delivering-care/opioids/10-ways-new-opioids-law-could-help-address-epidemic. Published 2018. Accessed January 8, 2020

[68] Patrick SW, Schumacher RE, Benneyworth BD, Krans EE, McAllister JM, Davis MM. Neonatal abstinence syndrome and associated health care expenditures: United States, 2000–2009. JAMA. 2012; 307(18):1934–1940

[69] Hudak ML, Tan RC, Committee on Drugs, Committee on Fetus and Newborn, American Academy of Pediatrics. Neonatal drug withdrawal. Pediatrics. 2012; 129(2):e540–e560

2 Practice Building Techniques

A. Michael Devane, Venkata Macha, Andrew J. Gunn, and J. David Prologo

2.1 Case Presentation

Uterine fibroid embolization (UFE) is an image-guided, minimally invasive procedure for women with symptomatic uterine fibroids. Despite multiple randomized clinical trials demonstrating its efficacy, UFE is not widely recognized among patients and referring physicians as a viable treatment option.[1] As an example, interventional radiologists (IRs) at the University of Alabama at Birmingham (UAB) performed approximately 25 UFEs in 2016 despite serving a metropolitan population of >1,000,000 people. The physicians in the group contacted colleagues from the Department of Obstetrics and Gynecology (Ob/Gyn) to discuss the possibility of giving lectures, hosting educational dinners, or creating a research collaboration. However, the number of UFE referrals did not increase significantly. To develop this practice, physicians in the group then began to work with UAB Hospital's Marketing Department to improve patient and physician awareness. First, they produced a podcast about UFE with the assistance of UAB Medcast, a free online repository of continuing medical education (CME) podcasts.[2] Next, a willing UFE patient from their practice volunteered to share her experience in the form of short educational video.[3] Soon after, a local news station picked up the video that led to an invitation for one of the IRs to appear for a live television interview. Slowly, patient self-referrals began to increase. Ob/Gyn physicians from UAB saw the video and the interview. This exposure eventually led to an invitation to give Grand Rounds and speak at their Department's annual CME event. Finally, these interactions led to the development of a regular uterine fibroid conference where IRs and Ob/Gyn physicians would meet to discuss cases and the relevant literature. Overall, these practice-building efforts have significantly improved the collaboration between the two groups of physicians. IR at UAB performed > 50 UFEs in 2019, representing a >100% increase in procedural volume.

2.2 Discussion

Practice building is a critical skill for IR in general, as referral patterns can vary widely, and awareness of image-guided procedures can be limited. Apart from the financial viability and professional satisfaction gained from practice expansion, the ability to improve the availability of image-guided procedures is an important goal for providing comprehensive patient care. As it involves integration of advanced interventional pain management to one's interventional radiology practice (and practice building overall), the pillars of a successful expansion include: procedural expertise, longitudinal patient care, education, personal branding, professional development, and service.

2.2.1 Procedural Expertise

Although this pillar may feel self-explanatory, it is fundamental and worthy of emphasis. The information contained in subsequent chapters of this text can provide a diverse background into both well-established and developing image-guided pain management procedures. The core of a successful practice is to provide safe, effective care tailored to specific patient needs, concerns, and goals. The practice of interventional radiology combines innovation with technical skills, imaging expertise, and clinical knowledge to positively impact patient care. Each consultation is an opportunity to both hone and demonstrate procedural expertise. Therefore, careful patient selection should be prioritized to minimize complications and unnecessary procedures.

2.2.2 Longitudinal Patient Care

Excellence in patient care begins with a thorough consultation in the clinic and continues throughout the patient's postprocedure course. The historical model of performing procedures by the IR, while other physicians promote patient care, is obsolete in today's health care environment. In 1968, Dr. Charles Dotter, widely known as the Father of Interventional Radiology, said, "If my fellow angiographers prove unwilling or unable to accept or secure for their patients the clinical responsibilities attendant on transluminal angioplasty, they will become high-priced plumbers facing forfeiture of territorial rights based solely on imaging equipment others can obtain and skill still others can learn."[4] IRs can no longer afford to cede patient evaluation, preprocedure consultation, and postprocedure care to others if they expect to build a robust referral base. In recognition of this, radiological societies such as the American College of Radiology, the Society of Interventional Radiology, and the American Society of Interventional and Therapeutic Neuroradiology have published practice standards for the clinical aspects of interventional radiology.[5,6] To this end, a dedicated ambulatory clinic is a necessity for longitudinal patient care. An ambulatory clinic provides dedicated space and resources for patient consultation and postprocedure care. Apart from patient care advantages, an ambulatory clinic can also serve as a means to facilitate referrals. For instance, a dedicated ambulatory clinic with associated staff provides patients and referring physicians with a single point of contact for the IR. For patients, this means that they do not have to rely on a primary care or specialty physician for a referral to IR since they can contact the clinic directly to set up a consultation. For referring physicians, a clinic can lower barriers for an IR referral. For example, a physician may be unsure if the patient needs a procedure. Previously, there was no consistent way for an IR to see the patient and provide opinion without scheduling a procedure. Additionally, a clinic provides the IR the opportunity to see the patient after the procedure, therefore removing that burden from the referring service. The physician who performed the procedure is best equipped to determine its efficacy based upon the patient's history and physical findings as well as deal with any potential complications. In our experience, the establishment of a dedicated ambulatory clinic for interventional radiology has been a critical driver of our practice-building efforts.[7]

2.2.3 Education

Many physicians bristle at the idea of their practice being marketed like a consumer product as images of distasteful television advertisements come to mind. Certainly, there are many examples of physicians who have used this form of marketing. In our opinion, the forms of physician marketing that will lead to respectable, long-term growth are more akin to educating the community. In this sense, community education may represent one of the most potent vehicles for highlighting your practice. Educating the community can take a variety of forms. First, with regards to referring physicians, education can take place during Grand Rounds, education dinner or lunches, medical symposia, CME courses, or multidisciplinary conferences. Referrers must be informed of the procedures that your practice offers that could benefit their patients.

Second, every practicing IR needs an online presence, including an interactive website. The website serves as a convenient mechanism to learn about interventional radiology and set up clinical consultations. This website could house scientific literature, descriptions of the types of conditions treated, and other educational links. If possible, an area for patients and referring physicians to submit questions is advantageous. Be sure to include contact information for the clinic as well as a generic email address.

Third, social media is a powerful platform for practice building. Sites such as Facebook, Twitter, Instagram, and LinkedIn are useful to engage with patients and other physicians. Patient advocacy groups are active in social media, and patients often seek information from those groups. Engaging with those groups to provide education about treatment options is an effective means of reaching those patients.[8] Social media can also be useful to stay in touch with interventional radiology colleagues and keep abreast of their techniques in treating pain.

Finally, traditional means of practice building such as television, newspaper, radio, and local magazines remain relevant but carry a financial cost. One report found that an 8-week advertisement in a local magazine selected based upon patient demographics yielded 35 clinic visits, 35 magnetic resonance imaging (MRI) examinations, 17 Uterine Artery Embolization (UAE), and 17 postprocedure MRI.[9] Group practices, industry, and hospitals may have funds to support these efforts.

2.2.4 Personal Branding

Everything we do each day is part of our personal brand, which defines our perception as a physician by patients and other doctors. Of everything discussed in this chapter, personal branding is, at the same time, the most crucial and straightforward concept. Personal branding is nearly entirely about authenticity and integrity. Classically, the "three A's" consisting of availability, affability, and ability are still valid. Although intuitive to successful physicians, it is something that we must continuously develop. Our everyday attitude and performance define who we are as doctors. However, personal branding extends beyond the physician as the attitude and bedside manner of the entire interventional radiology team (technologists, nurses, receptionists, and support staff) reflect the brand of the whole practice. Without a doubt, the digital age has indelibly changed personal branding.

A physician's online presence broadcasts its brand to a global audience. Online patient ratings and scoring of physicians are a new medium for patients to communicate their satisfaction or dissatisfaction. Undoubtedly, patients share their treatment experience via social media and online chats. Finally, IRs should seek to increase the number of personal interactions with referring physicians. The IR should attend multidisciplinary conferences to provide the IR voice to the local medical community. Be prepared to share your email and cell phone number with referring physicians to facilitate future communications. In total, these efforts will help to build your personal brand.

2.2.5 Professional Development

Professional development helps to ensure that patient care remains safe, up-to-date, and relevant. Awareness of patient outcomes in practice is requisite to professional development. Consequently, topics already addressed in this chapter, including longitudinal patient care and procedural expertise, can help with professional development. Utilizing evidence-based medicine and CME, a physician should always seek to improve the outcomes. The term "kaizen" refers to the Japanese business philosophy of continuous process improvement. After World War II, the Japanese industry was devastated. Dr. W. Edwards Deming went to Japan as a consultant for its economy and helped to turn the island nation into an industrial giant using "kaizen."[10] Although a detailed discussion of continuous process improvement is beyond the scope of this chapter, the spirit of "kaizen" is instructive for physicians, namely, the perpetual quest for personal improvement, sharpening of technical skills, and enhancing medical knowledge are rooted in this philosophy.

2.2.6 Service

Horst Schulze is a co-founder of the Ritz Carlton enterprise, which is widely recognized as the gold standard for customer service. Our customers, as we expand our interventional radiology practices into new domains, are the patients and the referring services. The connection between Horst Schulze and our practices lies in the ability to solidify relationships by "fulfilling the customer's expectations each and every time they make contact with us."[11]

For the IR, this translates to managing problems for the referring physicians and providing patients comfortable, seamless procedural experiences with appropriate efficacy. Regarding the former, affable responses to requests from referrers, appropriate and timely inpatient or outpatient consultations, and robust communication result in a satisfied customer. Oncologists, hospitalists, primary care referrers, and all other potential referring services are often multitasking, busy sources of business for the IR—who are relieved that we will manage the current patient problem from beginning to end. Likewise, the patients serve as satisfied customers who expand customer base by sharing their subjective experience.

When our intentions as operators are drawn to the experience of the referrer and the patient (in addition, of course, to objective clinical outcomes) the success and sustainability of our practices will flourish.

2.3 Summary

Practice-building skills are essential for an IR to develop a thriving practice, which requires attention to detail, continuous effort, and a patient-centered focus. The pillars of a successful pain management practice in interventional radiology include procedural expertise, longitudinal patient care, education, personal branding, professional development, and service.

A quote from Dr. Charles Dotter best concludes this chapter. "The angiographer who enters into the treatment of arterial obstructive disease can now play a key role, if he [she] is prepared and willing to serve as a true clinician, not just a skilled catheter mechanic. He [she] must accept the responsibility for the direct care of patients before and after the procedure; know them as patients, not just a blocked artery...However important radiological diagnosis, its ultimate object is treatment. We've come a long way in this direction, and if we go wisely, can go much further."[12]

References

[1] https://www.sirweb.org/globalassets/aasociety-of-interventional-radiology-home-page/patient-center/fibroid/sir_report_final.pdf. Accessed September 18, 2020

[2] https://www.uabmedicine.org/web/medicalprofessionals/medcast-home. Accessed September 18, 2020

[3] Greer T. Patient finds relief from abnormal menstrual cycles with minimally invasive hysterectomy alternative. The University of Alabama at Birmingham. https://www.uab.edu/medicine/news/latest/item/1652-patient-finds-relief-from-abnormal-menstrual-cycles-with-minimally-invasive-hysterectomy-alternative. Accessed September 18, 2020

[4] Funaki B. Top 5 reasons why you can't blame interventional radiologists for neglecting clinical duties for so long. Semin Intervent Radiol. 2006; 23(4): 303–304

[5] American College of Radiology, American Society of Interventional and Therapeutic Neuroradiology, Society of Interventional Radiology.. Practice guideline for interventional clinical practice. J Vasc Interv Radiol. 2005; 16(2 Pt 1):149–155

[6] Swischuk JL, Sacks D, Pentecost MJ, Mauro MA, Moresco K, Roberts AC, Lewis CA, Larson PA, Cardella JF, Dorfman GS, Darcy MD. Clinical practice of interventional and cardiovascular radiology: current status, guidelines for resource allocation, future directions. J Am Coll Radiol. 2004 Oct;1(10):720-7

[7] Siskin GP, Bagla S, Sansivero GE, Mitchell NL. The interventional radiology clinic: key ingredients for success. J Vasc Interv Radiol. 2004; 15(7):681–688

[8] Wadhwa V, Brandis A, Madassery K, et al. #TwittIR: understanding and establishing a Twitter ecosystem for interventional radiologists and their practices. J Am Coll Radiol. 2018; 15 1 Pt B:218–223

[9] Chrisman HB, Basu PA, Omary RA. The positive effect of targeted marketing on an existing uterine fibroid embolization practice. J Vasc Interv Radiol. 2006; 17(3):577–581

[10] Deming WE, Orsini JN. The Essential Deming: Leadership Principles from the Father of Quality Management. New York: McGraw-Hill; 2013

[11] Schulz H. Excellence Wins: A No Nonsense Guide to Becoming the Best in a World of Compromise. Zondervan; 2019

[12] Roberts AC. The 2004 Dr. Charles T. Dotter lecture: interventional radiology today—what would Charles Dotter say? J Vasc Interv Radiol. 2004; 15(12): 1357–1361

3 The Freestanding Outpatient Clinic

Aneesa Majid

3.1 Introduction

As you build your pain management service, the question will arise as to where you will provide your services. One option is in an outpatient office-based lab (OBL). This chapter will outline at a high level what you need to know and consider when deciding if you should include an OBL as part of your practice.

The OBL market in 2022 was valued at $10.3 billion. This is expected to grab at a compound annual growth rate (CAGR) of 7.52% from 2023 to 2030. Prior to the Covid -19 pandemic, 70% of surgical procedures were being performed in the outpatient settings. The pandemic has increased patient's desires to be treated in an outpatient setting rather than the hospital, which likely will accelerate the OBL market growth.

What are the advantages of performing procedures in an OBL or Ambulatory Surgical Center (ASC) versus a hospital outpatient department (HOPD)? For the physician, there is significant autonomy and control in an OBL or ASC. They are able to control their own schedule as well as the entire patient care process from scheduling through postprocedure care, becoming a stronger advocate for the patient.

Additional advantages include the following:
- Safety due to decreased morbidity and risk of nosocomial infections
- Efficiency due to decreased interruptions in patient flow
- Focused care due to singular focus by both doctors and staff
- Cost efficient due to reduced ancillary testing and overnight stays
- Satisfaction of patients, staff, and doctors
- Improved reimbursement for physicians[2]

3.2 Definitions

An OBL is defined as "facilities where the health professional routinely provides health examinations, diagnosis, and treatment of illness or injury on an ambulatory basis."[3] The location cannot be in a hospital, skilled nursing facility, military treatment facility, community health centers, state or local public health center, or intermediate care facility. Currently, there are just over 700 OBLs in the United States, increasing at a rate of 25 per month.[4] In states with corporate practice of medicine laws, such as California and Texas, these centers can only be owned by medical professionals. Generally, these facilities are regulated by the Medical Board or state. A certificate of need or special permit may not be needed, depending on the state. There is no special regulation from Medicare for participation as long as the billing provider and practice are Medicare participants. Some states may require state inspection or accreditation.

An ASC is defined by The Centers for Medicare and Medicaid Services (CMS) as "A freestanding facility (other than a physician's office) where surgical and diagnostic services are provided on an ambulatory basis." There are currently over 5,500 ASCs operating nationwide.[4] Nonmedical professionals and corporations can own these facilities. The operation and licensing are generally regulated by the state. Most states require a certificate of need and/or state licensing. In addition, there are strict layout and building requirements such as size of hallways, number of beds, parking, heating, ventilation and air conditioning (HVAC), and numerous other requirements. Finally, to receive payment from Medicare, the facility must have Medicare Deemed status.

To determine which option is best, one needs to look at what are the state regulations as well as what are the reimbursement rates, both private payer and Medicare, for the procedures one intends to perform at the facility. Some procedures may reimburse more in an OBL, some may reimburse more in an ASC, some may reimburse more in an HOPD. Many centers have chosen to use a hybrid model.

A hybrid model is when a center operates for some days as an ASC and some days as an OBL. This is a way to maximize reimbursement. However, it is often very difficult to retrofit an OBL to an ASC due to the stringent structural requirements. Thus, the recommendation when starting an outpatient clinic from scratch is to build or build-out the facility as an ASC.

In addition to the above considerations, specifically for pain management clinics, knowing and understanding all Centers for Disease Control and Prevention (CDC) and state regulations are extremely important. While the CDC provides guidelines, they in general support state regulations concerning pain management and opioids.

3.3 Financial Considerations

The financial outlay for an OBL/ASC is significant and includes the following.[5]

3.3.1 Setup Costs

- Costs will vary depending on whether you are leasing or buying the space and the approximate square footage.
- Costs will depend on whether you are collaborating as part of a larger multispecialty ASC or single specialty providing services for pain management as well as state regulations that determine whether an OBL, ASC, or hybrid model is best. Most often, pain management centers are ASCs.
- Build-out: This is one of the major costs of setting up a lab and is highly variable. If a practice already has a space, it may cost between $100,000 and $250,000 to build-out, possibly less. However, if it does not, exceeding $2,000,000 is easily possible. Costs in a build-out include, but is not limited to, cost of construction, architect fees, permits, and licensing, depending on state regulation.
- Equipment is the second major cost of the lab. The most expensive item will be the fluoroscopy unit. Other items include patient monitors, backup power, stretchers, crash cart, furniture, and office supplies. Some of the equipment cost may be decreased by purchasing refurbished units versus purchasing new. Even more important will be the service contracts for the equipment. Financing for equipment is often through leases or bank loans.

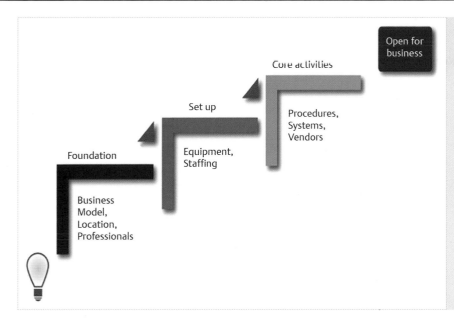

Fig. 3.1 Schematic demonstrating a stepwise approach to opening an outpatient office-based lab (OBL)/ASC.

Foundation
Business Model, Location, Professionals

Set up
Equipment, Staffing

Core activities
Procedures, Systems, Vendors

Open for business

- Supplies for procedures: The supplies needed will be determined by types of cases and physician preference.

3.3.2 Operating Costs

- Staffing: Both clinical and administrative staffing is needed. For clinical staff, a minimum of two registered nurses, a scrub tech, an X-ray tech, and possibly one to two medical assistants are needed. In addition, administrative staff for scheduling, coding, billing, prior authorization, and management of the clinic is necessary. Hiring the right staff is essential for a successful lab. The right staff will provide efficiency and determine the culture of the organization. Wrong hires will lead to turnover, increased expense, and a poor reputation of the clinic. Hiring staff is one of the important, if not *the* most important, decisions to be made.
- Supplies: In general, at least 2 weeks of supplies on hand is recommended. Various terms for equipment pricing exist including consignment, equipment kits, and capitated pricing.
- Equipment: Depending on how the equipment purchases were financed, monthly payments will be a part of the fixed operational costs.

3.3.3 Estimating Revenue

- Making realistic estimations of how many cases can be done in the lab per day and how long it will take to ramp up to this number is extremely important. A brand-new lab can take a minimum of 12 to 18 months to be near full capacity.
- Determine what the case mix will be.
- Determine what the average payment per case will be using the case mix and payer mix.

3.3.4 Additional Costs[6]

- Legal
- Financial planning

- Management company
- Billing company
- Marketing and branding, including a client referral management system (CRM) as well as personal marketing efforts to increase referral base

A good summary of the steps to open an OBL/ASC is summarized in ▶ Fig. 3.1.[7]

3.4 Personal Considerations

Transitioning to an outpatient-based practice has many rewards for the physician. The autonomy, the satisfaction of efficient workflow processes and improved patient care, and the control of one's daily schedule to name a few. However, the effort required to make a successful lab is often underappreciated.

In addition to the business knowledge that is acquired, the additional work to oversee and manage the operations as well as generating and building referrals to the practice is constant. An entrepreneurial mindset is needed as well as knowing what your strengths are and what or who is needed to fill in your gaps—knowledge or skill.

▶ Fig. 3.2 demonstrates what the physician's top priority is (▶ Fig. 3.2a) and all the aspects that must be successful and work together for a successful lab (▶ Fig. 3.2b).

A physician cannot do it all and must have help. Management companies and partnerships will be key to helping the lab to be successful. Indeed, it is a team process that leads to success. However, the physician is the head coach of the team, and the leadership of the physician will be key to its success.

3.5 Conclusion

Performing pain management procedures in an outpatient lab can be very rewarding personally, professionally, and financially. Success will require an increase in business knowledge, careful strategic and financial planning, strategic partnerships, and a well-curated excellent team. Key physician leadership

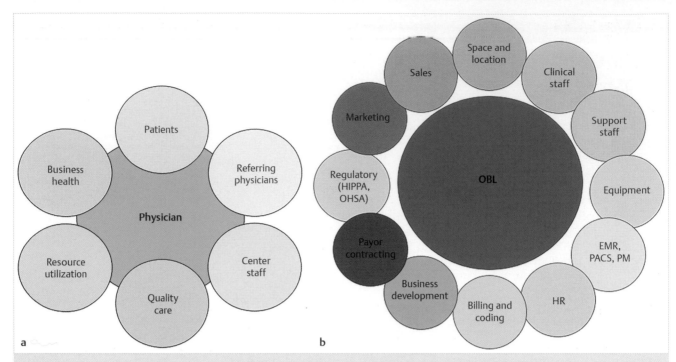

Fig. 3.2 (**a**) Figure demonstrating the priorities in opening an outpatient office-based lab (OBL)/ASC. (**b**) Figure demonstrating the aspects leading to opening a successful lab. EMR, Electronic Medical Record; HIPAA, Health Insurance Portability and Accountability Act; PACS, picture Archival Computer System; OSHA, The Occupational Safety and Health Administration; PM, Practice Management (Courtesy of Michael Cummings, MD, MBA and Mary Costantino, MD, Founder and Medical Director, Advanced Vascular Centers, Portland OR)

with an entrepreneurial mindset and work ethic will provide the culture needed to succeed.[8]

References

[1] U.S. Office-based Labs Market Size, Share & Trends Analysis Report. Grand View Research Market Analysis, December 2020 www.grandviewresearch.com

[2] Carr J. The Office-Based Interventional Suite: The Dread of Hospitals ... or the Future of Cardiovascular Contemporary Care. Cardiovascular Disease Management 4th Annual Symposium, Outpatient Endovascular and Interventional Society (OEIS), October 13–14, 2016

[3] Center for Medicare Services. Accessed July 5, 2023 at: https://medaxiom.com

[4] New ASC Revenue Sources via New Reimbursement Trends Related to OBLS. MedAxiom. October 4, 2020. New ASC Revenue Sources via New Reimbursement Trends Related to OBLs - MedAxiom.https://www.evtoday.com

[5] Kho H, Ahn S. Financial considerations for office based intervention labs. Endovascular Today, January 2014.https://www.evtoday.com

[6] Private Practice Models: Office Based Labs, SIR Private Practice Advisory Committee, Cummings and Costantino, December 3, 2020 educare.boston-scientific.com

[7] Key OBL Considerations, PV Podium, Boston Scientific educare.boston scientific.com

[8] Courtesy of Mary Costantino, MD, Founder and Medical Director, Advanced Vascular Centers, Portland OR

4 Lytic Vertebral Body Metastasis with Fracture

Anderanik Tomasian and Jack W. Jennings

4.1 Case Presentation

A 52-year-old man with renal cell carcinoma presented with painful T12 vertebral body osteolytic metastatic lesion with a minimally displaced pathologic fracture. The patient was presented at multidisciplinary tumor board. He had excellent Karnofsky performance status and life expectancy of greater than 6 months, and reported focal pain at the T12 vertebral level with no radicular symptoms. Physical examination revealed focal tenderness at the T12 vertebral level with no neurologic deficits. The Spine Instability Neoplastic Score (SINS) was 7. Multidisciplinary consensus was reached to proceed with percutaneous radiofrequency ablation (RFA) with vertebral augmentation in order to achieve local tumor control, pain palliation, and pathologic fracture stabilization.

In order to ablate the entire T12 vertebral body volume, simultaneous bipedicular RFA was performed under moderate sedation in an outpatient setting using a navigational bipolar RFA electrode system (▶ Fig. 4.1). RFA was initially performed along the anterior vertebral body to achieve an ellipsoid $3 \times 2 \times 2$ cm ablation volume for each electrode, followed by retraction of electrodes to cover the vertebral body posteriorly using identical ablation parameters. Medial articulation of RFA electrode tips was implemented in order to achieve overlapping coalescent ablation zones for improved efficiency. RFA was immediately followed by vertebral augmentation performed in standard fashion. The patient reported near-complete resolution of pain and was discharged home after 3 hours of monitoring.

4.2 Discussion

A multidisciplinary team approach, including radiation oncologists, medical oncologists, oncologic spine surgeons, and interventional radiologists, is recommended in the evaluation and treatment of patients with vertebral metastases.

Although external beam radiation therapy is currently considered the reference standard for local tumor control and pain palliation of spinal metastases, one should consider its limitations, particularly regarding efficacy in providing timely and adequate pain palliation.[1,2] These are important factors, particularly considering a diminished life expectancy in many of these patients.[1,2] Furthermore, radiation-resistant tumors and cumulative dose to the spinal cord that may limit further treatment, and/or tumor recurrence, lead to additional limitations.[3]

The morbidity associated with vertebral surgical interventions and patients' frequent poor underlying functional status limit the efficacy of these procedures, which are mainly considered for patients with neurologic compromise or spinal instability. Although the World Health Organization's analgesic ladder recommends opioids for initial management of cancer-related bone pain,[4] this approach remains suboptimal

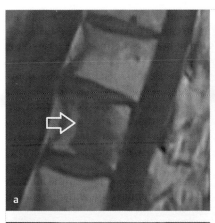
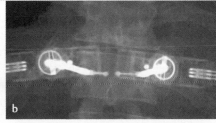
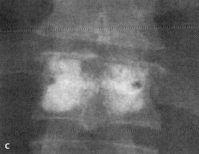
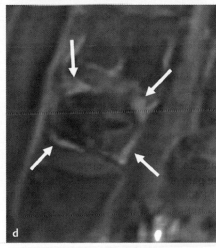

Fig. 4.1 A 52-year-old man with renal cell carcinoma and painful T12 metastatic lesion. Sagittal T1-weighted image **(a)** shows bone marrow-replacing lesion (arrow) within T12 vertebral body with subtle central vertebral body height loss compatible with pathologic fracture. Anteroposterior fluoroscopic image during simultaneous bipedicular radiofrequency ablation **(b)** shows medial articulation of electrode tips which are 5 to 10 mm apart (width of the spinous process as landmark). Anteroposterior fluoroscopic image **(c)** demonstrates post-ablation vertebral augmentation. Sagittal, T1-weighted, fat-saturated, contrast-enhanced magnetic resonance imaging (MRI) image obtained 12 months following treatment **(d)** shows local tumor control with enhancing granulation tissues along the periphery of ablation zone **(d, arrows)**. Note hypointense cement within the ablation cavity **(d)**.

due to common side effects of such medications, as well as frequent incomplete alleviation of pain.

4.2.1 Tumor Ablation Goals

Recent advances and evolution of percutaneous minimally invasive thermal ablation technologies, with or without vertebral augmentation, offer attractive options for certain subgroups of patients with spinal metastases. There are several distinct advantages of using this approach, including timely and durable pain palliation, excellent local tumor control rates, reinforcement of the treated vertebra, and short- and long-term improvement in functional status. These treatments occur without compromising adjuvant radiation or chemotherapy.[5,6,7,8,9,10,11,12,13]

4.2.2 Patient Selection Guidelines

The main factors used in determining a patient's eligibility to undergo percutaneous thermal ablation in the management of vertebral metastases include pain, performance status, life expectancy, degree of spinal stability, the presence of metastatic epidural spinal cord compression (MESCC), and the extent of extraosseous visceral metastases.[5,6,14] The validated and widely accepted Karnofsky Performance Status Scale is utilized in clinical practice to evaluate the patient's performance status.[15] In addition to performance status, spinal instability is evaluated based upon the Spinal Instability Neoplastic Score (SINS).[16] Scores for this metric range from 0 to 18, with higher scores translating into greater instability. Although no score exists to prompt surgical intervention, surgical evaluation for potential tumor resection and/or stabilization is typically performed in patients with SINS scores of 7 or higher. Percutaneous thermal ablation is relatively contraindicated in patients with spinal instability, depending on the degree of instability. Similar to operative interventions, no specific SINS threshold exists for thermal ablation techniques.

Although vertebral metastases complicated by central canal stenosis are typically managed by surgical intervention, thermal ablation may be considered as an alternative option in this patient population. Ablation is particularly useful in patients who are not surgical candidates, and is performed in the absence of spinal cord compression. It is important to note that in patients with central canal stenosis caused by tumor alone, thermal ablation may result in retraction or arrest of growth of the soft tissue component of the epidural tumor. However, ablation will not alleviate symptoms due to osseous retropulsion.

The National Comprehensive Cancer Network (NCCN) has incorporated percutaneous thermal ablation in the treatment of osseous metastases in its published guidelines. According to the latest NCCN guidelines for the treatment of cancer pain in adults (version 3.2019), thermal ablation may be considered for palliation of metastatic bone pain in the absence of oncologic emergency, when chemotherapy is inadequate and radiation therapy is contraindicated or not desired by the patient.[17]

The recently published American College of Radiology (ACR) Appropriateness Criteria describes specific recommendation in the treatment of vertebral metastases.[18] First, vertebral augmentation and thermal ablation may be appropriate in the treatment of asymptomatic pathologic spinal fractures with or without edema on magnetic resonance imaging (MRI). Second,

vertebral augmentation and thermal ablation procedures are usually appropriate in the treatment of pathologic spinal fracture with severe and progressive pain. Third, vertebral augmentation is usually appropriate and thermal ablation may be appropriate in the treatment of pathologic spinal fractures with spinal malalignment. The appropriateness category of "may be appropriate" is defined as, "The imaging procedure or treatment may be indicated in the specified clinical scenarios as an alternative to imaging procedures or treatments with a more favorable risk-benefit ratio, or the risk-benefit ratio for patients is equivocal." An appropriateness category of "usually appropriate" is defined as, "The imaging procedure or treatment is indicated in the specified clinical scenarios at a favorable risk-benefit ratio for patients."[18]

4.2.3 Thermal Ablation Modalities

Radiofrequency Ablation

RFA is mainly utilized in the treatment of vertebral metastases with the following imaging characteristics. First, tumors should be primarily osteolytic as the higher impedance of osteoblastic lesions renders RFA ineffective.[5,12,18] Second, lesions should have no or little extra-osseous components. Finally, tumors should be located in the posterior vertebral body (particularly centrally), where access is safe and feasible using navigational articulating electrodes.

The recent availability of navigational bipolar RFA electrodes offers several distinct advantages compared to traditional unipolar straight electrodes. These advantages are particularly beneficial in the treatment of vertebral metastases.[5,7,12] The first advantage of these newer devices is the bipolar electrode design, obviating the need for grounding pad placement and eliminating the risk of skin thermal injury. Second, real-time intraprocedural monitoring of the ablation zone size is made possible by the design including built-in thermocouples along the electrode shaft. Third, an electrode tip that can be articulated in different orientations through one skin/bone entry site, allowing treatment of difficult-to-access tumors. This is particularly important for tumors in the posterior central vertebral body. In addition, these articulating electrodes achieve larger ablation zones when using a transpedicular approach.[5,7,12] Finally, tissue char (carbonization) is minimized with the use of internally cooled electrodes.

There are recent consensus recommendations by the International Spine Radiosurgery Consortium in differentiating clinical target volume (CTV) from gross tumor volume (GTV) in order to account for marginal radiation therapy failures due to microscopic tumor infiltration. This differentiation has caused a paradigm shift in the management of vertebral metastases.[19] The consensus recommendation defines CTV (to be treated by stereotactic spine radiosurgery) to include GTV *plus* adjacent abnormal bone marrow signal intensity on MRI in order to account for microscopic tumor invasion. This finding on MRI accounts for subclinical tumor spread in marrow.[19]

Simultaneous bipedicular vertebral RFA is a novel technique that efficiently generates two confluent, coalescent, and overlapping ablation zones in close proximity to one another. This decreases the convective cooling effect (heat sink), the risk of thermal injury, and charring and impedance related issues[5]

(▶ Fig. 4.1). A more thorough ablation may be achieved using this approach, aligning with the stereotactic spine radiosurgery paradigm discussed above. This allows treatment of the entire vertebral body volume and pedicles, allowing for improved local tumor control rates and more durable pain palliation.[19]

Limitations of RFA include: ablation zone occult on computed tomography (CT); the use of monopolar systems in patients with metallic implants and pacemakers due to risk of skin thermal injury and pacemaker malfunction; heat-sink effect due to cerebrospinal fluid and vertebral venous plexus flow; procedure-related pain; and increased pain in the immediate post-ablation period. It should be recognized that the heat-sink effect along the posterior vertebral body and pedicles decreases the possibility of neural thermal injury.[5]

Microwave Ablation

Microwave ablation (MWA) is less susceptible to the heat-sink effect and variable tissue impedance than RFA, in theory resulting in a more uniform and larger ablation zone. This may allow for a more efficient ablation using a single antenna.[9,13] Other advantages of MWA include: efficacy in treatment of osteoblastic lesions; the lack of the need for grounding pads minimizing risk of skin thermal injury; a lack of contraindication in patients with metallic implants; and minimal risk of back-heating along the antennae seen in the latest generations of microwave devices.[9,13] It should be recognized that, similar to cryoablation described below, intact cortical bone does not serve as a barrier to microwave energy propagation. Another potential pitfall while using MWA is the rapid deposition of high power output (up to 100 Watts), which may be a disadvantage in the treatment of spinal tumors due to potential risk of neural thermal injury. Finally, the MWA zone is largely occult on CT with less distinct ablation zone boundaries compared with RFA and cryoablation, leading to a less predictable ablation zone.

Cryoablation

Cryoablation is characterized by an initial freezing cycle (approximately 10 minutes or longer, depending on tumor characteristics) immediately followed by an active thawing phase (commonly 5 minutes). A second freezing cycle (similar to the initial freezing cycle) is typically performed.[8] A temperature of −40 °C or lower must be achieved in order to guarantee reliable cell death.[8] Cryoablation is typically considered in the treatment of spinal metastases with the following features: vertebral body tumors with large soft tissue components; large tumors involving the posterior vertebral elements; paravertebral soft tissue tumors; and osteoblastic lesions.

Cryoablation has several distinct advantages over other ablation methods, most notably visualization of a low-density ice ball during ablation on CT. This allows for a more precise, and presumably safer, ablation procedure. Additional advantages include the simultaneous use of several cryoprobes to achieve additive overlapping and sculpted ablation zones, less intraprocedural and immediate postprocedural pain compared to heating ablation techniques, and the availability of MRI-compatible cryoprobes. Disadvantages of cryoablation include: the frequent lack of distinct visualization of an ice ball within osteoblastic

tumors (and at times normal bone); extended procedure length during ablation of larger tumors; the cost associated with use of multiple cryoprobes; and delay in cement augmentation during combined ablation–augmentation procedures, delayed in order to minimize interference with cement polymerization. It is also important to note that an intact vertebral cortex does not prevent expansion of the ice ball, which should be taken into consideration when cryoablating vertebral tumors.[8]

4.2.4 Thermal Protection

During thermal ablation of spinal metastases, proximity of the spinal cord and nerve roots to the ablation zone carries a significant risk of neural injury. Several techniques are available to minimize the risk of neural injury, classified as active and passive thermal protection techniques.[5,7,8,12,14]

Active thermal protection is typically achieved by techniques to provide thermal insulation. This includes hydrodissection with injection of warm or cool liquid in the epidural space or neuroforamina. For hydrodissections, ionic solutions should be avoided in order to avoid the creation of a plasma field and undesired energy propagation. In addition, pneumodissection with the injection of epidural/neuroforaminal carbon dioxide may also be performed. In clinical practice, active thermal protection is initiated once the ablation zone temperature reaches 45 °C (heat) and 10 °C (cold).[5,7,8,12,14]

Passive thermal protection strategies include patient feedback when performing the ablation under moderate sedation; real-time temperature monitoring by placement of thermocouples within the epidural space and/or neuroforamina; motor and somatosensory evoked potential amplitude monitoring; and electrostimulation of peripheral nerves for early detection of impending nerve injury.[5,7,8,12,14] Approaches to minimize skin thermal injury include precise assessment of ablation zone size and geometry, surface application of warm saline during cryoablation, and using bipolar RFA electrode systems.

4.2.5 Complications

The most important potential complication of thermal ablation of spinal metastases is thermal injury to the spinal cord and nerve roots. Most of these injuries are transient and are typically managed by transforaminal or epidural injection of steroids and the use of long-acting local anesthetics. There has been a recent report of a case of permanent bilateral lower extremity paralysis as well as bowel and urinary incontinence immediately following RFA (combined with vertebral augmentation) of lumbar spinal osseous metastasis. This complication was presumably due to thermal injury of bilateral lumbar ventral nerve roots.[20] Bone weakening and risk of ablation-related fracture are typically minimized in select patients with the use of concurrent vertebral augmentation. Cement leakage into the central canal/epidural space or neuroforamina may result in increased pain due to central canal or neuroforaminal stenosis, spinal cord compression, or potentially spinal cord thermal injury due to an exothermic effect of cement polymerization. Skin thermal injury remains a potential risk as well.

4.2.6 Vertebral Augmentation

Following thermal ablation of vertebral metastases, vertebral augmentation may be performed to better achieve pathologic fracture stabilization or as a preventative measure for further pain palliation in patients with persistent pain. Vertebral augmentation may also be used in patients with tumor progression on imaging despite maximum external beam radiation therapy, a contraindication to radiation therapy, or an insufficient response to systemic therapies and opioid administration (▶ Fig. 4.1).[5,6,7,11,12] Vertebral augmentation may not be necessary following thermal ablation of posterior vertebral elements only, or in the lower sacral spine segments. In patients with spinal instability (detailed below) and contraindications for surgery, vertebral augmentation may be performed with or without ablation in order to limit motion at the pathologic fracture site as well as prevent further vertebral body collapse and hopefully improve the patient's pain. Spinal stability is not completely achieved in such cases, and other therapies including surgical interventions should be considered.

References

[1] Goetz MP, Callstrom MR, Charboneau JW, et al. Percutaneous image-guided radiofrequency ablation of painful metastases involving bone: a multicenter study. J Clin Oncol. 2004; 22(2):300–306

[2] Lutz S, Berk L, Chang E, et al. American Society for Radiation Oncology (ASTRO). Palliative radiotherapy for bone metastases: an ASTRO evidence-based guideline. Int J Radiat Oncol Biol Phys. 2011; 79(4):965–976

[3] Gerszten PC, Mendel E, Yamada Y. Radiotherapy and radiosurgery for metastatic spine disease: what are the options, indications, and outcomes? Spine. 2009; 34(22) Suppl:S78–S92

[4] WHO's Cancer Pain Ladder for Adults. World Health Organization. www.who.int/cancer/palliative/painladder/en/. Published November 27, 2013. Accessed June 13, 2019

[5] Tomasian A, Hillen TJ, Chang RO, Jennings JW. Simultaneous bipedicular radiofrequency ablation combined with vertebral augmentation for local tumor control of spinal metastases. AJNR Am J Neuroradiol. 2018; 39(9): 1768–1773

[6] Wallace AN, Robinson CG, Meyer J, et al. The metastatic spine disease multidisciplinary working group algorithms. Oncologist. 2015; 20(10): 1205–1215

[7] Tomasian A, Gangi A, Wallace AN, Jennings JW. Percutaneous thermal ablation of spinal metastases: recent advances and review. AJR Am J Roentgenol. 2018; 210(1):142–152

[8] Schag CC, Heinrich RL, Ganz PA. Karnofsky performance status revisited: reliability, validity, and guidelines. J Clin Oncol. 1984; 2(3):187–193

[9] Fisher CG, DiPaola CP, Ryken TC, et al. A novel classification system for spinal instability in neoplastic disease: an evidence-based approach and expert consensus from the Spine Oncology Study Group. Spine. 2010; 35(22): E1221–E1229

[10] Swarm RA, Paice JA, Anghelescu DL, et al. Adult Cancer Pain, Version 3.2019, NCCN Clinical Practice Guidelines in Oncology. National Comprehensive Cancer Network. https://jnccn.org/view/journals/jnccn/17/8/article-p977.xml. Published 2019. Accessed December 21, 2019

[11] Shah LM, Jennings JW, et al. Expert Panels on Neurological Imaging, Interventional Radiology, and Musculoskeletal Imaging. ACR Appropriateness Criteria® management of vertebral compression fractures. J Am Coll Radiol. 2018; 15(11S):S347–S364

[12] Wallace AN, Tomasian A, Vaswani D, Vyhmeister R, Chang RO, Jennings JW. Radiographic local control of spinal metastases with percutaneous radiofrequency ablation and vertebral augmentation. AJNR Am J Neuroradiol. 2016; 37(4):759–765

[13] Tomasian A, Wallace A, Northrup B, Hillen TJ, Jennings JW. Spine cryoablation: pain palliation and local tumor control for vertebral metastases. AJNR Am J Neuroradiol. 2016; 37(1):189–195

[14] Kastler A, Alnassan H, Aubry S, Kastler B. Microwave thermal ablation of spinal metastatic bone tumors. J Vasc Interv Radiol. 2014; 25(9):1470–1475

[15] Callstrom MR, Dupuy DE, Solomon SB, et al. Percutaneous image-guided cryoablation of painful metastases involving bone: multicenter trial. Cancer. 2013; 119(5):1033–1041

[16] Bagla S, Sayed D, Smirniotopoulos J, et al. Multicenter prospective clinical series evaluating radiofrequency ablation in the treatment of painful spine metastases. Cardiovasc Intervent Radiol. 2016; 39(9):1289–1297

[17] Hillen TJ, Anchala P, Friedman MV, Jennings JW. Treatment of metastatic posterior vertebral body osseous tumors by using a targeted bipolar radiofrequency ablation device: technical note. Radiology. 2014; 273(1):261–267

[18] Khan MA, Deib G, Deldar B, Patel AM, Barr JS. Efficacy and safety of percutaneous microwave ablation and cementoplasty in the treatment of painful spinal metastases and myeloma. AJNR Am J Neuroradiol. 2018; 39(7): 1376–1383

[19] Cox BW, Spratt DE, Lovelock M, et al. International Spine Radiosurgery Consortium consensus guidelines for target volume definition in spinal stereotactic radiosurgery. Int J Radiat Oncol Biol Phys. 2012; 83(5):e597–e605

[20] Huntoon K, Eltobgy M, Mohyeldin A, Elder JB. Lower extremity paralysis after radiofrequency ablation of vertebral metastases. World Neurosurg. 2020; 133:178–184

5 Lytic Lesions Involving the Vertebral Body without Associated Fracture

Jason Levy

5.1 Case Presentation

A 79-year-old woman presented to the interventional radiology clinic with low back pain related to an L3 metastasis. She had a long history of metastatic ER-positive, HER-2 negative breast cancer with osseous metastases. Depending on activity, her pain level ranged from 5 to 10 out of possible 10. She was well known to the interventional radiology clinic from prior yttrium-90 therapy for liver metastases. Prior metastatic osseous therapy included multifraction external beam radiation to her right shoulder 4 months earlier, but no local spine therapy. The pain control regimen included oxycodone (10 mg by mouth every 4 hours) when necessary.

Physical examination demonstrated no signs of neuropathy and a normal motor and sensory examination of the lower extremities. Direct pressure on the spinous process produced mild discomfort. The pain was referred to bilateral superior hips, right worse than left. Ambulation was somewhat limited secondary to pain. Magnetic resonance imaging (MRI) revealed lytic metastases with enhancement at the posterior aspect of L3 (▶ Fig. 5.1).

The case was discussed at a multidisciplinary tumor board. Given the presence of a dominant lytic osseous metastasis and an inherent fracture risk, mechanical stabilization with tumor treatment was desired. Radiofrequency ablation (RFA) was chosen over radiation and cryoablation as the initial treatment option due to the ease of providing more optimal cement with this technology.

Preprocedure dexamethasone (10 mg) and ketorolac (15 mg) were administered intravenously. The procedure was performed with moderate sedation and analgesia utilizing Versed 3.5 mg and 100 µg fentanyl. Care was taken to maintain consciousness during the ablation portion of the procedure in order to get patient feedback. Bilateral transpedicular access was obtained to the L3 vertebral body, and coaxial radiofrequency probes were placed bilaterally to ablate the tumor in L3. A targeted ablation was performed in order to include the posterior margin of the vertebral body. Ablation was carried out for 15 minutes. Upon completion of the ablation, polymethylmethacrylate (PMMA) cement was placed in a coaxial fashion (▶ Fig. 5.2).

In the immediate postprocedure recovery period, an additional 15 mg of ketorolac was administered intravenously. Within 3 hours post-procedure, the patient was already reporting pain relief. By 3 days post-procedure her pain level had decreased to 1 out of possible 10. The pain relief sustained at 1 week, 1 month, and 6 months post-procedure.

5.2 Discussion

The spine is the most commonly affected site for metastatic bone cancer, often from breast, lung, prostate, or kidney primary tumors.[1] The most frequent complaint of patients with skeletal metastases is pain, which occurred in 79% of patients.[2] The pain can have a significant effect on quality of life.[3]

Skeletal metastases have two primary pain generators, mechanical and biologic. Mechanical pain is caused by vertebral instability and can be seen with lytic lesions even without a visible fracture. Mechanical pain is addressed by cement or instrument stabilization. Biological pain is caused by neurostimulating cytokines that stimulate nerve receptors. The release of cytokines occurs with osteoclastic-mediated bone resorption, and can be treated with ablation.[4,5]

Treatment goals for lytic vertebral body metastases are pain palliation, improvement in quality of life, preservation of neurologic function, and stabilization of mechanical structures. Tumor treatment and mechanical stabilization are paramount to preventing delayed skeletal events such as fracture or neurologic injury. By the time a patient presents to the interventional

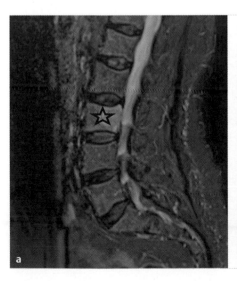
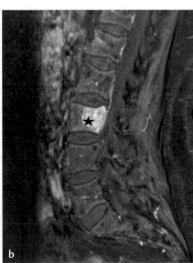

Fig. 5.1 Sagittal T2-weighted (T2W) short tau inversion recovery (STIR) image **(a)** and T1-weighted (T1W) post-gadolinium **(b)** magnetic resonance imaging (MRI) demonstrate posterior L3 metastases (stars).

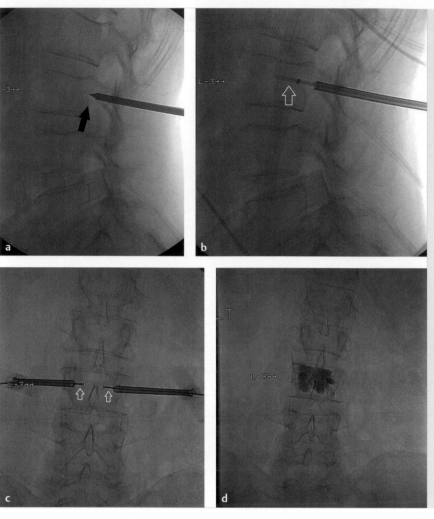

Fig. 5.2 **(a)** Lateral intraprocedural fluoroscopic image. Arrows point to the posterior vertebral cortex. The stylet is used to map the posterior extent of the ablation. When performed simultaneously through a coaxial bilateral transpedicular access, the ablation zone grows in a straight posterior line. **(b, c)** Lateral and anteroposterior (AP) fluoroscopic images demonstrating the coaxial radiofrequency ablation (RFA) probes (arrows). **(d)** AP view post polymethylmethacrylate (PMMA) cement.

radiology clinic, systemic options with chemotherapy, immunotherapy, or hormonal therapy have usually failed or provided insufficient relief. At this point local options with radiation therapy, surgery, and ablation are considered. The ideal therapy allows for rapid relief with minimal or no disruption from the systemic therapy protocol.

Both vertebral augmentation and RFA have been shown in prospective studies to provide rapid and sustained pain relief in vertebral body metastases.[6,7] The addition of RFA prior to cement augmentation has also been proposed to have a cavitary effect that will allow for a more predictable cement fill.[8] RFA in vertebral body metastases has been demonstrated to reduce the most consequential cement leaks, namely, venous leaks and those posterior to the vertebral body.[9]

External beam radiation therapy (EBRT) continues to be the most common radiation treatment for painful bone metastases, with increasing utilization of stereotactic body radiation therapy (SBRT). However, all forms of radiation are known to carry a significant risk of fracture of the treated vertebral body.[10] In a Memorial Sloan Kettering study, the risk of fracture with SBRT has been suggested to be as high as 39%.[11] Although thermal ablation is effective for pain and tumor control, similar to radiation therapy, it also further weakens the involved bone. When an axial loading weight-bearing bone is involved, there is a risk

of pathological fracture; in this setting, augmentation with cementoplasty is needed.

5.3 Companion Case

A 42-year-old woman was admitted to the hospital with severe debilitating pain. She had multifraction EBRT completed 1 week prior to admission for a T5 lytic metastasis from breast sarcoma. Prior to multifraction EBRT, she was fully functional and reported pain scores of 4 out of 10. Upon admission, however, she was unable to ambulate, she was off systemic therapy protocol and reported 10 out of 10 pain. She had a patient-controlled analgesia (PCA) Dilaudid pump for pain control. A sagittal computed tomography (CT) prior to radiation and sagittal short tau inversion recovery (STIR) with corresponding axial T2-weighted image (T2WI) after radiation demonstrated a new fracture (▶ Fig. 5.3).

Physical examination demonstrated no signs of neuropathy with normal motor and sensory examination of the lower extremities. Bladder and bowel control were intact. Her mobility was limited secondary to pain; due to this, her gait could not be assessed. Vertebral body RFA and cementoplasty were offered.

Preprocedure dexamethasone (10 mg) and ketorolac (15 mg) were administered intravenously. The procedure was performed

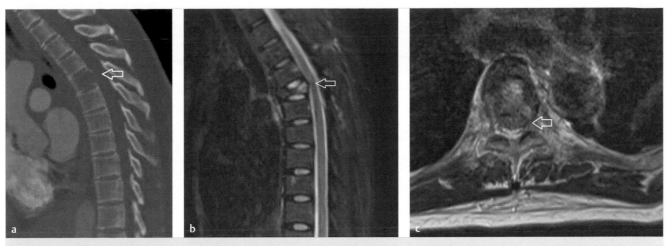

Fig. 5.3 (a) Pre-external beam radiation therapy (EBRT) computed tomography (CT) demonstrates lytic T5 metastasis (arrow). (b) Sagittal short tau inversion recovery (STIR) magnetic resonance imaging (MRI) showing radiation-induced T5 fracture now with retropulsion (arrow). (c) Axial T2-weighted image (T2WI) shows fracture with retropulsion (arrow).

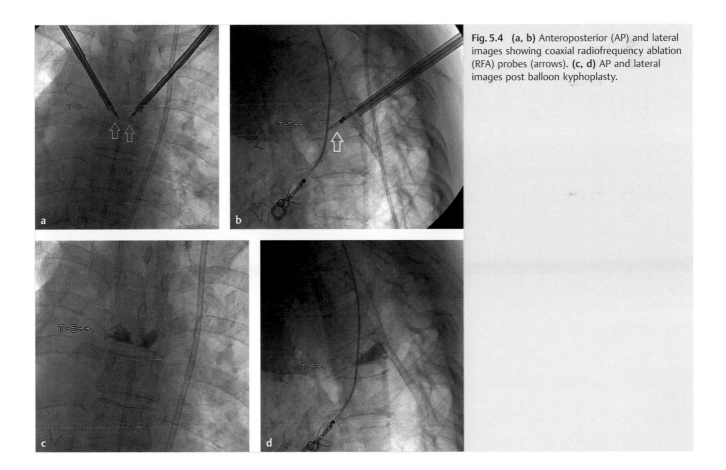

Fig. 5.4 (a, b) Anteroposterior (AP) and lateral images showing coaxial radiofrequency ablation (RFA) probes (arrows). (c, d) AP and lateral images post balloon kyphoplasty.

with monitored anesthesia care. Bilateral parapedicular access was obtained to the T5 vertebral body. Coaxial radiofrequency probes were placed bilaterally in order to ablate T5. A targeted ablation was performed to include the posterior margin of the vertebral body. Ablation was carried out for 11.5 minutes. Upon completion of the ablation, balloon kyphoplasty was performed in standard fashion (▶ Fig. 5.4).

The patient reported relief within 3 hours of the procedure. Her systemic therapy protocol was reinitiated the next morning, and she was able to ambulate and attend physical therapy. Her pain level was reduced to 1 out of 10 at 1 week, which was sustained at 6-month follow-up.

Preparing the goals of therapy is paramount prior to entering into any treatment plan. The goal of mechanical stabilization may be sacrificed with radiation, and can lead to a delayed skeletal event such as fracture. The risk is higher in patients with lytic metastases.[11,12] In fact, some authors have suggested mechanical stabilization before radiation in "high-risk" cases.[13,14] RFA and cement augmentation can be performed alone or in a combined approach with single or multiple fraction EBRT or SBRT.

References

[1] Nielsen OS, Munro AJ, Tannock IF. Bone metastases: pathophysiology and management policy. J Clin Oncol. 1991; 9(3):509–524

[2] Janjan N, Lutz ST, Bedwinek JM, et al. American College of Radiology. Therapeutic guidelines for the treatment of bone metastasis: a report from the American College of Radiology Appropriateness Criteria Expert Panel on Radiation Oncology. J Palliat Med. 2009; 12(5):417–426

[3] Nakatsuka A, Yamakado K, Maeda M, et al. Radiofrequency ablation combined with bone cement injection for the treatment of bone malignancies. J Vasc Interv Radiol. 2004; 15(7):707–712

[4] Rybak LD. Fire and ice: thermal ablation of musculoskeletal tumors. Radiol Clin North Am. 2009; 47(3):455–469

[5] Callstrom MR, Charboneau JW, Goetz MP, et al. Image-guided ablation of painful metastatic bone tumors: a new and effective approach to a difficult problem. Skeletal Radiol. 2006; 35(1):1–15 [serial online]

[6] Berenson J, Pflugmacher R, Jarzem P, et al. Cancer Patient Fracture Evaluation (CAFE) Investigators. Balloon kyphoplasty versus non-surgical fracture management for treatment of painful vertebral body compression fractures in patients with cancer: a multicentre, randomised controlled trial. Lancet Oncol. 2011; 12(3):225–235

[7] Guenette JP, Lopez MJ, Kim E, Dupuy DE. Solitary painful osseous metastases: correlation of imaging features with pain palliation after radiofrequency ablation—a multicenter American College of Radiology imaging network study. Radiology. 2013; 268(3):907–915

[8] Georgy BA, Wong W. Plasma-mediated radiofrequency ablation assisted percutaneous cement injection for treating advanced malignant vertebral compression fractures. AJNR Am J Neuroradiol. 2007; 28(4):700–705

[9] David E, Kaduri S, Yee A, et al. Initial single center experience: radiofrequency ablation assisted vertebroplasty and osteoplasty using a bipolar device in the palliation of bone metastases. Ann Palliat Med. 2017; 6(2):118–124

[10] Sze WM, Shelley M, Held I, Mason M. Palliation of metastatic bone pain: single fraction versus multifraction radiotherapy—a systematic review of the randomised trials. Cochrane Database Syst Rev. 2004(2):CD004721

[11] Rose PS, Laufer I, Boland PJ, et al. Risk of fracture after single fraction image-guided intensity-modulated radiation therapy to spinal metastases. J Clin Oncol. 2009; 27(30):5075–5079

[12] Cunha MV, Al-Omair A, Atenafu EG, et al. Vertebral compression fracture (VCF) after spine stereotactic body radiation therapy (SBRT): analysis of predictive factors. Int J Radiat Oncol Biol Phys. 2012; 84(3):e343–e349

[13] Massicotte E, Foote M, Reddy R, Sahgal A. Minimal access spine surgery (MASS) for decompression and stabilization performed as an out-patient procedure for metastatic spinal tumours followed by spine stereotactic body radiotherapy (SBRT): first report of technique and preliminary outcomes. Technol Cancer Res Treat. 2012; 11(1):15–25

[14] Gerszten PC, Germanwala A, Burton SA, Welch WC, Ozhasoglu C, Vogel WJ. Combination kyphoplasty and spinal radiosurgery: a new treatment paradigm for pathological fractures. J Neurosurg Spine. 2005; 3(4):296–301

6 Sclerotic Lesions Involving the Vertebral Body

William G. O'Connell, Nima Kokabi, and Aron Chary

6.1 Case Presentation

A 53-year-old Black woman with metastatic breast cancer presented to the interventional radiology (IR) clinic for evaluation of low back pain and progression of a compression fracture at T12. Her primary complaint was increasing pain in the mid- to lower back that radiated to her left side. She reported the pain as a maximum of 8/10, which improved to 5/10 with pain medication. She reported an inability to stand up straight without feeling pain, causing her to walk bent over. She was unable to cook or wash dishes because she could not stand up straight, and she was walking with a cane to prevent falling. She had a fentanyl patch for pain relief, and was also taking oral Abraxane. She had received palliative radiation therapy to C1-C3, T9-S11, the left femur, and whole-brain radiation for symptomatic metastasis

On physical examination, the patient had mid back tenderness on palpation. She had 5 + strength in proximal flexor and extensor muscles (hip and knee movements), as well as 5 + strength in foot dorsiflexion and plantar flexion. She ambulated hunched over with a cane.

Computed tomography (CT) imaging revealed a compression fracture at T12 as well as more subtle compression fractures involving T10, T11, L1, L2, and L5, which also contained sclerotic metastases. Additionally, the density of the spine overall was increased for a woman of her age, likely a result of previous radiation therapy (▶ Fig. 6.1).

The patient was scheduled for multilevel spine radiofrequency ablation (RFA) with kyphoplasty to treat the compressed vertebral bodies and dominant sclerotic metastases. The plan of care options outside of IR were maximized, including systemic therapy administered by oncology and external beam radiation therapy already completed by radiation oncology.

The patient successfully underwent RFA and kyphoplasty of T10, T11, T12, L1, L2, and L5 under general anesthesia on two separate procedures. She initially underwent treatment of T12, L2, and L5. Although there was some symptomatic improvement, this improvement was not as profound as expected. It was determined to treat T10, T11, and L1 (▶ Fig. 6.2), which was successfully performed 1 month after the initial vertebral augmentation procedures (▶ Fig. 6.3).

The patient did exceptionally well after the procedures with complete resolution of back pain to 0/10. She was able to reduce her pain medication and ambulate to perform her desired activities of daily living.

6.2 Discussion

Sclerosis is the pathological hardening of tissue, especially from overgrowth of fibrous tissue or an increase in interstitial tissue. Sclerosis involving the bone is related to abnormal bone mineralization and/or remodeling. Sclerotic bone lesions are best identified with ionizing radiation to confirm increased radiodensity, including radiographs, CT scans as well as positron

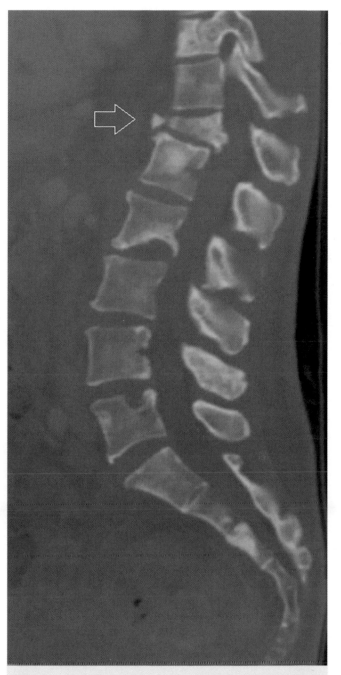

Fig. 6.1 Sagittal reconstructed computed tomography (CT) of the lower thoracic and lumbar spines demonstrating multiple sclerotic metastases. An associated severe compression fraction of the sclerotic T12 vertebral body (arrow).

emission tomography (PET)/CT scans. Nuclear medicine bone scans with Tc-99 m methylene diphosphonate (MDP) and occasionally magnetic resonance imaging (MRI) can identify bone lesions; however, increased radiodensity must be confirmed with radiographs or CT prior to labeling the lesion as sclerotic.

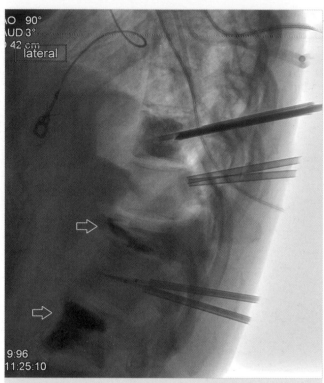

Fig. 6.2 Lateral fluoroscopic view during vertebral augmentation procedures at T10, T11, and L1. Cement from prior procedures at T12 and L2 is also noted (arrows).

Table 6.1 Common etiologies for sclerotic bone lesions

Normal
- Enostosis

Abnormal Bone Remodeling
- Paget's disease
- Sclerosing bone dysplasias
- Tuberosclerosis
- Osteopetrosis
- Osteopoikilosis
- Pyknodysostosis (hyperostosis of long bones)
- Osteopathia striata (metadiaphyses of long bones)
- Progressive diaphyseal dysplasia (periosteal and endosteal cortical thickening of long bones and calvaria)
- Hereditary multiple diaphyseal sclerosis (asymmetric cortical thickening of long bones)
- Hyperostosis corticalis generalisata (endosteal cortical thickening of long bones, skull, and facial bones)

Malignancy
- Prostate metastasis
- Breast cancer
- Treated metastases (e.g., post radiation therapy)

Infection

Degenerative Changes

Fractures, Usually Partially Healed

Osteochondroma

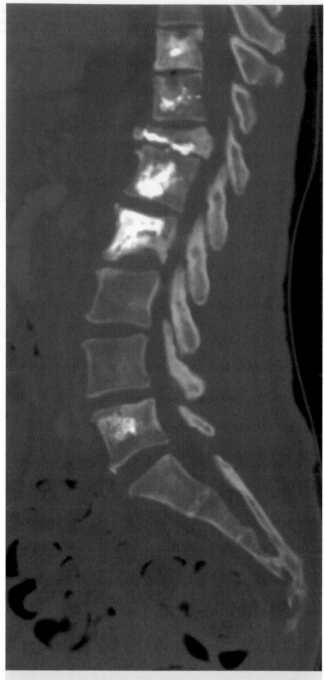

Fig. 6.3 Computed tomography (CT) imaging after ablation and kyphoplasty showing an appropriate treatment of T10, T11, T12, L1, L2, and L5 with deposition of polymethylmethacrylate mixed with barium in the vertebral bodies (compare to ▶ Fig. 6.1).

Evaluation of sclerotic bone lesions can be challenging. Sclerotic vertebral body lesions are caused by an assortment of medical conditions, including normal enostoses (▶ Table 6.1). Identifying the underlying cause of the sclerosis is essential prior to formulating a treatment plan. Incorporating the radiologic findings with the clinical picture is essential for accurate diagnosis and determining treatment goals. The sclerosis distribution, location, and change with time are all important factors. Ruling out active infection, acute cord compression, and unstable spine fractures is critical since these conditions might contraindicate a certain procedure. Additionally, the authors recommend against treating sclerotic lesions in the cervical spine unless these procedures are performed in conjunction with a credentialed spine surgeon.

Back pain related to sclerotic vertebral metastases is likely due to osseous disruption and micromovement at the fracture plane. Administering cement into the fracture will stabilize this micromovement and drastically improve the pain. Ablation is performed prior to administering cement to prevent inadvertent spread of malignancy into the paravertebral space. One of the unique challenges with treating sclerotic lesions is that the dense bone can be difficult to traverse/access. Additionally, it is often difficult to determine which levels are causing the pain; therefore, it might be necessary to treat all levels where there are obvious compression fractures as well as those levels that contain bulky metastatic disease.

7 Multiple Myeloma in the Spine

Faramarz Edalat, Aron Chary, William G. O'Connell, and J. David Prologo

7.1 Case Presentation

A 63-year-old woman with a remote history of breast cancer presented with severe upper back pain and a new T3 osteolytic lesion resulting in a vertebral body fracture. The patient underwent a biopsy of T3 demonstrating plasma cell neoplasm. She was subsequently evaluated by a neurosurgeon who deemed the fracture stable and deferred surgical intervention. She underwent radiotherapy, but despite a maximized opioid regimen still had persistent severe back pain. Contrast-enhanced magnetic resonance imaging (MRI) demonstrated a diffuse enhancing lesion within the T3 vertebral body and associated pathological compression fracture resulting in 50% height loss (▶ Fig. 7.1). The patient was referred to interventional radiology to discuss treatment options. A T3 vertebral body radiofrequency ablation (RFA) (OsteoCool RF Ablation System, Medtronic, Dublin, Ireland) and kyphoplasty were performed under general anesthesia with significant, durable pain relief on subsequent clinical follow-ups (▶ Fig. 7.2).

7.2 Discussion

Multiple myeloma (MM) is a hematological malignancy that primarily occurs in the elderly, with a median age at diagnosis of 65 to 74 years. A 5-year survival rate of 50% is generally reported.[1,2] According to the Surveillance, Epidemiology and End Results (SEER) program, there are an estimated 32,000 new cases of MM and 13,000 deaths from MM each year in the United States.[3] The pathophysiology of MM is defined as neoplastic plasma cells producing monoclonal immunoglobulins that can proliferate in the bone marrow, resulting in extensive osseous destruction and pathological fractures. Multiple myeloma is suspected in patients with bone pain and lytic osseous lesions, increased serum protein concentration, presence of serum or urine monoclonal protein, anemia, hypercalcemia, and/or acute renal failure.[4]

Skeletal involvement is the major feature of MM, often involving the central skeleton that can result in mechanical pain and pathological fracture in up to 70% of patients.[1] The biological basis of pathological fractures in patients with MM is increased osteoclast activation and osteoblast inhibition, which prevents fracture healing. Patients may concomitantly present with neurological symptoms of spinal cord compression or radiculopathy from nerve root compression by extramedullary plasmacytoma or bone fragments from vertebral body compression fracture (VBCFx). Patients often require urgent clinical and imaging evaluation. MRI with gadolinium contrast and/or (^{18}F)-fluorodeoxyglucose-positron emission tomography (PET) are mainstay of imaging in patients with MM. Contrast-enhanced MRI is highly sensitive for focal or diffuse pattern involvement of MM lesions in the skeleton. Additionally, given that bone scans detect osteoblastic activity only, this imaging modality is positive in only 20% of patients with MM.[5]

7.3 Clinical Approach

In approaching MM patients with spine involvement, particular attention is given to prevention or treatment of skeletal-related

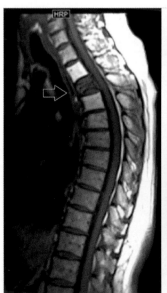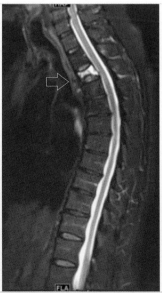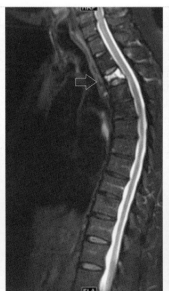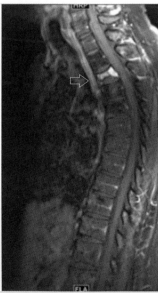

Fig. 7.1 Precontrast, sagittal T1 (upper left), T2 (upper right), T2-weighted, fat-saturated (lower left), and postcontrast, sagittal, T1-weighted, fat-saturated (lower right) images of the thoracic spine demonstrating T3 pathological compression fracture (arrows) with 50% height loss with vertebral body enhancement consistent with multiple myeloma involvement.

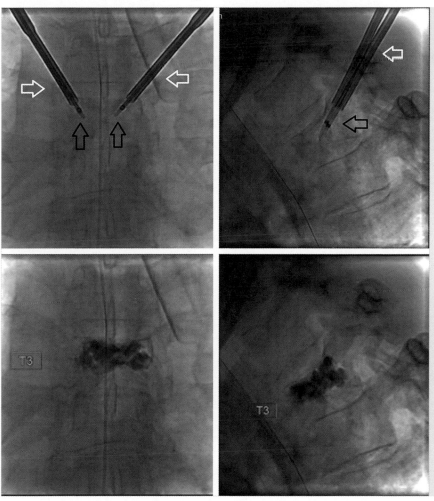

Fig. 7.2 Intraprocedural fluoroscopic images on anteroposterior (AP) and lateral views demonstrating bilateral vertebral body access cannulas (white arrows) and radiofrequency ablation (RFA) probes (black arrows) positioned within the vertebral body (upper images). AP and lateral fluoroscopic images of the thoracic spine after completion of kyphoplasty (bottom images).

events (SREs). SREs are defined as complications that occur as a result of a neoplastic process within the skeleton resulting in pain, namely, pathological fractures or spinal cord compression. Mainstay medical therapy for SREs includes chemotherapy, hematopoietic cell transplantation, and osteoclast inhibitors (e.g., bisphosphonates). In the setting of pathological VBCFx, however, medical therapy is often ineffective in providing timely pain relief and provides no benefit in fracture stabilization.[6]

The assessment of MM patients with VBCFx involves determining pain scores, performance scores, life expectancy, spinal stability, and presence or absence of neurological symptoms. Spinal stability can be evaluated based on the Spine Instability Neoplastic Score (SINS), with a score of ≥7 considered to put the patient at risk for spinal instability.[7] The goal of treatment in MM patients with VBCFx is fracture stabilization, pain relief, and improved quality of life (QoL). Patients with VBCFx are at increased risk for subsequent fractures due to abnormal sagittal imbalance and increased compressive forces on the anterior aspect of the spine. This can lead to progressive kyphotic angulation of the spine reducing lung function, which also leads to increased morbidity and mortality. Treatment planning is initiated after a multidisciplinary discussion with medical and radiation oncology, interventional radiology, and spinal surgery teams.

7.4 Percutaneous Treatments

Indications for percutaneous treatment include severe back pain that interferes with daily activities with an identified pain generator source from the vertebral body pathological fracture, without contraindications including uncorrectable coagulopathy, spinal instability, and presence of focal neurological symptoms. The procedure is performed under general anesthesia or moderate sedation with epidural anesthesia. Although a majority of procedures can be performed with fluoroscopy alone, cone-beam computed tomographic guidance can be used in complex cases.[8,9] The ablation modality used in MM patients with VBCFx is usually bipolar RFA which works with low-power generators resulting in predictable ablation zones in the bone. This decreases complications from overheating of nearby neural structures, as compared to the unpredictable larger ablation zones provided by monopolar RFA devices.[10] Bilateral vertebral body access is obtained with a working cannula through which RFA is performed followed by kyphoplasty in standard fashion. After the procedure, patients are subsequently evaluated in clinic on follow-up at 4 weeks.

Percutaneous thermal ablation of vertebral metastasis has been reported to be effective in pain reduction and local tumor control. RFA is the most common thermal ablation modality used in the treatment of spinal neoplastic disease. RFA uses an electrode that carries electromagnetic frequency current leading to a rise in temperature around the tip of the electrode causing cell death by coagulation necrosis.[11]

Percutaneous vertebral augmentation (VA) is performed with or without vertebral body ablation to prevent or stabilize pathological fractures. In a prospective study of 106 patients with MM and VBCFx treated with percutaneous vertebroplasty, there was a statistically significant decrease in pain scores after the treatment.[12] In a separate prospective, multicenter study of 100 patients with painful metastatic bone disease treated with RFA, followed by cementoplasty, there was a rapid and statically significant improvement in pain scores.[13] Of the 100 patients in this study, 87 patients had involvement of the thoracolumbar spine and 13 had involvement of the pelvis and/or sacrum. Finally, the Cancer Patient Fracture Evaluation (CAFE) was a multicenter, randomized controlled trial of 134 patients with cancer, 49 of whom had MM and one to three VBCFx, who were randomized to kyphoplasty or nonsurgical management.[14] Kyphoplasty was shown to be a safe and effective treatment for achieving rapid reduction in back pain in these patients.

References

[1] Anitha D, Baum T, Kirschke JS, Subburaj K. Risk of vertebral compression fractures in multiple myeloma patients: a finite-element study. Medicine (Baltimore). 2017; 96(2):e5825

[2] Kyle RA, Gertz MA, Witzig TE, et al. Review of 1027 patients with newly diagnosed multiple myeloma. Mayo Clin Proc. 2003; 78(1):21–33

[3] SEER Stat Fact Sheets: Myeloma https://seer.cancer.gov/statfacts/html/mulmy.html

[4] Rasch S, Lund T, Asmussen JT, et al. Multiple myeloma associated bone disease. Cancers (Basel). 2020; 12(8):E2113

[5] Hillengass J, Usmani S, Rajkumar SV, et al. International myeloma working group consensus recommendations on imaging in monoclonal plasma cell disorders. Lancet Oncol. 2019; 20(6):e302–e312

[6] Kyriakou C, Molloy S, Vrionis F, et al. The role of cement augmentation with percutaneous vertebroplasty and balloon kyphoplasty for the treatment of vertebral compression fractures in multiple myeloma: a consensus statement from the International Myeloma Working Group (IMWG). Blood Cancer J. 2019; 9(3):27

[7] Fisher CG, DiPaola CP, Ryken TC, et al. A novel classification system for spinal instability in neoplastic disease: an evidence-based approach and expert consensus from the Spine Oncology Study Group. Spine. 2010; 35(22): E1221–E1229

[8] Tsoumakidou G, Koch G, Caudrelier J, et al. Image-guided spinal ablation: a review. Cardiovasc Intervent Radiol. 2016; 39(9):1229–1238

[9] Tomasian A, Jennings JW. Vertebral metastases: minimally invasive percutaneous thermal ablation. Tech Vasc Interv Radiol. 2020; 23(4): 100699

[10] Cazzato RL, Auloge P, De Marini P, et al. Spinal tumor ablation: indications, techniques, and clinical management. Tech Vasc Interv Radiol. 2020; 23(2): 100677

[11] Barile A, Arrigoni F, Zugaro L, et al. Minimally invasive treatments of painful bone lesions: state of the art. Med Oncol. 2017; 34(4):53

[12] Anselmetti GC, Manca A, Montemurro F, et al. Percutaneous vertebroplasty in multiple myeloma: prospective long-term follow-up in 106 consecutive patients. Cardiovasc Intervent Radiol. 2012; 35(1):139–145

[13] Levy J, Hopkins T, Morris J, et al. Radiofrequency ablation for the palliative treatment of bone metastases: outcomes from the multicenter OsteoCool Tumor Ablation Post-Market Study (OPuS One Study) in 100 patients. J Vasc Interv Radiol. 2020; 31(11):1745–1752

[14] Berenson J, Pflugmacher R, Jarzem P, et al. Cancer Patient Fracture Evaluation (CAFE) Investigators. Balloon kyphoplasty versus non-surgical fracture management for treatment of painful vertebral body compression fractures in patients with cancer: a multicentre, randomised controlled trial. Lancet Oncol. 2011; 12(3):225–235

8 Painful Osseous Metastatic Disease I (Lytic, Non-Weight Bearing)

Dimitrios Filippiadis and Alexis Kelekis

8.1 Case Presentation

A 58-year-old man with oligometastatic sarcoma was referred to the interventional radiology (IR) department for directed therapy of a single metastatic lesion in the right glenoid. The patient was taking analgesics and opioids, and reported a pain score of 9/10 on numeric visual scale (NVS) units. Neurological examination demonstrated neither sensitive nor motor deficit affecting the right upper extremity. Computed tomography (CT) scan revealed a lytic lesion in the glenoid, while magnetic resonance imaging (MRI) showed a lesion of pathologic signal intensity with peripheral enhancement following contrast medium injection (▶ Fig. 8.1).

CT-guided microwave ablation (MWA) combined with standard cementoplasty was decided upon as first choice therapy. The lesion was approached via a percutaneous posterior transosseous route. Once the trocar was within the lesion, a microwave antenna was inserted coaxially. The trocar was withdrawn over the antenna in order to remain outside of the expected ablation zone and away from the antenna's active tip (▶ Fig. 8.2a). Based upon the lesion's size and the expected necrotic zone, an ablation session was performed according to the vendor's provided guidelines concerning energy and time. Once the ablation session was complete and following a 5-minute waiting period, the trocar was repositioned inside the lesion, the microwave antenna was removed, and cement injection was performed aiming to fill the lesion and extend the cement into normal bone. A CT scan after the therapeutic session evaluated cement dispersion inside the lesion and lack of extraosseous cement leakage (▶ Fig. 8.2b). The procedure was uneventful, and the patient was hospitalized overnight and discharged the next day.

Clinical examination the morning after ablation and cementoplasty revealed a pain score of 1/10 on NVS units (significant pain reduction of 8 NVS units); the residual pain was secondary to minor discomfort at the puncture sites.

8.2 Discussion

Pain is highly prevalent in cancer patients, reported in up to 70% of all patients. Cancer-related pain is undertreated in a very high percentage of these patients (56–82%), and inevitably results in a poor quality of life. Pharmaceutical agents (e.g., analgesics and opioids) have been the gold standard in the treatment of cancer pain.[1,2,3] Particularly in cases of metastatic bone disease and when a lytic lesion is present in a non-weight bearing region, thermal ablation of bone has emerged as an effective and essential tool, supplementing the role of surgery and radiotherapy.[4,5] Indications for this combined procedure include local tumor control or pain palliation in cases of lesions refractory to or unsuitable for conventional therapies.[4,5,6] Ablation techniques include radiofrequency ablation (RFA), MWA, cryoablation (CA), laser ablation (LA), and MRI-guided high intensity focused ultrasound (HIFU).[4,5,6,7]

Percutaneous ablation provides reduction in cancer pain due to the resultant necrosis of the tumor and the pain-sensitive periosteum, tumor volume decompression, reduction in nerve-stimulating cytokines, and inhibition of osteoclast activity.[4,5,6,8] Proper patient selection is based upon tumor characteristics, the patient's general health status, and the degree of periprocedural bone destruction.[6]

Ablation sessions are usually performed under general anesthesia or sedation. In order to avoid thermal injury in the adjacent nerve structures, active or passive thermoprotection techniques by means of thermal insulation, and temperature and neurophysiological monitoring are key elements during the procedure, especially in cases where there is close proximity (less than 1 cm distance) between the neural structure and the expected ablation zone.[9,10] Moreover, additional measures for skin protection should be taken when superficial tumors are involved (▶ Fig. 8.3).

In non-weight bearing locations and in order to provide structural support, ablation techniques can also be combined

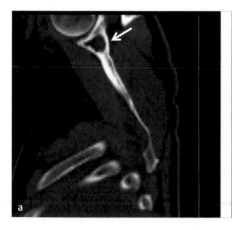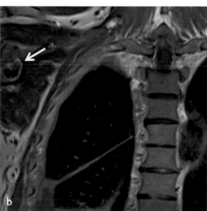

Fig. 8.1 (a) Computed tomography sagittal reconstruction showing a lytic intraosseous lesion of the right glenoid (white arrow). (b) T1-weighted magnetic resonance imaging (MRI) in coronal plane post gadolinium (Gd) injection demonstrating a lesion with low signal intensity and peripheral enhancement (white arrow).

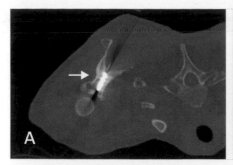
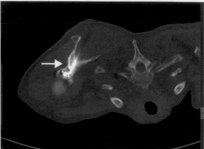

Fig. 8.2 (a) Computed tomography during ablation shows the microwave antenna inside the lesion (arrow). (b) Computed tomography following the procedure demonstrating the cement during the final stage of injection (arrow).

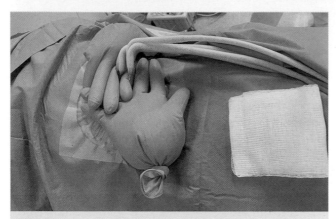

Fig. 8.3 Sterile gloves filled with warm saline are placed on the patient's skin during cryoablation of a superficially located lesion (different case than the patient presented in ▶ Fig. 8.1 and ▶ Fig. 8.2).

with cementation (vertebroplasty or osteoplasty), helping to prevent postprocedural osteonecrosis with subsequent pathological fractures.[11]

Numerous studies in the literature report on the efficient and safe role of thermal ablation techniques (RFA, MWA, CA, HIFU) in the treatment of painful bone metastases.[4,5,6,7,8,12] At the time of this writing, there is no consensus regarding the superiority of a particular ablation method in terms of treatment results and complications. The decision to use a particular technique is multifactorial, and takes into consideration the histology, location, and size of each tumor, the patient's comorbidities, and local practice.

References

[1] Filippiadis DK, Tselikas L, Tsitskari M, Kelekis A, de Baere T, Ryan AG. Percutaneous neurolysis for pain management in oncological patients. Cardiovasc Intervent Radiol. 2019; 42(6):791–799

[2] Coleman R, Body JJ, Aapro M, Hadji P, Herrstedt J, ESMO Guidelines Working Group. Bone health in cancer patients: ESMO Clinical Practice Guidelines. Ann Oncol. 2014; 25 Suppl 3:iii124–iii137

[3] van den Beuken-van Everdingen MH, Hochstenbach LM, Joosten EA, Tjan-Heijnen VC, Janssen DJ. Update on prevalence of pain in patients with cancer: systematic review and meta-analysis. J Pain Symptom Manage. 2016; 51(6):1070–1090.e9

[4] Filippiadis DK, Yevich S, Deschamps F, Jennings JW, Tutton S, Kelekis A. The role of ablation in cancer pain relief. Curr Oncol Rep. 2019; 21(12):105

[5] Yevich S, Tselikas L, Kelekis A, Filippiadis D, de Baere T, Deschamps F. Percutaneous management of metastatic osseous disease. Linchuang Zhongliuxue Zazhi. 2019; 8(6):62

[6] Gangi A, Tsoumakidou G, Buy X, Quoix E. Quality improvement guidelines for bone tumour management. Cardiovasc Intervent Radiol. 2010; 33(4):706–713

[7] Moynagh MR, Kurup AN, Callstrom MR. Thermal ablation of bone metastases. Semin Intervent Radiol. 2018; 35(4):299–308

[8] Kurup AN, Callstrom MR. Image-guided percutaneous ablation of bone and soft tissue tumors. Semin Intervent Radiol. 2010; 27(3):276–284

[9] Kurup AN, Schmit GD, Morris JM, et al. Avoiding complications in bone and soft tissue ablation. Cardiovasc Intervent Radiol. 2017; 40(2):166–176

[10] Garnon J, Cazzato RL, Caudrelier J, et al. Adjunctive thermoprotection during percutaneous thermal ablation procedures: review of current techniques. Cardiovasc Intervent Radiol. 2019; 42(3):344–357

[11] Prologo JD, Patel I, Buethe J, Bohnert N. Ablation zones and weight-bearing bones: points of caution for the palliative interventionalist. J Vasc Interv Radiol. 2014; 25(5):769–775.e2

[12] Prologo JD, Passalacqua M, Patel I, Bohnert N, Corn DJ. Image-guided cryoablation for the treatment of painful musculoskeletal metastatic disease: a single-center experience. Skeletal Radiol. 2014; 43(11):1551–1559

9 Painful Osseous Metastatic Disease I (Sclerotic)

Ernesto Santos and Juan C. Camacho

9.1 Case Presentation

A 63-year-old-woman, who was a former smoker, with a history of stage IV small cell lung carcinoma was found to have an isolated occipital metastasis. This lesion responded to erlotinib and stereotactic radiosurgery (2100 cGy). Several weeks later, there was progression of disease to bone (L2 and the right iliac bone). She underwent radiation therapy (RT) to L2 (2700 cGy) 10 months after initial presentation and to the right iliac bone (2700 cGy) 3 months later. She was started on osimertinib, but did not demonstrate any radiographic response from the radiated bone. Due to progression of disease in the bone metastases, she was re-irradiated (3500 cGy for each lesion) 8 months later. In another 2 months, she had systemic progression and received carboplatin + pemetrexed + pembrolizumab with mixed response on imaging. The patient developed a right lower extremity (RLE) L2 sensorimotor neuropathy due to RT to the iliac bone lesion; this was managed with physical therapy, oxydocone (5 mg Q8h), and Gabapentin (300 mg) with adequate control of her pain.

After 10 months (38 months after initial presentation), she was presented to the Thoracic Disease Management Team due to progression of disease in the right iliac bone and hip pain. The patient was not a candidate for RT and was referred to the anesthesia pain service and interventional radiology (IR). On presentation in the clinic, she reported 8/10 right hip and right groin biological pain with minimal mechanical component when walking. Her pain was constant and precluded restful sleep. She used a cane to assist in her balance. She had chronic RLE weakness (hip and knee flexion) and radiculopathy related to radiation-induced femoral nerve injury. She was on oxycodone 5 mg every 8 hours, lyrica 300 mg/day, and tramadol with constipation as a side effect. Computed tomography (CT) demonstrated a right iliac bone sclerotic lesion extending to the acetabular roof (▶ Fig. 9.1).

The main complaint of this patient was biological pain, so image-guided ablation was considered the procedure of choice

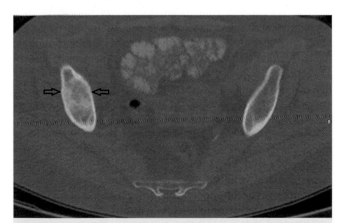

Fig. 9.1 Axial computed tomography (CT) image reveals a sclerotic lesion involving the right iliac bone in the supra-acetabular region (arrows).

to alleviate her pain and to improve her quality of life (QoL). Despite the acetabular roof being a weight-bearing area, the patient did not describe significant mechanical pain. Additionally, the lesion was sclerotic, so there was no need to combine cementoplasty with ablation. Given the sclerotic nature of the lesion, cryoablation is the recommended ablation technique (vs. radiofrequency ablation [RFA] and microwave ablation [MWA]) since the ice-ball can better penetrate the bone than RFA and MWA.

Image-guided cryoablation was performed under general anesthesia. No intraoperative nerve monitoring was used since the sciatic and femoral nerves were located away from the right iliac bone lesion. Two 11-G bone needles were placed into the sclerotic lesion under CT guidance and two cryoprobes were inserted in thetumor (▶ Fig. 9.2a-d). Two cycles of 8 minutes of freezing and 5 minutes of thawing were conducted.

Follow-up was performed in the IR clinic at 1 week, 1 month, and 6 months post-procedure. Her pain level was 4/10 at 1 week, and she required fewer opioids for pain control. She was on lyrica and acetaminophen at 1 month follow-up and her constipation resolved completely. Her QoL significantly improved at 6 months (3/10).

9.2 Discussion

After lung and liver, bone is the third most frequent site of metastasis. Prostate and breast carcinoma are responsible for many of the skeletal metastases (> 70%), reflecting both the high incidence and relatively long clinical course of these cancers.[1] Although the overall incidence of bone metastasis is not known, the relative incidence is high, particularly in patients with advanced disease: 70% of patients with breast and prostate, 60% with thyroid, 35% with lung, 40% with bladder, and 25% with renal cancers.[2] Patients with bone metastases can develop severe pain, impaired mobility, diminished QoL, pathologic fractures, or spinal cord compression.

Based on radiological features, bone metastases can be classified as lytic, blastic, or mixed. Sclerotic metastases are characterized by new bone formation and are particularly noted in patients with prostate and lung carcinoma, carcinoid tumors, and Hodgkin's lymphoma.[2]

Bone pain is the most common type of cancer-induced pain. Such pain can manifest as constant biological, movement-related (mechanical), or neuropathic pain; combinations of these types of pain are common. Patients with uncontrolled biological pain can usually benefit from RT or ablation. Cementoplasty or mechanical stabilization is typically used in patients with mechanical pain and can be performed in conjunction with image-guided ablation. The goals of image-guided percutaneous interventions in patients with painful osseous metastases are pain relief and increased mobility, improvement in QoL, mechanical stabilization of bone, and local tumor control.

There are several percutaneous ablation techniques developed in the last 30 years such as chemical ablation (alcohol or other sclerosant injection), RFA, MWA, cryoablation, laser

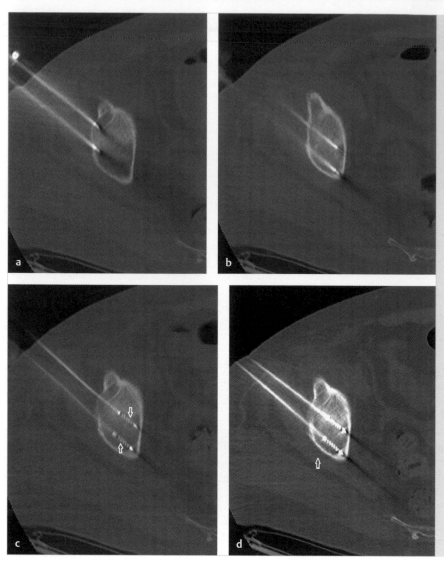

Fig. 9.2 (a–d) Placement of two parallel 11-G needles into the sclerotic lesion via an antero-lateral approach. The lesion was completely crossed with both metallic cannulas to allow cryoprobe placement in the sclerotic tumor. The bone needles were removed over a stiff wire and two peel-away sheaths were inserted over the wire. Two cryoprobes were advanced through the peel-away sheaths and centered in the sclerotic lesion (arrows) and cryoablation was performed. The ice-ball was not visualized within the sclerotic lesion but extended into the adjacent soft tissues (arrow).

ablation, irreversible electroporation, and high intensity focused ultrasound.[3] A multicenter study of 43 patients with painful osseous metastases was published by Goetz et al in 2004.[4] This landmark article reported significant pain reduction and decrease in the use of opioids after image-guided ablation. Since then, several prospective studies have confirmed image-guided bone ablation to be safe and effective in the treatment of painful osseous metastases.[5,6]

Preprocedural imaging is key in the evaluation and treatment planning for patients undergoing ablation procedures. CT imaging is helpful to identify the bone metastases and surrounding anatomical structures. Additionally, CT is the most common imaging technique used to guide and monitor the treatment outcome. Positron emission tomography (PET) CT scan helps to identify and target hypermetabolic lesions in patients with prior locoregional therapies (e.g., radiotherapy). Due to its excellent spatial resolution and tissue differentiation, MRI is the best imaging technique to identify neural structures.

Although there are no randomized trials comparing heating (RFA and MWA) versus freezing (cryoablation), it has been suggested that cryoablation may be more effective regarding pain response and requiring less procedural and postprocedural pain medications.[7]

Compared to lytic metastases, sclerotic osseous lesions are more difficult to treat. Handheld automatic drills may facilitate percutaneous access to allow needle placement and treatment of such metastases.[8] There are no studies published comparing which ablation technique (RFA, MWA, or cryoablation) is more efficient in treating patients with sclerotic osseous metastases. RFA can be optimized for treating painful sclerotic bone metastases by reducing power to avoid early impedance increases.[3] Despite that, RFA probes may not be capable of achieving ablative temperatures in extremely sclerotic metastases because of the lack of water content and associated impedance.[9] MWA has also been used in the treatment of osteoblastic metastases with favorable early results.[10] With cryoablation, the ice-ball can penetrate deeply into bone, which may allow more complete treatment of painful osteoblastic metastases.[11] The cryoablation zone can be monitored in real time because of the visibility of the ice-ball as a well-marginated, low-attenuation area on CT in patients with osteolytic metastases. The ice-ball is also seen on MRI, with the outer edge of the ice-ball corresponding to 0 °C.[11]

The ice-ball is not visible in dense bone and has to be extrapolated based on the extension of the hypodensity into the adjacent soft tissue.[9] Similar to RT and surgery, the ice-ball should extend beyond the tumor margin to prevent recurrence, particularly in patients with oligometastatic disease. For this reason, cryoablation may be the technique of choice for osteoblastic metastases. There are many different types of cryoprobes available depending on the desired volume and shape of the ice-ball, and multiple cryoprobes can be used simultaneously. In the case presented here, cryoablation was clinically effective in this patient with a right iliac bone sclerotic lesion; however, visualization of the ice-ball was poor in the bone when CT guidance was used. In this case, the ice-ball was only visualized in the adjacent soft tissues (▶ Fig. 9.2a-d).

References

[1] Cecchini M, Wetterwald A, Pluijm G, Thalmann G. Molecular and biological mechanisms of bone metastasis. EAU Update Series. 2005; 3:214–226

[2] Macedo F, Ladeira K, Pinho F, et al. Bone metastases: an overview. Oncol Rev. 2017; 11(1):321–327

[3] Gangi A, Buy X. Percutaneous bone tumor management. Semin Intervent Radiol. 2010; 27(2):124–136

[4] Goetz MP, Callstrom MR, Charboneau JW, et al. Percutaneous image-guided radiofrequency ablation of painful metastases involving bone: a multicenter study. J Clin Oncol. 2004; 22(2):300–306

[5] Callstrom MR, Dupuy DE, Solomon SB, et al. Percutaneous image-guided cryoablation of painful metastases involving bone: multicenter trial. Cancer. 2013; 119(5):1033–1041

[6] Hurwitz MD, Ghanouni P, Kanaev SV, et al. Magnetic resonance-guided focused ultrasound for patients with painful bone metastases: phase III trial results. J Natl Cancer Inst. 2014; 106(5):dju082

[7] Zugaro L, DI Staso M, Gravina GL, et al. Treatment of osteolytic solitary painful osseous metastases with radiofrequency ablation or cryoablation: a retrospective study by propensity analysis. Oncol Lett. 2016; 11(3):1948–1954

[8] Wallace AN, Chang RO, Tomasian A, Jennings JW. Drill-assisted, fluoroscopy-guided vertebral body access for radiofrequency ablation: technical case series. Interv Neuroradiol. 2015; 21(5):631–634

[9] Kurup AN, Morris JM, Callstrom MR. Ablation of musculoskeletal metastases. AJR Am J Roentgenol. 2017; 209(4):713–721

[10] Khan MA, Deib G, Deldar B, Patel AM, Barr JS. Efficacy and safety of percutaneous microwave ablation and cementoplasty in the treatment of painful spinal metastases and myeloma. AJNR Am J Neuroradiol. 2018; 39(7):1376–1383

[11] Kurup AN, Callstrom MR. Ablation of skeletal metastases: current status. J Vasc Interv Radiol. 2010; 21(8) Suppl:S242–S250

10 Painful Neoplastic Disease of the Head and Neck

Uei Pua, Ming-Yann Lim, Siu Cheng Loke, and Amit Anand Karandikar

10.1 Introduction

Recurrent head and neck tumors, while traditionally treated with a primarily palliative intent, have seen a recent trend toward more aggressive treatment strategies such as salvage surgery and radiation therapy. In tandem, there is a growing interest in exploring percutaneous ablation as a minimally invasive alternative in patients unfit for surgery or radiation. The purpose of this chapter is to explore the current status and illustrate the pertinent technical aspects of percutaneous ablation in recurrent head and neck tumors.

10.2 Background

Recurrence of head and neck tumors after initial successful treatment of the index head and neck cancer (HNC) poses a significant clinical challenge. It occurs in two main scenarios. First, it may present as locoregional recurrence after treatment of the index tumor; it is known that 50 to 60% of HNC patients develop a recurrence within 2 years of the index surgery.[1] Alternatively, a secondary primary malignancy (SPM), which is histologically and geographically distinct from the index tumor, can occur. Cumulative risk of developing an SPM in the HNC population in 20 years is reported to be around 36%.[2] The most common sites of SPM after an HNC remains in the head and neck region (35–73%), followed by lung (15–32%) and esophagus (9%).[2,3,4] SPM typically may occur decades after treatment of the index tumor, and is postulated to be a result of "field cancerization" related to common etiological factors (e.g., human papillomavirus infection, smoking), which were also present during the first cancer occurrence. Less well studied is that of radiation-induced SPM in which patients receiving high doses of radiation for the index tumor are thought to be at increased risk of developing SPM with a long latency period.[5]

Although recurrent HNC traditionally portends a poor prognosis and is treated primarily with palliative intent or best supportive care, recent data have shown that survival benefits can be conferred by adopting a more aggressive approach.[1,6] This is in part due to improved patient selection and evolved surgical care,[1,6] resulting in re-appraisal of the treatment paradigms of recurrence in the head and neck region. This has spurred growth in interest among interventional radiologists to develop techniques to complement the change of mindset in this area.[7,8,9,10]

10.3 Current Treatment Strategies

A detailed discussion of the current treatment of recurrent HNC is beyond the scope of this chapter. Briefly, the standard of care for recurrent HNC is salvage surgery requiring wide resection with R0 margins, and myocutaneous flap reconstruction to cover large postoperative defects. The choice of surgery is site-dependent (e.g., laryngectomy for hypopharyngeal recurrences or mandibulectomy for mouth/tongue recurrence) with the attendant morbidity taken into consideration. Radiation therapy is an accepted treatment alternative in case surgical treatment is contraindicated, with platinum-based chemotherapy reserved for palliative intent.[1,2,3,4,5,6]

Challenges, however, exist as these patients are not treatment naïve. Salvage surgery can be highly morbid (up to 16% major complication and 2.7% mortality rates),[11] if not impossible due to previous surgery or encroachment on critical structures (e.g., carotid artery). In addition, if adjuvant radiotherapy is contraindicated due to dose limitation there is a high chance of locoregional recurrence. Morbidity from conventional radiation therapy such as speech or swallowing impediment is present in up to 43% of patients[12]; additionally, cumulative radiation dose from prior treatment may have reached toxicity levels for adjacent critical structures (e.g., brainstem).[1,2,3,4,5,6,12] Although the literature about this remains scarce, percutaneous ablation under ultrasound, computed tomography (CT) or magnetic resonance (MR) guidance has been used to fill this treatment gap for local tumor control and palliation.[7,8,9,10]

10.4 Ablative Modalities in the Head and Neck

The goal of ablation is primarily palliation, with local tumor control (debulking) and symptom relief (e.g., bleeding or bulk symptoms) as the main aim. To this end, subtotal ablation, where residual tumor in intentionally left, is often an accepted end-point.

The most commonly used ablation technologies are radiofrequency ablation (RFA) and cryoablation.[7,8,9,10] There is a general trend of using cryoablation in the deep spaces of the neck, as real-time ice-ball monitoring of the ablation zone in relation to critical structures is feasible on cross-sectional imaging such as CT and magnetic resonance imaging (MRI).[9,10] Although both MRI and CT have the ability for multiplanar assessment of the ablation zone, MRI has the distinct advantage of multiplanar needle guidance, allowing for real-time access trajectories beyond the axial plane limitation of CT.[10]

RFA is still widely used in more superficial areas such as in the thyroid bed (visceral space) and cervical nodal stations (▶ Fig. 10.1a–d).[7] This is due to the ability to monitor the ablation "storm-cloud" under ultrasound guidance. A distinct advantage of RFA over cryoablation is the ability of cautery by the RFA probe to stop bleeding. This is particularly useful in palliation of bleeding tumors.

At the authors' institution, all ablations are performed under general anesthesia with endotracheal or, when present, endotracheostomy intubation (▶ Fig. 10.1b). Prophylactic antibiotics coverage for oral and skin organisms is routinely administered. Postprocedural imaging (CT or MRI) is performed at 6 weeks, and then every 3 months thereafter (▶ Fig. 10.2).

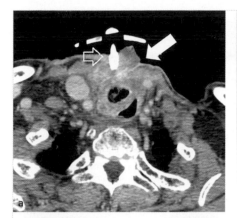

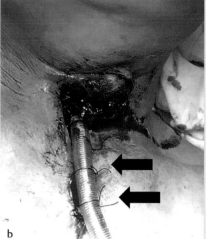

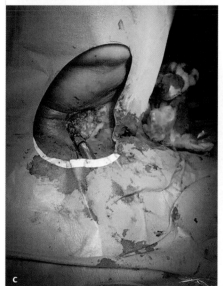

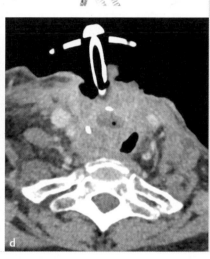

Fig. 10.1 A 67-year-old woman with recurrence of anaplastic thyroid cancer with invasion into the left internal jugular and trachea. She underwent total thyroidectomy, modified left radical neck dissection with tracheostomy creation, and adjuvant radiotherapy. She developed a local recurrence over the tracheostomy site 1 year later; her primary symptom was recurrent contact bleeding with eight episodes of blood transfusions treated with cautery, and a persistent melena-like foul smell due to bacteria breakdown of blood products around the tracheostomy site. (**a, b**) Preablation computed tomography (CT) and photograph showing the exuberant tumor mass encompassing the tracheostomy with bleeding. CT demonstrates the tumor (**a**, solid arrow) encroaching on the tracheostomy tube (open arrow). Note the use of the armored endotracheostomy tube (kink resistant) that is anchored with sutures to the chest wall to prevent dislodgement during ablation (**b**, arrows). This is the standard for all patients undergoing ablation with tracheostomies. Ablation was performed using "moving shot technique" with Viva RF system (STARmed, Seoul, Korea) under ultrasound guidance to achieve subunits of echogenic foci along the retracting RF probe. The 18-G monopolar ablation probe has a 1-cm active tip with a short shaft of 10 cm for ease of control. (**c**) Postablation photograph demonstrating complete cessation of bleeding and a devitalized tumor. (**d**) CT performed 6 weeks after ablation shows tumor retraction away from the tracheostomy site but with residual tumor (subtotal ablation; compare to **a**). The patient nevertheless did not have any recurrence of bleeding symptoms.

10.5 Considerations in Planning and Performing Ablations in HNC

10.5.1 Anatomy and Planning

Postoperative anatomy, in particular reconstructive flaps, poses unique challenges. The altered anatomy and irregular shape of recurrent tumors require ablation planning in a multidisciplinary setting with requisite in-depth knowledge of postoperative HNC anatomy.

Vascular structures need to be identified preprocedurally to prevent major hemorrhage. Besides the carotid space and vertebral artery, branches of the external carotid arteries must be identified using an arterial phase cross-sectional study before the procedure. For reconstructive flaps, the pedicle artery should be identified whenever possible (▶ Fig. 10.2b). However, sacrifice of the pedicle artery is acceptable once the flap has completely incorporated onto the recipient site.

Cranial nerves within the vicinity or invaded by tumor can usually be ablated as existing nerve palsy is already often present, and post-treatment palsies are generally considered an acceptable side effect of salvage surgery or radiation. This outcome must be communicated clearly to the patient.

Probe placement can be difficult since tumors are often infiltrative and irregular in shape. The authors typically use the "2 × 1 rule," where probes are placed 2 cm apart from each other and 1 cm from the tumor margin. Instead of extensive preprocedure planning, as is performed with ablation of tumors, the mid-level or the widest dimension of the tumor in the axial plane is identified on CT and probes are inserted as needed to fulfill the 2 × 1 rule in that plane. Following this, cranial and caudal probes are inserted in the axial planes up to 2 cm away from the mid-level probes to cover the entire tumor (▶ Fig. 10.2c, d). Often, additional probes are needed after the first freeze cycle due to incomplete tumor coverage. All probes are then reactivated for another two freeze–thaw cycles (i.e., total of three freeze–thaw cycles for the first set of probes). In the authors' experience, an additional freeze cycle achieves an additional 10 to 15% increase in ice-ball diameter. Progression of ice-ball is monitored at 3 minutes interval (▶ Fig. 10.3). As a caveat, although the tumoricidal −20 to −40 °C isotherm is 5 to 10 mm inside the margin of visualized ice-ball, ablation must be terminated once the advancing ice-ball reaches a critical structure (e.g., brain). The lack of a complete ablative margin and potential incomplete ablation in this scenario represent an accepted limitation of this technique.

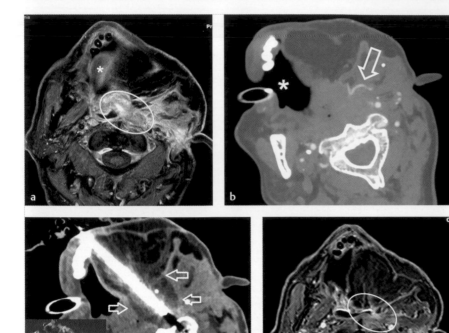

Fig. 10.2 A 70-year-old man post salvage maxillomandibulectomy and parotidectomy for radiation-induced carcinoma with recurrence of squamous cell carcinoma in the myocutaneous flap. He was referred for salvage ablation for impending airway obstruction. (a) Contrast-enhanced axial magnetic resonance imaging (MRI) demonstrates the cancer recurrence (white circle). Note the position of the tongue (*) in contact with the tumor. (b) Preprocedural computed tomography (CT) angiography showing the vascular structures in the area of operation and the pedicle artery supplying the flap (white arrow). Oral packing was performed to displace the tongue from the ablation site (*, compare with a). (c) Intraprocedural CT showing ice-ball formation (arrows) and the three-probe array in the coronal reformat (inset). (d) Contrast-enhanced MRI at 6 months showing complete regression of the mass (circle—compare with a).

10.5.2 Access and Probe Trajectory

The authors prefer a percutaneous route even in deeper structures, even when alternative routes such as transoral may present a more direct path. This is in part due to the familiarity to position probes using axial anatomy on CT fluoroscopy as well as the theoretical advantage of avoiding contamination of the ablated tumor bed by oral flora through the access punctures.

Tumors in superficial spaces such as the submandibular (▶ Fig. 10.3), sublingual, buccal, and parotid spaces can be accessed directly under CT and/or ultrasound guidance. Tumors in deeper spaces such as the masticator and parapharyngeal spaces are routinely accessed through a retromaxillary (masticator space lesions) or the retromolar trigone approach (parapharyngeal space) (▶ Fig. 10.4).

Access through a myocutaneous flap can be performed once the flap has completely healed. Although often a heterogenous and "bizarre" appearance is seen on cross-sectional imaging (▶ Fig. 10.2a and ▶ Fig. 10.3b), except potential bleeding from pedicle artery injury, flaps are usually devoid of critical structures such as nerves and therefore can be traversed safely. This helps in providing many potential trajectories for multiple probes to treat nonsuperficial tumors (▶ Fig. 10.2a–d).

10.5.3 Ablation Parameters and Monitoring

Conventional power and time-based progression algorithms for ice-ball progression are seldom directly applicable in HNC. This may be due to different cold-sink factors in the neck region when compared to abdominal visceral and, in particular, in reconstructive flaps that are relatively hypovascular compared to native tissues. As such, a "go slow, go long" approach can be used by starting with 30% freezing power with 10% increments every 2 minutes while monitoring the ice-ball formation (▶ Fig. 10.3). In the authors' experience, a maximum of 50% power will usually suffice based on the needle positioning above. The usual dual freeze–thaw cycle (10:8:10:8 minutes) ensues, repeating the highest power reached in the first cycle.

Ice-ball monitoring is particularly important when ablating near critical structures (▶ Fig. 10.5a–c) and the ablation shape could be modeled safely by switching off the respective probes just before the ice-ball encroaches upon the structure (▶ Fig. 10.5c).

10.6 Special Considerations

10.6.1 Carotid Space

Tumor involvement of the carotid artery commonly occurs with tumors involving the parapharyngeal space. The risk of carotid blow-out should be determined and includes circumferential tumor involvement, neck dissection with the stripping of the vasa vasorum, direct contact with saliva, and prior radiation with a cumulative dose greater than 70 Gy.[13,14]

Carotid blow-out syndrome (CBS) can occur as an exposed carotid artery found incidentally on imaging (Type 1), clinical episodes of bleeding ("sentinel bleed") that resolve with wound packing and pressure (Type 2 or "impending blow-out"), and carotid hemorrhage that is rapidly fatal (Type 3). History suggestive of Type 2 CBS must be excluded, as ablation is likely to

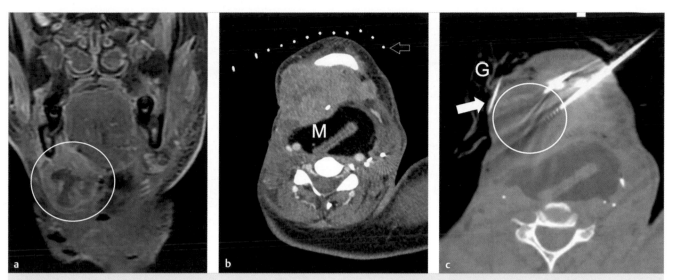

Fig. 10.3 A 42-year-old woman with stage 4C hypopharyngeal squamous cell carcinoma, post total laryngopharyngectomy with bilateral neck dissection and anterolateral thigh flap reconstruction of the pharynx. She underwent radiation and systemic therapy and had recurrence in the right submandibular flap region, causing pain and mass symptoms. (a) Preprocedure contrast-enhanced coronal magnetic resonance (MR) showing the tumor recurrence on the flap (white circle). (b) Preoperative arterial phase axial computed tomography (CT). The "M" marks the muscular flap reconstruction of the neopharynx that underwent denervation-related atrophy with fat infiltration, giving rise to the fat attenuation appearance. A planning grid (arrow) was applied to aid probe insertion. (c) Intraprocedural CT showing skin protection with the creation of artificial subcutaneous emphysema using a 23-G needle (white arrow) and warm saline-soaked gauze (G). The patient demonstrated significant improvement in pain score with ablation (Visual Acuity Score reduction from 8/10 to 3/10).

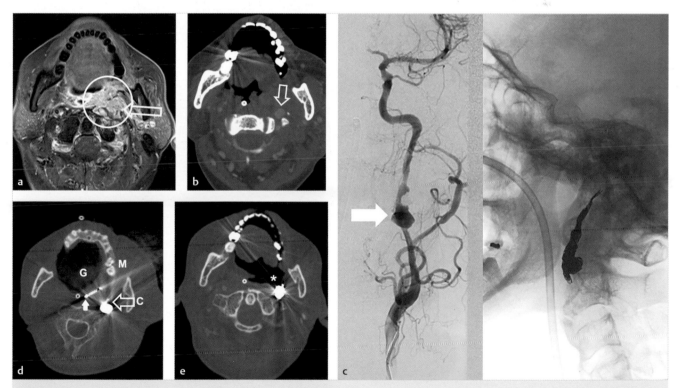

Fig. 10.4 A 72-year-old man with recurrent nasopharyngeal carcinoma with circumferential involvement of the carotid space and invasion into the retropharyngeal space. He had prior nodal resection and adjuvant radiotherapy 4 years previously. He was referred for symptoms of trismus and gagging with impending airway compromise. Symptoms of recurrent small episode bleed (Type 2 carotid blow-out) were treated with packing, and ablation was deferred. (a) Axial, contrast-enhanced magnetic resonance imaging (MRI) demonstrating tumor recurrence (circle and arrow). (b) Computed tomography (CT) angiography performed 3 days later when he presented with massive bleeding. CT confirmed a pseudoaneurysm arising from the internal carotid artery, consistent with Type 3 carotid blow-out (white arrow). (c) Pre- and post-emergency coiling of the left internal carotid artery (white arrow showing pseudoaneurysm). (d) The patient underwent cryoablation for symptomatic control 2 weeks following the embolization procedure. CT showing two cryoablation probes inserted via a retromolar (solid arrow showing one of the two probes). This is the standard approach to the parapharyngeal space, between the last mandibular molar (M) and the mandibular condyle (C). To prevent frost injury, the tongue was displaced by inserted gauze (G) using a McGill forceps. Note the position of the second cryoablation probe which is in contact with the embolization coils (open arrow). Severe hypotension and bradycardia were encountered during ablation which resolved when the second probe was switched off. (e) CT obtained 4 months post ablation showed complete debulking of the tumor (*, compare with a).

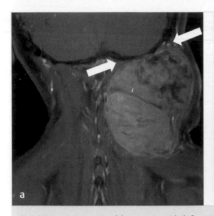
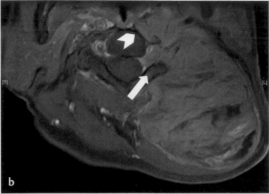
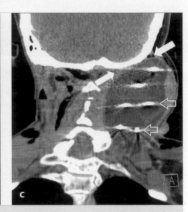

Fig. 10.5 A 66-year-old woman with left paraspinal synovial tumor with extension in the prevertebral space, referred for palliative ablation for bulk symptoms. She had recurrence 3 years after surgical resection and was deemed unsuitable for radiotherapy; she refused salvage surgery. (**a**) Contrast-enhanced coronal magnetic resonance imaging (MRI) showing the large enhancing mass abutting the occipital bone and cerebellum (white arrows), which forms the limit of the ablation margin. (**b**) Axial MRI demonstrating extension of the tumor to involve the left neuroforamen (arrow) and prevertebral space (arrowhead). (**c**) Composite coronal computed tomography (CT) showing the six cryoablation probe array with ice-ball formation (open arrows show two of the probes) 8 minutes into the first cycle. The most cranial probe was deactivated at this time as the ice-ball approached the left occipital bone (solid arrows) and threatened the cerebellum. Ablation was continued with the rest of the probes. This case highlights the need for judicious monitoring of the ablation using CT.

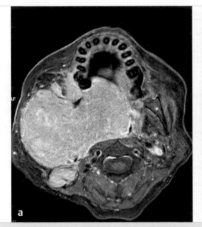
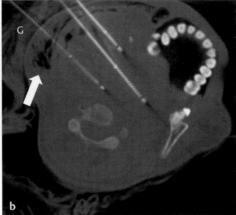

Fig. 10.6 A 62-year-old woman with a recurrent right middle cranial fossa meningioma with lung metastases. She underwent resection of the meningioma involving a right craniotomy, right parotidectomy, and mandibulectomy with a left anterolateral myocutaneous flap reconstruction. She was referred for palliative ablation for symptoms of dysphagia. (**a**) Contrast-enhanced magnetic resonance imaging (MRI) of the recurrence showing tumor extending from the region of the reconstruction into the oropharyngeal space with compression of the esophagus. (**b**) Axial computed tomography (CT) during ablation involving six cryoablation probes, each ablating at two locations (only three probes are shown). Artificial subcutaneous emphysema (white arrow) was created together with the use of warm saline-soaked gauze for dermal protection (G).

further weaken the surrounding structures supporting the diseased carotid artery and precipitate a Type 3 CBS. Because of this, a Type 2 CBS is considered a contraindication for ablation. In such patients, CT angiography should be performed to exclude the presence of a pseudoaneurysm, and if present prophylactic carotid artery embolization may be considered in well-collateralized patients before performing the ablation procedure (▶ Fig. 10.4b, c).

Additionally, as the vagus nerve and the carotid body reside within the carotid space, due to severe vagal stimulation cold conduction through the carotid artery or embolization coils (▶ Fig. 10.4c, d) can lead to hemodynamic instability during ablation.[9] Therefore, close intraprocedural monitoring of vital signs is crucial when ablating around the carotid space or when

the cryoablation probe is in direct contact with the embolization coils (▶ Fig. 10.4d, white arrow). Temporary cessation of ablation usually resolves the episode, and resumption of the ablation is often possible.

10.6.2 Frost Protection

Due to the superficial location of many tumors, to displace the dermis from the underlying ice artificial subcutaneous emphysema may be created by using 5 to 10 cc of air injected through a 23-G needle (arrows in ▶ Fig. 10.3c and ▶ Fig. 10.6b). In addition, standard skin warming using warm saline-soaked gauze should be considered ("G" in ▶ Fig. 10.3c and ▶ Fig. 10.6b).

The tongue is at risk of frost injury if it is in contact with the ice-ball during ablation involving the oral cavity, oropharynx, and hypopharynx. Being a mobile structure, after securing the endotracheal tube the tongue can be intentionally displaced away from the ablation site with oral packing using gauze (▶ Fig. 10.2b and ▶ Fig. 10.4d). During general anesthesia the tongue falls and contact the posterior wall of the oropharynx, so for deeper locations such as ablation in the parapharyngeal space a laryngoscope is used to displace the tongue anteriorly and a McGill forceps used to position a gauze between the flaccid tongue and the back of the throat (▶ Fig. 10.4d).

10.7 Summary

Although currently in the early stages of development, there is increasing interest among the ablation community for ablation of HNC; further studies are needed to define its role in this patient population. Ablation potentially presents a minimally invasive alternative in this group of treatment-refractory patients, and where treatment options are often limited, it may allow for local tumor control and palliation.

References

[1] Mehanna H, Kong A, Ahmed SK. Recurrent head and neck cancer: United Kingdom National Multidisciplinary Guidelines. J Laryngol Otol. 2016; 130 (S2) Suppl 2:S181–S190

[2] Chuang SC, Scelo G, Tonita JM, et al. Risk of second primary cancer among patients with head and neck cancers: a pooled analysis of 13 cancer registries. Int J Cancer. 2008; 123(10):2390–2396

[3] Denaro N, Merlano MC, Russi EG. Follow-up in head and neck cancer: do more does it mean do better? A systematic review and our proposal based on our experience. Clin Exp Otorhinolaryngol. 2016; 9(4):287–297

[4] Grégoire V, Lefebvre JL, Licitra L, Felip E, EHNS-ESMO-ESTRO Guidelines Working Group. Squamous cell carcinoma of the head and neck: EHNS-ESMO-ESTRO Clinical Practice Guidelines for diagnosis, treatment and follow-up. Ann Oncol. 2010; 21 Suppl 5:v184–v186

[5] Ng SP, Pollard C, III, Kamal M, et al. Risk of second primary malignancies in head and neck cancer patients treated with definitive radiotherapy. NPJ Precis Oncol. 2019; 3:22

[6] Jayaram SC, Muzaffar SJ, Ahmed I, Dhanda J, Paleri V, Mehanna H. Efficacy, outcomes, and complication rates of different surgical and nonsurgical treatment modalities for recurrent/residual oropharyngeal carcinoma: a systematic review and meta-analysis. Head Neck. 2016; 38(12):1855–1861

[7] Lim HK, Baek JH, Lee JH, et al. Efficacy and safety of radiofrequency ablation for treating locoregional recurrence from papillary thyroid cancer. Eur Radiol. 2015; 25(1):163–170

[8] Brook AL, Gold MM, Miller TS, et al. CT-guided radiofrequency ablation in the palliative treatment of recurrent advanced head and neck malignancies. J Vasc Interv Radiol. 2008; 19(5):725–735

[9] Guenette JP, Tuncali K, Himes N, Shyn PB, Lee TC. Percutaneous image-guided cryoablation of head and neck tumors for local control, preservation of functional status, and pain relief. AJR Am J Roentgenol. 2017; 208(2): 453–458

[10] Gangi A, Cebula H, Cazzato RL, et al. "Keeping a cool head": percutaneous imaging-guided cryo-ablation as salvage therapy for recurrent glioblastoma and head and neck tumours. Cardiovasc Intervent Radiol. 2020; 43(2):172–175

[11] Temam S, Koka V, Mamelle G, et al. Treatment of the N0 neck during salvage surgery after radiotherapy of head and neck squamous cell carcinoma. Head Neck. 2005; 27(8):653–658

[12] Denaro N, Russi EG, Adamo V, Merlano MC. State-of-the-art and emerging treatment options in the management of head and neck cancer: news from 2013. Oncology. 2014; 86(4):212–229

[13] Lu HJ, Chen KW, Chen MH, et al. Predisposing factors, management, and prognostic evaluation of acute carotid blowout syndrome. J Vasc Surg. 2013; 58(5):1226–1235

[14] Chen YJ, Wang CP, Wang CC, Jiang RS, Lin JC, Liu SA. Carotid blowout in patients with head and neck cancer: associated factors and treatment outcomes. Head Neck. 2015; 37(2):265–272

11 Painful Soft Tissue Metastases

Anderanik Tomasian and Jack W. Jennings

11.1 Case Presentation 1

A 74-year-old woman with metastatic high-grade spindle cell sarcoma presented with a progressively enlarging painful right deltoid intramuscular metastatic lesion. The patient was discussed in the multidisciplinary tumor board. Physical examination showed tender, firm, and nonmobile mass in right shoulder girdle soft tissue as well as limited passive and active range of motion of the shoulder girdle. The neurovascular examination was normal.

Imaging with magnetic resonance imaging (MRI) (▶ Fig. 11.1a) demonstrated a solid, enhancing right deltoid intramuscular metastatic lesion. Given the size of the tumor, cryoablation was selected to achieve local tumor control and pain palliation.

Cryoablation was performed under moderate sedation in an outpatient setting. A total of four cryoprobes were positioned within the tumor with inter-probe distances of 15 to 20 mm (▶ Fig. 11.1b). The initial freezing cycle was 13 minutes and 30 seconds, followed by 8-minute active thawing phase, a second freezing cycle of 10 minutes and 20 seconds, and a final 8-minute thawing phase. Thermal protection of the skin was performed with a skin surface application of warm saline. The patient reported near-complete resolution of pain, and local tumor control was achieved (▶ Fig. 11.1c).

11.2 Case Presentation 2

A 55-year-old woman with metastatic lung adenocarcinoma presented with a progressively enlarging left shoulder girdle metastatic lesion, and intractable pain minimally relieved by oral and intravenous pain medications. She also demonstrated severely limited range of motion, limiting her activities of daily living and functional independence. The patient was admitted for pain palliation. Physical examination revealed a large mass with limited active and passive motion of the shoulder girdle, mildly decreased muscle strength of the upper extremity (due to disuse), and an intact neurovascular system.

Imaging with computed tomography (CT) (▶ Fig. 11.2a) demonstrated a large, heterogeneously enhancing soft tissue metastatic lesion involving the left shoulder girdle musculature, with extension to the subcutaneous adipose tissues. Given the large size and complex geometry of the lesion, as well as lack of critical nerves in the vicinity, microwave ablation was performed. Cryoablation would have been an appropriate alternative choice.

Microwave ablation was performed under moderate sedation. Two 13-gauge microwave antennae were positioned within the cranial component of the tumor (approximately 2 cm apart), and microwave ablation was performed at 75 to 100 Watts for a total of 10 minutes, achieving overlapping 4 × 4 cm ablation zones (▶ Fig. 11.2b, c). The antennae were retracted, and a second ablation was performed using identical parameters to cover the entire cranial half of the tumor. The antennae were subsequently removed and placed within the caudal half of the tumor, and two sets of ablations were performed with identical parameters to cover the entire caudal half of the tumor. In order to minimize skin thermal injury, ablation zone margins were always kept greater than 2 cm from the skin surface. The patient described substantial pain relief following microwave ablation; there were no complications, and the patient was discharged on oral analgesics as needed.

11.3 Discussion

Over the past two decades, there have been substantial advancements in minimally invasive percutaneous thermal ablation techniques used in the treatment of musculoskeletal metastases.

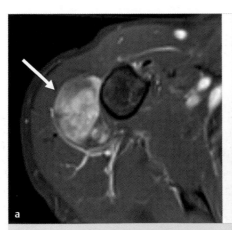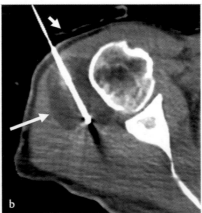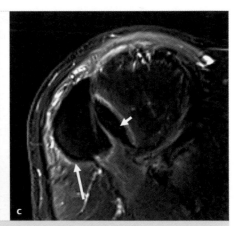

Fig. 11.1 (a) Axial, T1-weighted, fat-saturated, contras-enhanced magnetic resonance (MR) image demonstrates a solid enhancing right deltoid intramuscular metastatic lesion abutting the humeral head (arrow). (b) Axial computed tomographic (CT) image during cryoablation demonstrates placement of a cryoprobe within the tumor (one of four cryoprobes used), and the hypoattenuating ice-ball (long arrow) encompassing the tumor volume and extending beyond tumor boundaries to achieve adequate local tumor control. Note the intraosseous component of the ice-ball within the humeral head is largely CT-occult. Thermal protection of the skin with surface application of warm saline was performed (short arrow). (c) Axial, post-contrast, subtraction magnetic resonance image (MRI) performed 5 months following cryoablation shows local tumor control with nonenhancing ablated tumor volume (long arrow). Note osteonecrosis of the adjacent humeral head (short arrow).

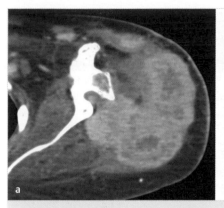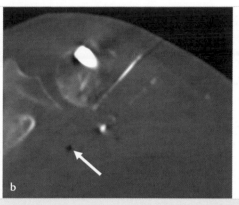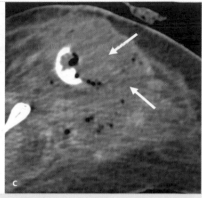

Fig. 11.2 (a) Axial computed tomography (CT) shows a large heterogeneously enhancing soft tissue metastatic lesion involving the left shoulder girdle musculature with extension to the subcutaneous adipose tissues. There is tumor involvement of the proximal humerus and scapular glenoid as well as the glenohumeral joint (not shown). (b) Axial CT image during microwave ablation demonstrates placement of two microwave antennae within the cranial half of the soft tissue metastatic lesion. Note intratumoral gas from tissue vaporization (arrow). Due to tumor involvement of the glenohumeral joint, residual articular cartilage thermal protection was not attempted. (c) Axial, contrast-enhanced CT image immediately following microwave ablation shows largely CT-occult ablation zone, intratumoral gas from tissue vaporization, and nonenhancing ablated tumor (arrows).

These treatments include bone and soft tissue lesions, and may be performed in conjunction with (or supplemented by) adjuvant radiation therapy, chemotherapy, or surgery. Such minimally invasive techniques offer several distinct advantages, including timely and durable pain palliation, excellent local tumor control rates, and short- and long-term improvement in patient's functional status.[1,2,3,4,5,6,7,8,9]

In patients with soft tissue metastatic disease, percutaneous thermal ablation treatment goals include pain palliation and/or local tumor control. Relief is noted in the majority of the patients when: there is persistent pain or imaging evidence of tumor progression despite maximized radiation therapy; radiation therapy is contraindicated or not desired by the patient; or there is an insufficient response to systemic therapies and analgesics. Additionally, in select patients, soft tissue oligometastases (fewer than five lesions) may be approached with a curative intent.

A multidisciplinary approach is recommended for evaluation and treatment of patients with musculoskeletal soft tissue metastases, typically including radiation oncologists, medical oncologists, oncologic surgeons, and interventional radiologists. Such a multidisciplinary approach ensures that each patient benefits from the latest advances in each medical discipline, while concurrently having a clear treatment plan among the multiple specialists.

The main factors determining a patient's eligibility to undergo percutaneous thermal ablation for management of soft tissue metastases include pain, extent of systemic metastatic disease, performance status, life expectancy, and presence of metastatic epidural spinal cord compression in large paraspinal tumors with central canal compromise.[1,2,3,4,5,6,7,8,9,10,11,12,13]

For management of musculoskeletal metastases, the National Comprehensive Cancer Network (NCCN) has incorporated percutaneous thermal ablation in published guidelines. In accordance with the latest NCCN guidelines for adult cancer pain (version 3.2019), percutaneous thermal ablation may be considered for palliation of pain caused by soft tissue metastases in the absence of oncologic emergency when chemotherapy is inadequate and radiation therapy is contraindicated or not desired by the patient.[10]

11.3.1 Thermal Ablation Techniques

Various percutaneous thermal ablation modalities have been successfully utilized in the treatment of soft tissue metastases, including cryoablation, radiofrequency ablation (RFA), and microwave ablation.[1,2,3,4,5,6,7,8,9] Each of these modalities has distinct advantages and disadvantages.

11.3.2 Cryoablation

In cryoablation, the initial freezing cycle (commonly 10 minutes) is immediately followed by a thawing phase (commonly 5–8 minutes), and typically followed by a second freezing cycle (commonly 10 minutes).[1,2,3,4,6,7,9,12,13] A temperature of −40 °C or lower must be achieved to guarantee reliable cell death.[14] The peripheral margin of the hypoattenuating ice-ball on CT typically corresponds to 0 °C, and therefore extension of the ice-ball beyond the neoplastic tissue boundary by at least 3 to 5 mm is recommended to ensure adequate treatment.[1,2,3,4,6,7,9,12,13] Cryoablation is typically used for treatment of soft tissue metastases with the following features: large tumors with complex geometry and paravertebral soft tissue metastases (▸ Fig. 11.1).

Cryoablation has several distinct advantages including visualization of the hypoattenuating ice-ball on CT, simultaneous use of several cryoprobes to achieve additive overlapping ablation zones (inter-cryoprobe distance of 1 to 1.5 cm is commonly implemented),[1,2,3,4,6,7,9,12,13] less intraprocedural and immediate postprocedural pain compared with heating ablation techniques, and the availability of MRI-compatible cryoprobes. Disadvantages of cryoablation of soft tissue metastases include extended procedure length in larger tumors and cost associated with use of multiple cryoprobes.

11.3.3 Microwave Ablation

Various microwave ablation zones may be obtained by using the latest generations of antenna technology.[5,15] Microwave ablation is commonly utilized in the treatment of soft tissue metastases with the following characteristics: large tumors with complex geometry and soft tissue metastases in the absence of adjacent critical soft tissue structures (▶ Fig. 11.2).

The advantages of microwave ablation include less susceptibility to the heat-sink effect and variable tumor tissue impedance, conceivably resulting in a more uniform and larger ablation zone as well as heightened efficiency, lack of need for grounding pads and minimized risk of skin thermal injury, simultaneous use of several antennae to achieve additive overlapping ablation zones, lack of contraindication in patients with metallic implants, and minimal risk of back-heating phenomena in recently introduced antennae.[5,15]

Disadvantages of microwave ablation include a largely occult ablation zone on CT, less distinct ablation zone margins compared with RFA and cryoablation, as well as potential overheating of the surrounding as a result of rapid delivery of high-power output (up to 100 Watts).

11.3.4 Radiofrequency Ablation

Substantial advances in radiofrequency equipment design technology, including the recent introduction of navigational bipolar RFA electrodes, offer distinct advantages in comparison with traditional unipolar straight electrodes. First, navigation of the electrode tip, which can be oriented in different directions from a single skin entry site, allows treatment of challenging-to-access tumors, achieving larger ablation zones and resulting in significant time savings. Second, real-time accurate intraprocedural monitoring of ablation zone size is made possible by built-in thermocouples along the electrode shaft. Finally, the bipolar electrode design obviates the need for grounding pad placement, thereby eliminating the risk of thermal injury of the skin.[6,7,11]

RFA is mainly utilized rather than cryoablation or microwave ablation in the treatment of soft tissue metastases that are: smaller tumors with favorable geometric morphology and difficult to access.

For soft tissue metastases, ablation of the entire volume of hyperintensity on fluid-sensitive sequences and enhancement on MRI, plus at least an additional 3-mm margin, is typically recommended to account for microscopic tumor spread, as well as to achieve improved patient outcomes.[6,7] Limitations of RFA include a CT-occult ablation zone, heat-sink effect due to adjacent blood vessels, and, in cases of hypervascular metastases, diminished efficiency in the treatment of larger soft tissue tumors with complex geometry. Relative contraindication for use of monopolar electrodes includes patients with metallic implants and pacemakers (due to risk of thermal injury of the skin and pacemaker malfunction). Potential complications include intraprocedural pain, and, occasionally, increased pain during the immediate post-ablation period.[3,6,7,9]

11.4 Thermal Protection and Complications

Percutaneous soft tissue thermal ablation carries a potential risk of undesired injury to adjacent vital structures, particularly nerves, vital organs such as bowel and lung, vessels, and skin. Knowledge of the pertinent adjacent neural anatomy is crucial and can minimize inadvertent thermal injury.[16] Several passive and active thermal protection strategies may be implemented to minimize the risk of thermal injury.[2,3,6,7,9,10,11,12] Passive thermal protection strategies include assessing patient's feedback when ablating under moderate sedation (particularly heat-based ablation), real-time temperature monitoring by placement of thermocouples adjacent to the structures at risk (such as nerves), motor and somatosensory evoked potential amplitude, latency monitoring when ablating under general anesthesia, and electro-stimulation of peripheral nerves for early detection of impending nerve injury.[2,3,6,7,9,10,11,12] Active thermal protection may be performed prophylactically, and is recommended when temperature reaches 45 °C (heat) or 10 °C (cold). Active thermal protection may be achieved by displacement of the structure at risk and/or thermal insulation using hydrodissection with injection of warm or cool liquid surrounding the structure at risk (ionic solutions should be avoided during RFA to avoid creation of plasma field and undesired energy propagation), pneumo-dissection with carbon dioxide injection, and balloon interposition. Approaches to minimize thermal injury of skin include precise assessment of ablation zone size and geometry, subcutaneous active thermal protection, surface application of warm saline during cryoablation, and use of bipolar radiofrequency electrode systems.

References

[1] McMenomy BP, Kurup AN, Johnson GB, et al. Percutaneous cryoablation of musculoskeletal oligometastatic disease for complete remission. J Vasc Interv Radiol. 2013; 24(2):207–213

[2] Wallace AN, McWilliams SR, Connolly SE, et al. Percutaneous image-guided cryoablation of musculoskeletal metastases: pain palliation and local tumor control. J Vasc Interv Radiol. 2016; 27(12):1788–1796

[3] Kurup AN, Morris JM, Callstrom MR. Ablation of musculoskeletal metastases. AJR Am J Roentgenol. 2017; 209(4):713–721

[4] Littrup PJ, Bang HJ, Currier BP, et al. Soft-tissue cryoablation in diffuse locations: feasibility and intermediate term outcomes. J Vasc Interv Radiol. 2013; 24(12):1817–1825

[5] Aubry S, Dubut J, Nueffer JP, Chaigneau L, Vidal C, Kastler B. Prospective 1-year follow-up pilot study of CT-guided microwave ablation in the treatment of bone and soft-tissue malignant tumours. Eur Radiol. 2017; 27(4):1477–1485

[6] Ma Y, Wallace AN, Waqar SN, et al. Percutaneous image-guided ablation in the treatment of osseous metastases from non-small cell lung cancer. Cardiovasc Intervent Radiol. 2018; 41(5):726–733

[7] Vaswani D, Wallace AN, Eiswirth PS, et al. Radiographic local tumor control and pain palliation of sarcoma metastases within the musculoskeletal system with percutaneous thermal ablation. Cardiovasc Intervent Radiol. 2018; 41(8):1223–1232

[8] Barral M, Auperin A, Hakime A, et al. Percutaneous thermal ablation of breast cancer metastases in oligometastatic patients. Cardiovasc Intervent Radiol. 2016; 39(6):885–893

[9] Kurup AN, Callstrom MR. Expanding role of percutaneous ablative and consolidative treatments for musculoskeletal tumours. Clin Radiol. 2017; 72(8):645–656

[10] Swarm RA, Paice JA, Anghelescu DL, et al. BCPS. Adult cancer pain, version 3.2019, NCCN Clinical Practice Guidelines in Oncology. J Natl Compr Canc Netw. 2019; 17(8):977–1007

[11] Tomasian A, Hillen TJ, Chang RO, Jennings JW. Simultaneous bipedicular radiofrequency ablation combined with vertebral augmentation for local tumor control of spinal metastases. AJNR Am J Neuroradiol. 2018; 39(9):1768–1773

[12] Tomasian A, Wallace A, Northrup B, Hillen TJ, Jennings JW. Spine cryoablation: pain palliation and local tumor control for vertebral metastases. AJNR Am J Neuroradiol. 2016; 37(1):189–195

[13] Callstrom MR, Dupuy DE, Solomon SB, et al. Percutaneous image-guided cryoablation of painful metastases involving bone: multicenter trial. Cancer. 2013; 119(5):1033–1041

[14] Weld KJ, Landman J. Comparison of cryoablation, radiofrequency ablation and high-intensity focused ultrasound for treating small renal tumours. BJU Int. 2005; 96(9):1224–1229

[15] Deib G, Deldar B, Hui F, Barr JS, Khan MA. Percutaneous microwave ablation and cementoplasty: clinical utility in the treatment of painful extraspinal osseous metastatic disease and myeloma. AJR Am J Roentgenol. 2019; 27:1–8

[16] Kurup AN, Morris JM, Schmit GD, et al. Neuroanatomic considerations in percutaneous tumor ablation. Radiographics. 2013; 33(4):1195–1215

12 Cryoneurolysis I

J. David Prologo and Zohyra E. Zabala

12.1 Case Presentation

A 37-year-old woman with metastatic breast cancer presented to interventional radiology (IR) with low back pain and right lower extremity pain and weakness. Prior to presentation, the patient had undergone multiple pain management therapies, including: L5 segmental radiation; multipronged medication therapy, including intravenous ketamine; and outpatient steroid injections. These treatments had minimal effect. The patient was being followed in the palliative care clinic, still lived independently at home, and expressed a desire to have better pain control.

On physical examination, the patient reported 9/10 pain that was exacerbated by movement. She could not identify anything that eased her pain. She had 4 + strength in her proximal flexion and extension muscles (hip and knee movements), and 5 + strength in her foot dorsiflexion, plantar flexion, inversion, and eversion. Her gait was guarded but steady. Imaging revealed neoplastic involvement of the L5 vertebral body and right lumbosacral trunk (▶ Fig. 12.1).

Plan of care options outside of interventional radiology had been exhausted. Given that there was no discernable fracture in the L5 vertebral body, cryoablation was offered as the most likely intervention to provide the patient relief from low back pain.

As in this case, the adjacent exiting nerve roots may be included in the planned ablation zone or targeted directly. In this case, a second probe was directed specifically to target the lumbosacral trunk (▶ Fig. 12.2). The procedures were performed with the patient under general anesthesia. Each location underwent two 8-minute freeze cycles separated by a 3-minute passive thaw.

During postanesthesia recovery, the patient expressed increased pain in her right lower extremity that was worse when compared to her pain level prior to the procedure. Her exacerbated symptoms necessitated hospital admission and implementation of a patient-controlled analgesia (PCA) pump for pain control. After 18 hours, the patient's pain subsided but she continued to report substantial weakness in her right lower extremity and an unsteady gait. Physical and occupational therapies were consulted. The patient was discharged within 24 hours with associated arranged home physical therapy and ankle-foot-orthosis (AFO) brace. At 15 days post-procedure, the patient reported a 90% reduction in pain, an improvement that lasted for the remainder of her life (5 months). Over the same period, the patient's hip flexor strength returned, and foot dorsiflexion and eversion and inversion improved to 2 + strength. She continued to use a walker for balance assistance.

12.2 Discussion

Medicinal use of the analgesic properties of cold dates back to Hippocrates in 460 BC.[1,2] Avicenna of Persia subsequently reported the use of cold to decrease pain related to surgery, and physicians in Napoleon's army noted decreased pain during amputation in soldiers exposed to extreme cold.[3] Modern-day implementation of device-mediated cold to target pain generators began with a landmark report by Lloyd et al in 1976, during which investigators targeted a variety of peripheral nerves in 64 patients using a gas-cooled cryoprobe guided by an integrated nerve stimulator. These authors noted that compared to other methods of nerve interruption, cryoneurolysis had the advantages of reversibility, repeatability, and decreased incidence of complications such as neuroma formation or neuritis.[4]

The integration of advanced imaging guidance through interventional radiology has unlocked a myriad of potential applications for this technology using a percutaneous approach. Nerve targets residing deep in the body may be targeted percutaneously without surgery using needle probes. The use of computed tomography (CT) as an imaging modality also offers the unique advantages of direct ablation zone visualization, precise targeting, and less procedure-related pain when compared to heat mediated or chemical agents.[5,6,7] In the setting of painful neoplastic disease, nerves may be targeted to interrupt the transmission of pain signals from a painful lesion (see Chapter 21) or as in this case targeted when directly involved by tumor.

The rationale for targeting involved nerves in the setting of painful metastatic disease follows from the mechanism of cryoneurolysis. Exposure of peripheral nerves to cold results in cessation of conduction, dissolution of microtubules, and subsequent Wallerian degeneration, a sequence that is dependent on temperature, time, and nerve diameter. Palliation follows from complete interruption of nerve function and longer ablation times ($\geq$ 8 minutes × 2), which is necessary to ensure the appropriate injury and avoid partial ablation—a condition that may result in pain, allodynia, and/or incomplete or only short-term relief.[2,8,9,10]

The postprocedure course for patients who undergo percutaneous image-guided targeted cryoneurolysis requires special consideration. First, it is not uncommon for patients to experience acute worsening of their symptoms or development of new pain in the distribution of the original symptoms immediately following the procedure. This phenomenon is likely due to a combination of acute nerve injury, central sensitization, and interruption of a baseline medical regimen for the procedure. Managing patient expectations prior to the procedure is helpful, including discussion about a probable short-term post-procedure admission and the use of PCA until the discomfort subsides. Operators can expect the symptoms to resolve during the 24 hours following the procedure.

Second, if the targeted nerve is a motor nerve or mixed motor and sensory nerve, the procedure will induce weakness in the supplied musculature.[10,11] Prospective management of the weakness must include physical and occupational therapy treatment plans, as well as availability of necessary prostheses. For example, targeting of the sciatic nerve or peroneal nerve (or, as in this case, the lumbosacral trunk) is expected to induce dorsiflexion compromise, commonly called "foot drop." Patients with foot drop may improve functionality during recovery with an AFO brace. Preprocedure discussion with physical medicine and rehabilitation collaborators may prove helpful. Activation

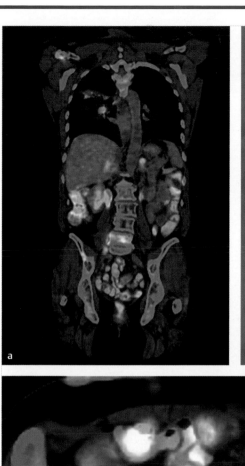
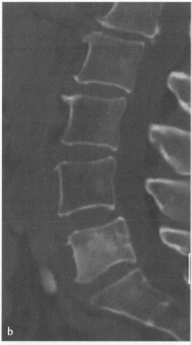
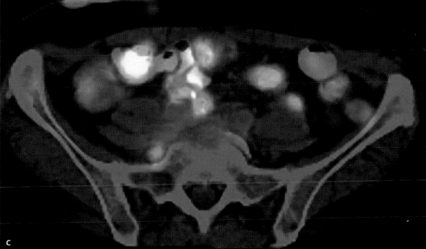

Fig. 12.1 Coronal (**a**) and axial (**c**) positron emission and sagittal computed tomography (CT) (**b**) reconstruction demonstrate neoplastic involvement of the L5 vertebral body and adjacent exiting nerve roots and lumbosacral trunk.

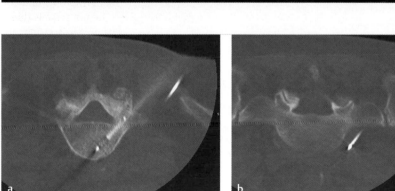

Fig. 12.2 Intraprocedural images demonstrating placement of cryoablation probes (**a**) in a transpedicular fashion to target tumor involvement of L5, and (**b**) in the proximal portion of the lumbosacral trunk.

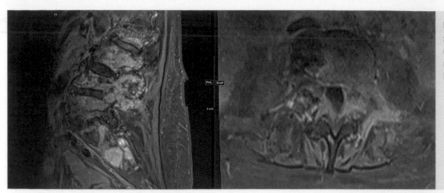

Fig. 12.3 Postcontrast, fat-saturated, T1-weighted, sagittal and axial magnetic resonance imaging (MRI) images demonstrating abnormal enhancement of soft tissue and involvement of L4 and the left L4 exiting nerve root.

of the affected musculature will occur according to nerve regeneration rates of 1 to 2 mm/day.[10]

12.3 Companion Case

A 57-year-old woman with metastatic urothelial cancer presented with intractable pain and weakness involving the left L4 dermatome. The symptoms had been present for 18 months. She had undergone two separate radiation regimens for a total of 36 treatments to the affected area, which was the maximal therapy she could undergo. Review of recent magnetic resonance imaging (MRI) images revealed metastatic disease involving the posterior elements of L4 and the adjacent exiting nerve root (▶ Fig. 12.3). The patient reported 10/10 pain that was not relieved by anything she could identify. Physical examination demonstrated movement limited by pain of the affected extremity and an unsteady gait (she required walker assistance for ambulation). A preprocedure discussion with the patient was undertaken regarding the management of immediate postprocedure pain, should it manifest, and certain weakness induced by the ablation.

After induction of general anesthesia, a single cryoablation probe was placed percutaneously in a left transpedicular fashion such that the predicted ablation zone would include the exiting nerve root and neoplasm involving the left pedicle (▶ Fig. 12.4). Two 10-minute freezes were undertaken, separated by a 3-minute thaw.

The patient recovered with immediate postprocedure pain relief and was discharged later the same day. As expected, she developed weakness in the distribution of L4 (hip flexion and foot dorsiflexion) requiring continued use of her walker for safe ambulation. The patient was followed up in interventional radiology clinic 20 days after the procedure and reported her pain as 2/10, which remained for 4 months until she expired.

12.4 Conclusion

Targeting of nerves directly affected by neoplasm using imaging guidance for percutaneous cryoablation offers patients and referrers unique options for palliation of pain in the setting of metastatic disease. Relief follows from direct cryoablation and destruction of the tumor cells as well as exposure of the involved nerve to cold temperatures for adequate amounts of time to induce conduction cessation, microtubule dissolution,

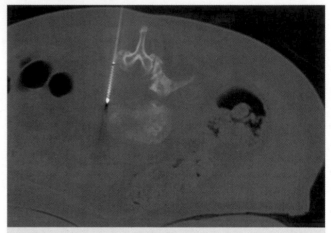

Fig. 12.4 Single, axial, intraprocedural computed tomography (CT) image from a palliative percutaneous cryoneurolysis procedure demonstrating positioning of the cryoablation probe along the left L4 pedicle, adjacent to the affected nerve.

and Wallerian degeneration. Important postprocedure considerations include potential short-term pain exacerbation and mid- to long-term predictable weakness and recovery in the supplied musculature.

References

[1] Cooper SM, Dawber RP. The history of cryosurgery. J R Soc Med. 2001; 94(4): 196–201

[2] Ilfeld BM, Preciado J, Trescot AM. Novel cryoneurolysis device for the treatment of sensory and motor peripheral nerves. Expert Rev Med Devices. 2016; 13(8):713–725

[3] Trescot AM. Cryoanalgesia in interventional pain management. Pain Physician. 2003; 6(3):345–360

[4] Lloyd JW, Barnard JDW, Glynn CJ. Cryoanalgesia. A new approach to pain relief. Lancet. 1976; 2(7992):932–934

[5] Prologo JD, Patel I, Buethe J, Bohnert N. Ablation zones and weight-bearing bones: points of caution for the palliative interventionalist. J Vasc Interv Radiol. 2014; 25(5):769–775.e2

[6] Thacker PG, Callstrom MR, Curry TB, et al. Palliation of painful metastatic disease involving bone with imaging-guided treatment: comparison of patients' immediate response to radiofrequency ablation and cryoablation. AJR Am J Roentgenol. 2011; 197(2):510–515

[7] Allaf ME, Varkarakis IM, Bhayani SB, Inagaki T, Kavoussi LR, Solomon SB. Pain control requirements for percutaneous ablation of renal tumors: cryoablation versus radiofrequency ablation—initial observations. Radiology. 2005; 237 (1):366–370

[8] Hsu M, Stevenson FF. Wallerian degeneration and recovery of motor nerves after multiple focused cold therapies. Muscle Nerve. 2015; 51(2): 268–275

[9] Chhabra A, Ahlawat S, Belzberg A, Andreseik G. Peripheral nerve injury grading simplified on MR neurography: as referenced to Seddon and Sunderland classifications. Indian J Radiol Imaging. 2014; 24(3):217–224

[10] Prologo JD, Johnson C, Hawkins CM, et al. Natural history of mixed and motor nerve cryoablation in humans—a cohort analysis. J Vasc Interv Radiol. 2020; 31(6):912–916.e1

[11] Cornman-Homonoff J, Formenti SC, Chachoua A, Madoff DC. Percutaneous cryoablation for the management of chronic pain secondary to locally recurrent rectal cancer with bowel and nerve root involvement. J Vasc Interv Radiol. 2018; 29(9):1296–1298

13 Cryoneurolysis II—No Direct Nerve Involvement

Amgad M. Moussa, Ernesto Santos, and Juan C. Camacho

13.1 Case Presentation

A 56-year-old man presented to the outpatient clinic with a large, painful left chest wall mass. The patient rated the pain at 8/10, dull and aching in character, exacerbated by coughing, and relieved by changing his position. He stated that he had a longstanding history of a small "knot" in his left lateral chest, but he only sought medical advice when he noticed that it had enlarged significantly in size over the past several months and became painful.

Computed tomography (CT) of the chest revealed a large soft tissue mass involving the left anterolateral chest wall and an associated left pleural effusion (▶ Fig. 13.1). The patient underwent image-guided biopsy of the chest wall mass, which confirmed pathological diagnosis of chondrosarcoma. Sampling of the left pleural fluid revealed malignant cells; a left tunneled pleural drainage catheter was placed (▶ Fig. 13.2). Given the patient's identified structural source of pain (▶ Fig. 13.3), an ultrasound-guided nerve block was performed in the same setting, where 4 cc of bupivacaine and 1 cc of triamcinolone were injected using a 22-gauge needle at each of the T8, T9, T10, and T11 posterior intercostal spaces to relieve his chest pain (▶ Fig. 13.4). The objective was to provide temporary pain relief and to perform a preliminary assessment of the patient's response to a potential cryoneurolysis.

Follow-up after 48 hours revealed that the patient's chest wall pain was controlled (rated 3/10 at worst) and responding well to acetaminophen. Following the patient's good response to intercostal nerve block, cryoneurolysis of the same nerves was performed 1 week later.

Under CT guidance, cryoablation probes were advanced along the inferior border of the posterior 8th, 9th, 10th, and 11th ribs in order to get access to the costal groove. Accurate positioning of the probes was confirmed with multiplanar reformats of CT images, and two freeze and an active thaw cycles (3 minutes and 1 minute, respectively) were performed. To prevent possible skin damage, subcutaneous pneumo-dissection was accomplished prior to cryoneurolysis by advancing a 19-gauge needle into the subcutaneous tissues and injecting 100 cc of room air (▶ Fig. 13.5 and ▶ Fig. 13.6). Clinical follow-up for up to 5 months after the procedure confirmed resolution of the pain with no need for pain medication except for use of occasional acetaminophen as rescue therapy.

13.2 Discussion

The first reported use of cryoablation for pain control was in 1974, when Nelson et al reported that intraoperative cryoablation of the intercostal nerves led to decreased use of analgesics after thoracotomy.[1] The initial use of cryoneurolysis in the intraoperative setting, under direct visualization and percutaneously utilizing anatomic landmarks or neurostimulation, showed it to be a safe and effective tool in pain management but limited in its applications.[1,2,3,4] With the development of imaging modalities and evolution of use of image guidance, interventional radiologists are now able to target deeper nerves, expanding the applications of cryoneurolysis.[5,6,7,8]

The mechanism of cryoneurolysis relies on inducing nerve damage through a mixture of damage to the vasa vasorum, endoneural edema, and dissolution of microtubules, culminating in cessation of axonal transport and decreased pain sensation.[9] Cryoneurolysis can be applied in cases where direct nerve involvement is the cause of the pain, and therefore can be used to target the site of nerve involvement. In cases where no direct nerve involvement is noted, it can be used to target the nerve "upstream" and prevent transmission of pain signals (as in the case presented here).

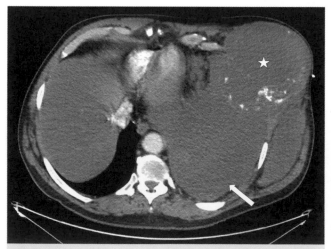

Fig. 13.1 Contrast-enhanced computed tomography (CT) of the chest demonstrating a large left anterior chest wall mass with chondroid matrix (star) and associated malignant left pleural effusion (arrow).

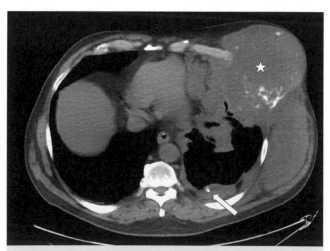

Fig. 13.2 Noncontrast computed tomography (CT) of the chest redemonstrates the known large left anterior chest wall chondrosarcoma (star) and the tip of the tunneled left pleural catheter (arrow).

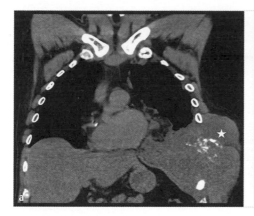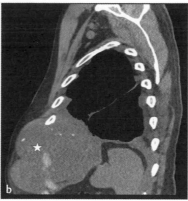

Fig. 13.3 Coronal (**a**) and sagittal (**b**) reformats of the noncontrast computed tomography (CT) of the chest demonstrate the dimensions of the chest wall mass (stars) and associated erosion of the left seventh rib.

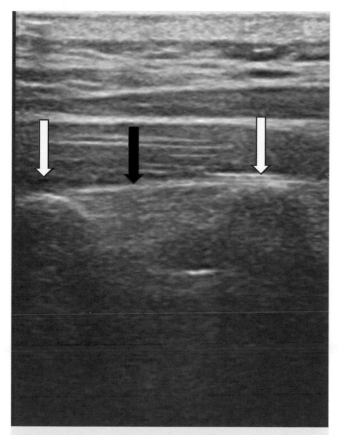

Fig. 13.4 Ultrasound image using a 9 MHz linear ultrasound probe showing transverse view of the ribs (white arrows) and the visualized intercostal spaces (black arrow). A 22-gauge needle (not shown) was used under real-time ultrasound guidance to inject 4 cc of bupivacaine and 1 cc of triamcinolone at the costal groove of the 8th, 9th, 10th, and 11th ribs. Following injection, fluid was noted in the costal groove.

Prior to cryoneurolysis, a preliminary assessment of the patient's response to the procedure can be measured by the response to local nerve block in the same location. This is done under image guidance, using a 22-gauge or 25-gauge needle, and a mixture of anesthetics and steroids. A patient who does not respond to the nerve block is unlikely to respond to cryoneurolysis.[3,9,10] Although the use of neurostimulation to reproduce the pain allows accurate identification of the nerves responsible for pain transmission from the lesion, it is not often used and knowledge of sensory dermatomes often suffices.[3]

Cryoneurolysis can be performed under monitored sedation using fentanyl and midazolam, although it is preferable to use minimal sedation when using neurostimulation as patient's cooperation is required.[9,10] Compared to radiofrequency or alcohol ablation, the procedure-related pain is low.[11] The imaging modality of choice for guidance depends on the target and operator's preference, with fluoroscopy, ultrasound, CT, and magnetic resonance imaging (MRI) being used.[5,7,9,12] Once the cryoablation probe is in position, one or two alternating freeze–thaw cycles are usually performed, the lengths of which vary according to the required size of the ablation zone. The ablation zone can be visualized in real time by monitoring the ice-ball formation.[6,10,12]

Overall, the outcomes of cryoneurolysis are promising, with several studies reporting variable decreases in pain scores and/or analgesic use following the procedure. Yoon et al reported a 6-point and 3.2-point decrease in mean pain scores at 1 month and 1 year, respectively, in patients who underwent cryoneurolysis for chronic peripheral neuropathic pain.[10] Prologo et al reported a 0.8-point decrease in mean pain scores at 7 days and a 3.9-point decrease at 45 days in patients who underwent cryoneurolysis for phantom limb pain.[12] The initially low improvement in pain following cryoneurolysis can be explained by the presence of an inflammatory reaction at the site of cryoneurolysis, which induces pain and may require anti-inflammatory medications.[12] The decrease in the efficacy of cryoneurolysis at long-term follow-up can be explained by regrowth of the nerve, which takes several months, owing to the preserved epineurium and perineurium.[10] However, it is safe to repeat the treatment if the pain recurs.[10]

Cryoneurolysis has a low reported complication rate, with most studies reporting minor or no complications following the procedure. Reported complications include pain or infection at the site of the cryoablation, with one study reporting a prolonged cerebrospinal fluid (CSF) leak after cryoablation of sacral and coccygeal nerves.[13] The use of image guidance decreases the potential risk of bleeding or organ injury during probe placement and increases the safety of the procedure. The safety, efficacy, and repeatability of cryoneurolysis make it a very useful tool in pain management.

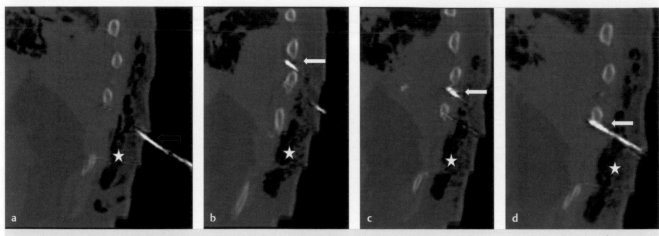

Fig. 13.5 Sagittal reconstructions of computed tomography (CT) of the chest done to confirm adequate positioning of the cryoablation probes (white arrows). (**a**) A 19-gauge needle (blue arrow) used to inject room air into the subcutaneous tissues (stars) to displace the skin away from the ablation zone and prevent skin injury. (**b–d**) Cryoablation probes in the 9th, 10th, and 11th intercostal spaces (white arrows) prior to cryoablation.

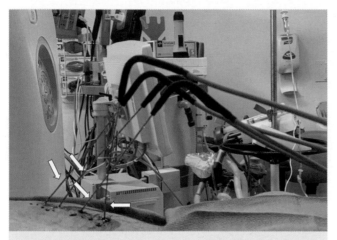

Fig. 13.6 Photograph from the procedure room with the ablation probes (arrows) in position prior to cryoneurolysis.

References

[1] Nelson KM, Vincent RG, Bourke RS, et al. Intraoperative intercostal nerve freezing to prevent postthoracotomy pain. Ann Thorac Surg. 1974; 18(3): 280–285

[2] Radnovich R, Scott D, Patel AT, et al. Cryoneurolysis to treat the pain and symptoms of knee osteoarthritis: a multicenter, randomized, double-blind, sham-controlled trial. Osteoarthritis Cartilage. 2017; 25(8):1247–1256

[3] Moesker AA, Karl HW, Trescot AM. Treatment of phantom limb pain by cryoneurolysis of the amputated nerve. Pain Pract. 2014; 14(1):52–56

[4] Tanaka A, Al-Rstum Z, Leonard SD, et al. Intraoperative intercostal nerve cryoanalgesia improves pain control after descending and thoracoabdominal aortic aneurysm repairs. Ann Thorac Surg. 2020; 109(1):249–254

[5] Bonham LW, Phelps A, Rosson GD, Fritz J. MR imaging-guided cryoneurolysis of the sural nerve. J Vasc Interv Radiol. 2018; 29(11):1622–1624

[6] Ilfeld BM, Gabriel RA, Trescot AM. Ultrasound-guided percutaneous cryoneurolysis providing postoperative analgesia lasting many weeks following a single administration: a replacement for continuous peripheral nerve blocks? A case report. Korean J Anesthesiol. 2017; 70(5):567–570

[7] Prologo JD, Lin RC, Williams R, Corn D. Percutaneous CT-guided cryoablation for the treatment of refractory pudendal neuralgia. Skeletal Radiol. 2015; 44 (5):709–714

[8] Yarmohammadi H. Mortell K, Prologo JD, Azaar N, Haaga J, Nakamoto DA. Percutaneous Efficiency and safety of percutanous CT-guided cryoablation of celiac plexus in treating intractable pain caused by pancreatic cancer. J Vasc Interv Radiol, 24(4): S131

[9] Trescot AM. Cryoanalgesia in interventional pain management. Pain Physician. 2003; 6(3):345–360

[10] Yoon JHE, Grechushkin V, Chaudhry A, Bhattacharji P, Durkin B, Moore W. Cryoneurolysis in patients with refractory chronic peripheral neuropathic pain. J Vasc Interv Radiol. 2016; 27(2):239–243

[11] Erinjeri JP, Clark TWI. Cryoablation: mechanism of action and devices. J Vasc Interv Radiol. 2010; 21(8) Suppl:S187–S191

[12] Prologo JD, Gilliland CA, Miller M, et al. Percutaneous image-guided cryoablation for the treatment of phantom limb pain in amputees: a pilot study. J Vasc Interv Radiol. 2017; 28(1):24–34.e4

[13] Bittman RW, Peters GL, Newsome JM, et al. Percutaneous image-guided cryoneurolysis. AJR Am J Roentgenol. 2018; 210(2):454–465

14 Celiac Plexus Neurolysis

Aron K. Chary and William G. O'Connell

14.1 Case Presentation

A 63-year-old man with stage IV metastatic pancreatic head adenocarcinoma was presented at a multidisciplinary pain conference. The patient initially presented to the Emergency Department (ED) with intractable abdominal pain. A 3.2 × 2.1 cm pancreatic head mass was discovered on computed tomography (CT) of the abdomen and pelvis. There was extension of disease surrounding the adjacent vasculature, with multiple retroperitoneal para-aortic and retrocaval lymph nodes. A few subcentimeter hypodense lesions were also present within the liver. The patient was discharged with oral pain medication and a follow-up consultation with oncology for further staging evaluation of the presumed pancreatic carcinoma.

Further workup and consultation with the oncologist revealed that the patient had been suffering from significant (8/10) abdominal pain for 4 to 5 weeks before finally presenting to the ED. The pain was minimally relieved by the oral pain medication prescribed in the ED. A palliative care consultation followed, allowing for further medical pain management optimization. Breakthrough pain, however, was still persistent. The prescribed pain medication regimen induced significant fatigue, nausea, constipation, and somnolence. A consultation was arranged with interventional radiology for further interventional pain management.

On physical examination, the patient reported 9/10 pain centrally within the region of the lower abdomen, with subjective "propagation" of pain "deep toward the spine." He could not identify any position or activity that mitigated the pain. The pain was constant, independent of the time of day or food consumption. Despite a fairly aggressive oral pain medication regimen, the degree of relief was minimal with reported debilitating side effects including constipation, nausea, and somnolence. The patient was somewhat tender to deep palpation within the central abdomen.

A recent staging magnetic resonance imaging (MRI) examination of the abdomen and pelvis revealed a large pancreatic head mass with para-aortic and retrocaval adenopathy. A few small nodular lymph nodes were also noted to extend posteriorly into the bilateral retrocrural space. Evaluation of the region of the celiac plexus demonstrated an adequate window bilaterally for posterior needle access (▶ Fig. 14.1).

Care options outside of interventional radiology had been maximized. Due to the clinical and imaging presentation, the patient was deemed an ideal candidate for CT-guided celiac plexus neurolysis. Cryoablation was chosen by the operator in this instance (vs. chemical neurolysis with ethanol). The procedure was performed with the patient under general anesthesia. The patient was placed in the prone position on the CT gantry. One probe was placed into the celiac plexus on each side (two probes in total), utilizing a posterior paravertebral antecrural approach. A total of two 10-minute freeze cycles separated by a 5-minute passive thaw cycle were performed (▶ Fig. 14.2).

▶ Fig. 14.3 demonstrates similar findings and cryoprobe placement in a second patient with pancreatic carcinoma.

14.2 Companion Case

An 83-year-old man with history of stage IV biliary adenocarcinoma status post pylorus-sparing Whipple procedure 4 years prior with known recurrence. The patient was initiated on further chemotherapy regimen. He subsequently developed recurrent cholangitis from biliary obstruction for which a right-sided internal–external biliary drain was placed. During the course of multiple hospital admissions for recurrent cholangitis, the patient developed progressively worsening abdominal pain. Despite aggressive medical management with narcotics and intermittent biliary drain exchanges, the abdominal pain persisted and the patient experienced a further decline in his quality of life from opiate-induced side effects. During one of the patient's hospital admissions, interventional radiology was consulted for further assistance with abdominal pain management.

At the time of the consultation, physical examination demonstrated generalized weakness with reported 10/10 central and deep epigastric pain. The pain was neither worsened nor relieved by ingestion of food or positioning. The patient reported having been fairly active in the previous few months leading up to the admission, but at the time of the examination he could barely walk due to intractable pain. CT of the abdomen and pelvis demonstrated sequelae from a pylorus-sparing Whipple procedure without apparent bulky tumor disease; however, progression was suspected on the basis of lab and tumor markers. CT-guided chemical neurolysis was offered due to lack

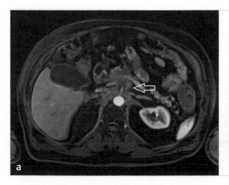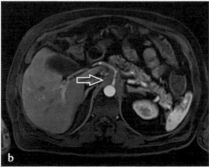

Fig. 14.1 Axial contrast-enhanced magnetic resonance imaging (MRI) images in the arterial phase through the level of the celiac axis and superior mesenteric artery (SMA). **(a)** Neoplastic soft tissue extension from pancreatic carcinoma infiltrating the celiac axis origin, with extension along the expected location of the celiac plexus (arrow). **(b)** Further soft tissue infiltration along the SMA origin infiltrating the expected celiac plexus distribution (arrow).

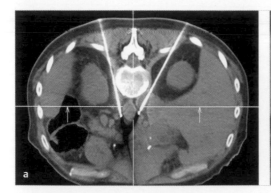

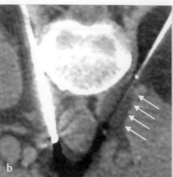

Fig. 14.2 Intraprocedural computed tomography (CT) images demonstrating posterior placement of bilateral cryoablation probes into the celiac plexus. (a) Cryoprobe needle placement bilaterally just lateral to the aorta between the celiac axis and superior mesenteric artery (SMA) origins. (b) Magnified view of the right-sided (prone position) probe ice-ball during one of the freeze cycles (arrows).

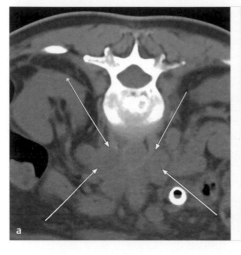

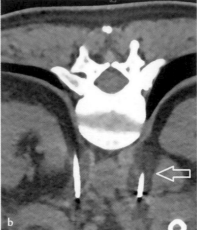

Fig. 14.3 Ancillary case of a patient with pancreatic cancer with bulky retroperitoneal adenopathy undergoing celiac plexus cryoablation. (a) Prone noncontrast computed tomography (CT) image demonstrating bulky aortocaval adenopathy just posterior and inferior to the pancreatic head mass (arrows). (b) Bilateral cryoprobes just inferior to the bulky adenopathy at the level of the superior mesenteric artery (SMA) with early intraprocedural ice-ball formation (arrow). Ethanol use was less favored due to concern for nodal inhibition from chemical dispersion throughout the plexus.

of infiltrative retroperitoneal disease and good window for ethanol dispersion.

The procedure was performed with the patient in the prone position on the CT gantry after intubation with general anesthesia (▶ Fig. 14.4a). Bilateral 22-guage × 15 cm Chiba needles were placed into the bilateral celiac plexi via a posterior (dorsal) paravertebral approach under CT guidance. Approximately 10 mL (5 mL per side) of diluted iodinated contrast (30:1 saline to iodinated contrast) was injected to evaluate dispersion within the nerve plexus and to exclude vascular infiltration. With each needle 20 mL of 100% ethanol was then injected for a total of 40 mL of ethanol. Postneurolysis CT imaging demonstrated good dispersion of the ethanol with contrast displacement and no evidence of immediate complication (▶ Fig. 14.4b). The patient recovered in the postanesthesia recovery unit for 2 hours and then returned to his inpatient room.

The patient was seen approximately 4 hours after the procedure, once the effect from anesthesia had begun to dissipate. He reported 0/10 pain on initial assessment; he continued to be pain free for many months. He was able to return to many of his normal daily activities and was immediately able to wean off the narcotic regimen. Of note, the patient did experience the well-known procedure-related side effect of diarrhea. Although very common with celiac plexus ethanol neurolysis, diarrhea is usually transient lasting only 2 to 3 days. In this particular case, the diarrhea was significant and lasted 2 to 3 weeks, requiring gastrointestinal and infectious

disease consultations to optimize supportive medical care. The diarrhea ultimately resolved without further metabolic derangement.

14.3 Discussion

Abdominal pain is a debilitating problem in many patients with upper abdominal malignancy, and affects quality of life, prognosis, and overall survival of the patients.[1,2] Management of cancer-related abdominal pain can be quite challenging and requires a multidisciplinary approach. High-dose narcotics and nonsteroidal anti-inflammatory drugs (NSAIDs) have conventionally been the mainstay of treatment in this population; however, this often contributes to adverse effects that further worsen the patient's quality of life. In search of alternative methods of alleviating abdominal pain symptoms without further compromising quality of life, neurolytic sympathetic block has evolved as an excellent localized supplementary treatment that is efficient, reproducibly effective, and relatively simple to perform.[3]

The neurologic symptom of cancer-induced pain from the upper abdominal organs is transmitted by special visceral afferent fibers that are relayed from the splanchnic nerves through the celiac plexus.[4] By disrupting the nociceptive impulses at the level of the celiac plexus or splanchnic nerves, alleviation of intractable pain associated with abdominal malignancy can be achieved.[5] Neurolysis refers to the permanent destruction of

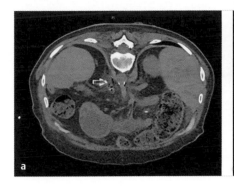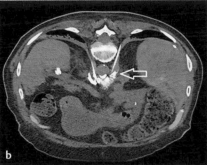

Fig. 14.4 Intraprocedural noncontrast computed tomography (CT) images through the celiac plexus. (a) Contrast dispersion of a test injection of very dilute iodinated contrast from the bilateral 22-gauge Chiba needles, showing contrast disseminated around the expected location of the celiac plexus (arrow). No intravascular spread was visualized. (b) Post-ethanol injection CT image demonstrates the expected appearance of dispersed ethanol around the celiac plexus. This often has the appearance of low density "gas bubbles," as ethanol has a similar attenuation to air.

the nerve plexus by interrupting the sympathetic nervous system at the ganglion level, which can be performed with chemical solution (e.g., ethanol) or thermal ablation (heat or cold).

Percutaneous celiac plexus neurolysis has been shown to have long-term improvement in abdominal pain with decreased narcotic usage in 70 to 90% of patients.[6] Image-guided celiac plexus neurolysis is most commonly performed utilizing multidetector CT.[6] This modality allows for accurate, safe, and selective targeting of the celiac plexus with anatomic identification of surrounding adjacent structures.

14.3.1 Anatomy of the Celiac Plexus

The celiac plexus is a network of nerve ganglia located adjacent to the aorta between the origins of the celiac trunk and superior mesenteric artery, typically located between T12 and L1. One of its main component is preganglionic sympathetic efferent nerve fibers, which derive from the greater splanchnic (T5–T9), lesser splanchnic (T10–T11), and least splanchnic (T12) nerves.[6] This network of ganglia relay preganglionic sympathetic and parasympathetic efferent fibers, as well as visceral sensory afferent fibers, to the viscera of the upper abdomen. The liver, gallbladder, pancreas, spleen, adrenal glands, kidneys, stomach, and distal esophagus to the distal transverse colon transmit nociceptive impulses via these visceral sensory afferent fibers.[7]

Due to advancements in multidetector CT technology, the celiac plexus is frequently identified on diagnostic abdominal CT.[8] On axial CT images, the bilateral ganglia often demonstrate a discoid or lobulated configuration that can resemble the limbs of the adjacent adrenal gland and diaphragmatic crus.[8] The right celiac ganglion is often located between the inferior vena cava (IVC) and right diaphragmatic crus, anteromedial (ventromedial) to the medial limb of the right adrenal gland. Zhang et al[9] described the location of the right celiac ganglion as residing just posterior (dorsal) to the angle formed by the left renal vein as it enters the IVC. The left celiac ganglion is consistently seen just medial and inferior (caudal) to the medial limb of the left adrenal gland and lateral to the left diaphragmatic crus.[8] The three-dimensional configuration of the plexus drapes along the anterolateral (ventral) region of the aorta between the celiac axis and SMA.

14.3.2 Technical Approach

There are several approaches to access the celiac plexus when performing neurolysis. The modality used, patient position,

needle location, and laterality are dependent on the mechanism of neurolysis, operator preference, and anatomic considerations. Anatomic considerations include body habitus, quantity of retroperitoneal fat, proximity of adjacent and surrounding organs, and degree of tumor/lymph node infiltration in the setting of abdominal malignancy. Anterior and posterior approaches are most commonly chosen utilizing CT guidance; however, percutaneous ultrasound, endoscopic ultrasound (EUS), and fluoroscopic guidance have also been described.[7]

In the anterior (ventral) approach, a needle is inserted through the abdominal wall directly anterior (ventral) to the level of the celiac plexus. Utilizing this method, various abdominal structures are often traversed including stomach, small bowel, liver, and pancreas. Traversal of these organs is generally well-tolerated.[7] The posterior (dorsal) approach requires prone positioning, with usually two needles inserted bilaterally through the paraspinous musculature into the region of the celiac plexus. Although this approach often necessitates placement of two needles, takes slightly more time, and requires the patient to lie in the prone position, for many operators targeting the ganglia is more accurate and selective due to precise placement into the nerve plexus (and lack of intervening organ traversal). CT guidance is also able to accurately depict anatomic variations of the celiac trunk or regional distortion that can result from tumor spread.[10] Another key benefit of CT is the ability to depict the extent of distribution of the neurolytic agent within the antecrural space via a test injection of diluted contrast. This also allows evaluation of contrast migration into adjacent structures or leakage into the peritoneal cavity.[10] In addition, alternative mechanisms of neurolysis (e.g., thermal ablation) can be safely performed using CT, taking advantage of precise targeting, direct ablation zone visualization, and usually less procedure-related pain when compared to chemical agents.[11]

14.3.3 History of Chemical Neurolysis for Celiac Plexus Ablation

Traditional agents used to achieve permanent neurolysis of the celiac plexus include ethanol and phenol.[10,12] Ethanol works through immediate precipitation of endoneural lipoproteins and mucoproteins within nerve ganglia, leading to leakage of cholesterol, phospholipid, and cerebroside from the neurilemma.[10,12] At ethanol concentration of above 50%, irreversible damage to neurons occurs, with the degree of destruction dependent on the distribution of ethanol within the celiac plexus.[10] Ethanol has been known to cause significant transient pain upon injection; hence, some authors recommend adding a long-acting local anesthetic such as bupivacaine to the ethanol cocktail in order to achieve injection-related pain control.[6] Very dilute iodinated contrast material (30 mL normal saline to 1 mL of iodinated contrast) has also been recommended in order to help visualize the distribution of ethanol prior to injecting the chemical neurolytic.[6,10] Given the more frequent use of general anesthesia to assist with blood pressure lability during the procedure, the authors' institutional preference is to administer 20 mL of pure 100% ethanol through bilaterally placed 22-gauge Chiba needles (total of 40 mL 100% ethanol) following to a test injection of diluted contrast via a posterior approach.

Chemical neurolysis of the celiac plexus using ethanol is well-studied and has proven to be an effective means for pain palliation in the setting of painful pancreatic adenocarcinoma.[13] Reported potential adverse side effects related to ethanol injection include: nontarget distribution, transient intractable diarrhea, cardioneurologic dysfunction, blood pressure lability, bleeding, or a combination of these sequelae.[13] This technique is also limited by bulky infiltrative tumors that can impede the dissemination and distribution of injected fluid, often rendering the procedure less effective and necessitating repeat interventions.[13]

14.3.4 Cryoneurolysis for Celiac Plexus

As previously alluded to, CT guidance has emerged as a favorable modality for celiac plexus neurolysis due to its precise targeting, real-time monitoring of needle placement, and utility in employing more advanced ablative techniques such as thermal ablation.[13] CT-guided cryoneurolysis was first reported by Mortell et al,[14] in which nine patients with pancreatic adenocarcinoma successfully underwent the procedure with only one minor complication. In patients with bulky tumor disease, retroperitoneal lymph nodes, or in whom ethanol neurolysis had failed previously, CT-guided cryoneurolysis may be the preferred treatment compared to a liquid neurolytic agent.[13]

14.4 Conclusion

Celiac plexus neurolysis is a safe and effective intervention for palliative pain management in patients with intractable abdominal pain due to malignant and nonmalignant etiologies. Image guidance allows for selective nerve ganglia targeting with controlled neurolysis via chemical or thermal ablation. Recent global initiatives for addressing the opioid crisis and providing patients with additional options for pain control have sparked interest in alternative forms of pain management. In patients with upper abdominal malignancies, celiac plexus neurolysis is effective in both eliminating the source of intractable abdominal pain and mitigating the effects of pharmacologic induced deterioration.[15]

References

[1] de Oliveira R, dos Reis MP, Prado WA. The effects of early or late neurolytic sympathetic plexus block on the management of abdominal or pelvic cancer pain. Pain. 2004; 110(1–2):400–408

[2] Wong GY, Schroeder DR, Carns PE, et al. Effect of neurolytic celiac plexus block on pain relief, quality of life, and survival in patients with unresectable pancreatic cancer: a randomized controlled trial. JAMA. 2004; 291(9):1092–1099

[3] Thompson GE, Moore DC, Bridenbaugh LD, Artin RY. Abdominal pain and alcohol celiac plexus nerve block. Anesth Analg. 1977; 56(1):1–5

[4] Loukas M, Klaassen Z, Merbs W, Tubbs RS, Gielecki J, Zurada A. A review of the thoracic splanchnic nerves and celiac ganglia. Clin Anat. 2010; 23(5): 512–522

[5] De Cicco M, Matovic M, Balestreri L, Fracasso A, Morassut S, Testa V. Single-needle celiac plexus block: is needle tip position critical in patients with no regional anatomic distortions? Anesthesiology. 1997; 87(6):1301–1308

[6] Kambadakone A, Thabet A, Gervais DA, Mueller PR, Arellano RS. CT-guided celiac plexus neurolysis: a review of anatomy, indications, technique, and tips for successful treatment. Radiographics. 2011; 31(6):1599–1621

[7] Nitschke AM, Ray CE , Jr. Percutaneous neurolytic celiac plexus block. Semin Intervent Radiol. 2013; 30(3):318–321

[8] Wang ZJ, Webb EM, Westphalen AC, Coakley FV, Yeh BM. Multi-detector row computed tomographic appearance of celiac ganglia. J Comput Assist Tomogr. 2010; 34(3):343–347

[9] Zhang XM, Zhao QH, Zeng NL, et al. The celiac ganglia: anatomic study using MRI in cadavers. AJR Am J Roentgenol. 2006; 186(6):1520–1523

[10] Wang PJ, Shang MY, Qian Z, Shao CW, Wang JH, Zhao XH. CT-guided percutaneous neurolytic celiac plexus block technique. Abdom Imaging. 2006; 31(6):710–718

[11] Prologo JD, Patel I, Buethe J, Bohnert N. Ablation zones and weight-bearing bones: points of caution for the palliative interventionalist. J Vasc Interv Radiol. 2014; 25(5):769–775.e2

[12] Titton RL, Lucey BC, Gervais DA, Boland GW, Mueller PR. Celiac plexus block: a palliative tool underused by radiologists. AJR Am J Roentgenol. 2002; 179 (3):633–636

[13] Bittman RW, Peters GL, Newsome JM, et al. Percutaneous image-guided cryoneurolysis. AJR Am J Roentgenol. 2018; 210(2):454–465

[14] Mortell K, Yarmohammadi H, Brocone M, Haaga J, Nakamoto D. Percutaneous CT-guided cryoablation of the celiac plexus in the palliative treatment of pancreatic cancer. J Vasc Interv Radiol. 2014; 25:817.e815

[15] Raj PP, Lou L, Erdine S, et al, eds. Interventional Pain Management: Image-Guided Procedures. 2nd ed. Philadelphia: Saunders Elsevier; 2008

15 Intrathecal Pain Pumps

Sudheer Potru, Sunil Agarwal, and Vinita Singh

15.1 Case Presentation

A 70-year-old woman with metastatic lung cancer presented with extensive osseous metastases throughout the thoracic, lumbar, and sacral spine. She had a history of multiple hospital admissions for intractable back pain, and also demonstrated radicular right leg pain in the L5 distribution. She described her pain as throbbing, aching, and stabbing, and rated it as 5/10 at rest and 10/10 with any movement. On physical examination, she had decreased strength in bilateral plantarflexion and dorsiflexion at the ankles, and spinal tenderness around the L5 level. In addition to severe degenerative disease, magnetic resonance imaging (MRI) of her lumbar spine (▶ Fig. 15.1) demonstrated a pathologic compression fracture of the L3 vertebral body with retropulsion of bone and epidural tumor resulting in moderate to severe spinal canal narrowing. There were additional mild compression fracture deformities at L1 and L5. There was also epidural tumor demonstrated as indicated above.

The patient received external palliative radiation, which was helpful, but she still continued to have debilitating pain. Her pain was unresponsive to oral medications including opioids (extended release morphine 60 mg twice per day, immediate release morphine 30 mg four to six times per day), steroids, and high-dose gabapentin. Moreover, she started to experience sedation, delirium, and constipation from her medication regimen, limiting any increase in dose.

The patient underwent continuous epidural infusion trial for possible intrathecal (IT) pump insertion; this trial resulted in 80 to 90% pain relief. Due to success of the epidural infusion trial, placement of an IT pump was performed.

The optimal location of the IT pump was determined by the patient (the left side of the abdomen at the beltline) (▶ Fig. 15.2). For the procedure, she received general anesthesia and was placed in the right lateral decubitus position with appropriate padding of pressure points. After surgical prep and drape, a 3-cm incision was made at the inferomedial aspect of the L3 interspace lateral to the midline, and a pocket was created at the level of the fascia in the abdomen. A 17-gauge spinal needle was advanced to the subarachnoid space at the L2–L3 level, and the IT catheter was inserted under fluoroscopic guidance until the tip of the catheter was positioned at the T10 vertebral level. The needle was removed and the catheter was anchored to the fascia using a 2–0 silk purse-string suture.

The pump pocket was prepared for pump insertion. A tunneling device was used to access the pump pocket from the spinal incision and the IT catheter was threaded along the tunnel and attached to the pump. Incisions were closed using standard technique. The IT pump was set to deliver hydromorphone 0.1 mg/day and bupivacaine 0.5 mg/standard day, which was slowly increased over the course of several days during hospitalization to hydromorphone 0.3 mg/day and bupivacaine 1.5 mg/day. She was allowed additional IT boluses for breakthrough pain via the patient therapy manager device. This provided excellent pain relief (pain scores 0 to 3 on a 10 point scale) for the remainder of her life, such that she was able to discontinue all her oral pain medications. Unfortunately, her disease continued to progress rapidly and she died several weeks later in hospice.

15.2 Discussion

15.2.1 Historical Context of Intrathecal Drug Delivery

Spinal anesthesia and analgesia date back to 1898, when August Bier first described administration of cocaine into his own IT space as well as that of six patients who underwent lower extremity surgery.[1] Although further discoveries and advances in this subfield took place for the next 80 years, it was not until the early 1970s that infusion pumps were developed to continuously administer IT medications.[2,3] IT morphine was first used in 1979 by Wang et al to treat intractable cancer pain.[4] In 1981, the use of an implantable intrathecal drug delivery system (IDDS) was first described involving an IT catheter connected to a motor-powered pump placed in the subcutaneous tissue.[5] Externally programmable, battery-powered IDDS pumps were introduced in 1991, allowing for noninvasive dose changes to IT medications using a wireless programming device.[6] The external programmer in modern devices has allowed for a more convenient and practical means to modify a therapeutic plan based on relevant clinical criteria, including changes in pain or spasm, side effects to medications, or other issues.[7]

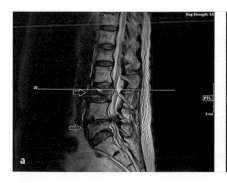
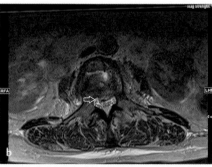

Fig. 15.1 Sagittal (**a**) and axial (**b**) magnetic resonance imaging (MRI) images of the lumbar spine showing multiple compression fractures (open arrows, **a**) and epidural tumor burden (open arrow, **b**).

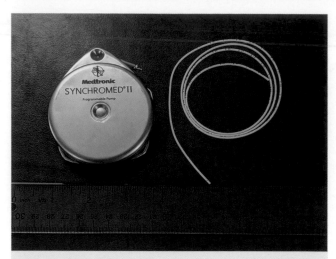

Fig. 15.2 Sample pump and catheter.

15.2.2 Implant Considerations (Patient Selection, Indications/Contraindications, and Trialing)

Current guidelines suggest careful consideration of disease-specific indications and patient characteristics when selecting IT drug delivery candidates. The Food and Drug Administration (FDA) has approved IT therapy for patients with moderate to severe trunk and limb pain, intractable pain, and/or intractable spasm that have failed more conservative treatment.[8,9,10] In 2017, the Polyanalgesic Consensus Conference (PACC) provided further updated disease-specific indications for IT therapy; these indications cover a wide variety of conditions including: severe axial neck or back pain, failed back surgery syndrome, visceral or somatic abdominal and/or pelvic pain, extremity pain, complex regional pain syndrome (CRPS), trunk pain including post-herpetic neuralgia and post-thoracotomy syndromes, cancer pain, and systemic opioid analgesic therapy complicated by intolerable side effects.[11] In all cases, but particularly among patients with cancer pain, providers should consider the stage of the disease, other interventions attempted, and the patient's life expectancy.[12] Currently, IT therapy is recommended in cancer patients with a life expectancy of at least 6 months.[13]

Many characteristics contribute to patient selection for IT therapy, including previous opioid or antispasmodic exposure and sensitivity, pain type and location, psychological factors, and patient's social support. A careful history of present illness, psychosocial evaluation, and physical examination of the patient are recommended before consideration for IT therapy.[12] IT therapy can be used to treat localized, diffuse, and global pain; however, current evidence for IT therapy in treating global pain is still not well established.[12] Patients should be assessed for risk factors that contribute to bleeding, infection, and cardiopulmonary limitations to determine their ability to mitigate complications from the procedure and tolerate the therapy over time. Practitioners should anticipate developing a long-term partnership with the patient and discuss appropriate expectations prior to initiation of IT therapy; this discussion is an excellent time to review the patient's psychological status and to ensure appropriate psychosocial support. This part of patient selection process is particularly critical, as failure to heed device alarms or follow-up at appropriate time intervals for refill can result in life-threatening withdrawal or complications as indicated later in this chapter. Cancer patients seeking palliative treatment may not require as extensive psychological screen as patients who are likely to live longer, but they may still benefit from counseling regarding chronic illness and overall treatment goals.

Although practice varies among clinicians, many operators perform a trial of IT drug delivery prior to implantation of an IT pump. An IT trial is performed to elucidate goals for pain relief and functional improvement, demonstrate reduction in systemic opioid use, and test for potential adverse reactions to IT medications.[14] Currently, there is no consensus on trialing technique, drug combination, or particular outcome that defines an efficacious trial, although many operators use 50% improvement in pain or spasm severity as an indicator of success following implantation. Bolus injection or admission for continuous multi-day catheter infusion at either epidural or IT sites are the currently accepted trialing techniques.[14] However, IT or epidural trial is not mandatory for implantation and potentially may not be suitable for all patients, such as those with multilevel spinal instrumentation, severe medical comorbidities, or chronic anticoagulation therapy. Despite the lack of consensus on trialing in the literature, experts agree that patients who undergo IT trial should be monitored appropriately for at least 24 hours, given the concern for respiratory depression particularly if opioids are used.[13]

15.2.3 Technical Considerations

Although cerebrospinal fluid (CSF) dynamics are not completely understood, current theories recognize that the rate of dispersion in the CSF cannot be attributed to diffusion alone, but may be attributed to pulsatile flow with oscillatory displacement.[12,15,16] IT pumps use either continuous-flow or variable-flow mechanisms, such as peristalsis, fluorocarbon propellant, osmotic pressure, and piezoelectric disk benders to deliver drugs to the receptor sites in the dorsal horn of the spinal cord.[11,12] Propellant pumps, such as the Codman 3000 (J&J Medical Devices, New Brunswick, NJ) and the Medtronic Isomed (Minneapolis, MN), are not battery-dependent, while programmable pumps, such as the Medtronic Synchromed II and the Flowonix Prometra II (Mt. Olive, NJ), rely on a battery that must be replaced within shorter time intervals.[9,10,11,12] Programmable pumps have variable drug delivery mechanisms and provide patients with the ability to control dosing by using a patient-held programmer. The Medtronic Synchromed II system uses a peristaltic rotor system of internal tubing to administer medication from the reservoir to the external catheter system, while the Flowonix Prometra II pump uses a valve-gated bellow for drug delivery.[9,10,11,12] Drug refill for implanted pumps is recommended every 1 to 3 months, with some anecdotal evidence suggesting up to 180 days depending on the drug dose, concentration, and patient factors.[16]

15.2.4 Programming and Refilling

Programming of the IT pump involves use of a specific pump programming device produced by the manufacturer. The programming device receives inputs of solution concentration and requested daily dose and calculates the rate of solution infusion automatically; this can be updated if the dose or solution is changed (by altering concentration or by addition or subtraction of another agent). In addition, most newer pumps' programming devices allow the practitioner to adjust the rate of the continuous IT infusion and set a dose for patient-controlled boluses for breakthrough pain.

Refilling the pump requires both a new, sterile compounded IT solution and utilization of the manufacturer-produced pump refill kit. Although the kit varies slightly between manufacturers, it typically contains two sizes of needles, a particle filter, multiple syringes, and often a small plastic template of the device that can be placed on the skin to assist in locating the access port (▶ Fig. 15.3).[9,10,11]

The refill process is as follows. After the initial interrogation of the pump is performed with the wireless programmer, the concentration and amount of the new solution should be checked against the indwelling solution. The overlying skin is sterilized, landmarks of the pump are used to guide placement of the refill kit needle into the access port, the indwelling solution is drained and removed (completely), and the fresh solution is attached and injected. After this, the pump is reprogrammed to reflect the updated concentration and amount of solution injected.[9,10,11]

If there is concern about pump–catheter connection or pump functionality, fluoroscopy can be used to complete a sideport myelogram, where the solution is aspirated back from the catheter via the pump sideport and contrast is injected to determine if the connection is appropriate and if the catheter is still in the IT space.

15.2.5 Medication and Dose Selection

Recommendations regarding medication use are outlined in the PACC guidelines. The choice of medication used for IT trial and within the implanted pump depends on several factors: type of pain (e.g., neuropathic, nociceptive, malignant) or spasm; patient's comorbidities and likely ability to tolerate side effects; and cost of compounded IT medication.[12]

Currently, only morphine, baclofen, and ziconotide (N-type calcium channel blocker used exclusively in the IT space) are approved by the FDA for IT therapy and are considered first-line treatment as monotherapy. IT hydromorphone is widely used clinically and is awaiting FDA approval at this time. Although numerous other options exist (including but not limited to fentanyl, sufentanil, bupivacaine, clonidine, midazolam, ketamine, and octreotide) and while IT medications are frequently combined in clinical practice, this is not routinely recommended if first-line, on-label therapies have not been tried and failed or are not otherwise contraindicated.[12]

In terms of starting dose, many clinicians adhere to the PACC guideline of initiating continuous infusion therapy at no greater than 50% of the trial rate, monitoring for side effects, and then uptitrating slowly to the appropriate dose to assist with pain or spasticity while minimizing the adverse effects.[12,17]

Complications relating to IT medication administration are similar to those with oral or systemic medication administration, although delivery directly to the IT space may limit some of these manifestations. That said, the ratio of IT potency to oral potency can sometimes exceed 100:1, meaning that even small IT doses can still result in adverse effects.[12,18]

Failure to refill the pump prior to solution depletion or any situation in which either portion of the drug delivery system (pump or catheter) fails or in which medication is not appropriately delivered to the IT space can result in some form of withdrawal. Depending on the identity and dose of the medication, this may simply present as loss of pain control or other potentially problematic or catastrophic consequences.

15.2.6 Complications

Complications related to IT therapy can be a result of: medication as described above; surgical procedure and technique; or device and catheter malposition or malfunction.

Local surgical complications include pain at the site of the implanted pump (typically self-limited) or local infection at the pump or catheter site, which may only require antibiotic therapy for a limited time. However, significant infection could potentially necessitate removal of a portion (if not all) of the system if the infection does not clear or if wound dehiscence occurs. In addition, peri-catheter CSF leaks due to a loose purse-string suture during pump placement can increase the risk of infection or postdural puncture headache, which can often be severe enough to require epidural blood patch.[18]

Although very rare overall, pump-related complications include the so-called "pump dump" (in which all the medication in the pump is delivered into the CSF quickly, potentially resulting

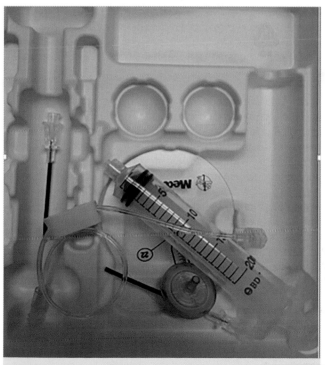

Fig. 15.3 Sample refill kit.

in overdose), stall or stoppage of the device due to electronic malfunction, stoppage due to MRI interference, or an undetected decreased flow rate due to low battery life. Unintentional injection of medication into the subcutaneous pocket containing the device or into the sideport (direct access to CSF) can also result in overdose.[18,19]

Catheter-related complications include direct neurologic trauma with the needle or catheter during placement itself, mechanical trauma to the catheter (with associated kinks, shears, or breaks), catheter malposition outside the IT space, and catheter-tip granuloma formulation. IT catheter-tip granuloma can result in neurologic sequelae, particularly if it is large; this complication is typically associated with very high concentrations of IT injectate and usually develops over several months.[18]

The most serious and feared complication of IT drug delivery is neurologic injury, including granuloma as previously described, as well as direct neurologic trauma with the needle or catheter. Spinal cord injury, nerve injury, and cauda equina injury have all been described during implantation of the IT catheter and pump placement. Spinal infection or hematoma, while usually rare, can result in rapid catastrophic injury or even death, particularly if expanding and left untreated.[19]

Strategies to avoid the above complications include thorough patient screening during selection, precise needle/catheter placement using fluoroscopic guidance (with entry ideally below the level of the spinal cord), proper surgical technique, and regular and careful interrogation and refill of the pump in a clinically appropriate and timely fashion.[18,19]

15.3 Companion Case

The abovementioned complications lead us to the additional case of a 32-year-old woman with history of chronic abdominal and pelvic pain secondary to advanced endometriosis. This pain was refractory to multiple surgical interventions. After trials of physical therapy, numerous medications, and interventional modalities, she underwent a 5-day IT catheter trial with morphine, which was successful in relieving > 70% of her pain but resulted in some adverse effects. She underwent a successful pump and catheter implantation with the Medtronic SynchroMed II pump in the buttock and Medtronic Ascenda 8782 IT catheter.

Over time, the patient's pain was eventually controlled with IT hydromorphone and clonidine, and she was able to return to work and care for her family effectively. However, over the course of several months, she began to complain of increasing abdominal and pelvic pain despite no change in her IT medication dose. She related no history of fall or trauma. Despite increases in medication via the pump, the pain began to escalate and became intolerable for her. She underwent repeat pelvic examinations from her gynecologist and abdominal computed tomography (CT) scans that demonstrated no change in her underlying disease burden.

Without progression of her disease her increasing pain was thought to be due to pump or catheter malfunction. Use of the programming device demonstrated no change in her dose or problems with medication delivery, and the volume of solution remaining in the pump at the time of refill was consistent with the expected amount.

With pump malfunction ruled out, the patient was brought to the fluoroscopy suite for a sideport myelogram to confirm catheter position in the IT space. Aspiration of CSF was limited but attempts to inject radiocontrast through the sideport proved very difficult due to high pressure within the delivery system. With radiocontrast injection, the patient did not experience any pain, as might be expected for a catheter-tip granuloma. At this point, with very high pressure on injection, catheter kink was suspected, and the patient underwent a CT scan of the thoracic and lumbar spines that demonstrated a severe 140-degree kink in the IT catheter (► Fig. 15.4). Upon direct visualization in the operating room the following week, the catheter was indeed found to be severely kinked and unsalvageable, so it was removed, and a new catheter was placed and tunneled to the in situ IT pump in the buttock. As the medication was appropriately titrated back to the patient's previous dose over several weeks, her pain level gradually returned to baseline and she returned to her usual activities of daily living.

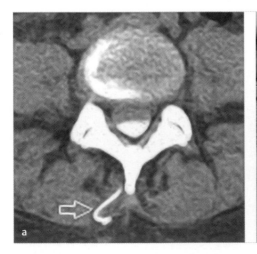
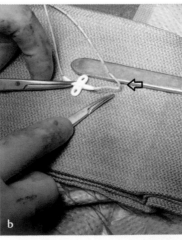

Fig. 15.4 Computed tomography (CT) scan (**a**) and intraoperative image (**b**) demonstrating kinked catheter (arrows), just above the anchor.

15.4 Conclusions

It bears noting that management of pain via an IT pump requires great care and meticulous attention to detail on the part of the clinician, and appropriate support and follow-up on the part of the implanted patient. As noted, patient compliance is crucial to ensure follow-up at appropriate time intervals for refill to prevent medication withdrawal symptoms.[18] For the clinician, given the potentially disastrous complications that could occur, proper placement of the pump and catheter during initial implantation is critical to success. In addition, the period of refill and reprogramming is also important, as the difference of even a single decimal place change involving programming can result in clinically significant and potentially life-threatening withdrawal or overdose.[10]

The challenges with managing IT pumps have led many clinicians to move away from their use, but their utility in refractory pain conditions remains clear, particularly in the cancer population when prescription opioids often prove insufficient for management of severe pain or result in intolerable side effects. Experienced implanters and users of this interventional modality have seen it dramatically improve certain patients' lives, allowing some patients to substantially reduce or entirely discontinue prescription oral opioid use. In this age of the opioid epidemic in the United States and with its associated scrutiny regarding prescription opioid use, the importance of this cannot be overstated.

References

[1] Bier A. Attempts over Cocainisirung of the Ruckenmarkers. Langenbecks Arch Klin Chir Ver Dtsch Z Chir. 1899; 51:361–369 [in German]

[2] Pert CB, Snyder SH. Opiate receptor: demonstration in nervous tissue. Science. 1973; 179(4077):1011–1014

[3] Blackshear PJ, Rohde TD, Prosl F, Buchwald H. The implantable infusion pump: a new concept in drug delivery. Med Prog Technol. 1979; 6(4):149–161

[4] Wang JK, Nauss LA, Thomas JE. Pain relief by intrathecally applied morphine in man. Anesthesiology. 1979; 50(2):149–151

[5] Onofrio BM, Yaksh TL, Arnold PG. Continuous low-dose intrathecal morphine administration in the treatment of chronic pain of malignant origin. Mayo Clin Proc. 1981; 56(8):516–520

[6] Wallace M, Yaksh TL. Long-term spinal analgesic delivery: a review of the preclinical and clinical literature. Reg Anesth Pain Med. 2000; 25(2):117–157

[7] Prager JP. Neuraxial medication delivery: the development and maturity of a concept for treating chronic pain of spinal origin. Spine. 2002; 27(22):2593–2605, discussion 2606

[8] Ripamonti CI, Santini D, Maranzano E, Berti M, Roila F, ESMO Guidelines Working Group. Management of cancer pain: ESMO Clinical Practice Guidelines. Ann Oncol. 2012; 23 Suppl 7:vii139–vii154

[9] Codman, a division of Johnson & Johnson. Implantable infusion pumps. http://www.codmanpumps.com/Products_pumps_overview.asp. Accessed October 9, 2020

[10] Medtronic plc. Targeted drug delivery. Indications, safety and warnings. Synchromed II. http://professional.medtronic.com/pt/neuro/idd/ind/index.htm#.VorVwVKkx-A. Accessed October 9, 2020

[11] Rauck R, Deer T, Rosen S, et al. Accuracy and efficacy of intrathecal administration of morphine sulfate for treatment of intractable pain using the Prometra(®) Programmable Pump. Neuromodulation. 2010; 13(2):102–108

[12] Deer TR, Pope JE, Hayek SM, et al. The Polyanalgesic Consensus Conference (PACC): Recommendations on Intrathecal Drug Infusion Systems Best Practices and Guidelines. Neuromodulation. 2017; 20(2):96–132

[13] Chambers WA. Nerve blocks in palliative care. Br J Anaesth. 2008; 101(1):95–100

[14] Deer TR, Prager J, Levy R, et al. Polyanalgesic Consensus Conference–2012: recommendations on trialing for intrathecal (intraspinal) drug delivery: report of an interdisciplinary expert panel. Neuromodulation. 2012; 15(5):420–435, discussion 435

[15] Hsu Y, Hettiarachchi HD, Zhu DC, Linninger AA. The frequency and magnitude of cerebrospinal fluid pulsations influence intrathecal drug distribution: key factors for interpatient variability. Anesth Analg. 2012; 115(2):386–394

[16] Hettiarachchi HD, Hsu Y, Harris TJ , Jr, Penn R, Linninger AA. The effect of pulsatile flow on intrathecal drug delivery in the spinal canal. Ann Biomed Eng. 2011; 39(10):2592–2602

[17] Knight KH, Brand FM, Mchaourab AS, Veneziano G. Implantable intrathecal pumps for chronic pain: highlights and updates. Croat Med J. 2007; 48(1):22–34

[18] Staats P S. Complications of intrathecal therapy. Pain Medicine. 2008; 9(Issue suppl_1):S102–S107

[19] Awaad Y, Rizk T, Siddiqui I, Roosen N, McIntosh K, Waines GM. Complications of intrathecal baclofen pump: prevention and cure. ISRN Neurol. 2012; 2012:575168

16 Osteoporotic Fracture I (Minimal Height Loss Vertebroplasty)

Danoob Dalili, Nicolas Theumann, Nicolas Amoretti, Daniel E. Dalili, Amanda Isaac, and Jan Fritz

16.1 Case Presentation

A 73-year-old woman presented with persistent localized pain to the lower thoracic region (On a background history of osteoporosis). Her pain was localized to the spinal region with no radicular symptoms. A magnetic resonance imaging (MRI) study of the thoracolumbar spine was performed, demonstrating an acute fracture at T9 corresponded to her symptoms (▶ Fig. 16.1). The patient presented to the angiography suite and a transpedicular vertebroplasty (VP) was performed in standard fashion (▶ Fig. 16.2). Preprocedural pain was 9/10 on the visual analog numerical score; immediate postprocedural pain was 1/10 which resolved completely after 1 week.

16.2 Discussion

Vertebroplasty was first described by Galibert and Deramond in 1984[1] to treat cervical hemangiomas. Since then the technique has evolved, with high-level evidence that advocates its benefits for treating both traumatic[2] and pathological fractures that may be secondary to osteoporosis,[3] aggressive intraosseous hemangiomata,[4] myeloma,[4,5] or lytic metastases.[6]

It is believed that an estimated 1.5 million Americans suffer osteoporotic fractures each year. A similar incumbrance of disease has been observed in the United Kingdom, with epidemiological studies proposing that one in two women and one in five men aged over 50 years will suffer an osteoporotic fracture, the majority of which are vertebral fractures, in their lifetime.[7,8] Vertebral body fractures are the most common type of osteoporotic fracture,[9,10] typically occurring in the mid-thoracic (T7–T8) and thoracolumbar (T12–L1) regions.[11] Vertebral fractures often cause significant and long-standing complications. The majority of vertebral compression fractures (up to 84%) are associated with pain lasting at least 4 to 6 weeks,[12] and one-third of the patients experience chronic back pain, kyphosis, and height loss as a result.[8,12,13] Vertebral fractures lead to further morbidity and mortality secondary to decreased mobility precipitating in breathing difficulties, deep vein thrombosis, skin ulcers, and pulmonary emboli as well as secondary kyphosis which impedes pulmonary function[14] and causes progressive frailty.[7,15] According to a 2020 study, the economic burden of osteoporosis-related fracture is significant, costing approximately $17.9 billion and £4 billion per annum in the USA and the UK,[8] respectively. Accurate and early diagnosis and treatment of vertebral fractures within a dedicated algorithm is therefore key to optimize outcomes in this vulnerable cohort of patients.

16.2.1 Diagnosis

Initial imaging remains plain film radiography (in the absence of radicular or cauda equina symptoms).[5] Traditional imaging protocols for screening include lateral weight-bearing radiographs of the thoracolumbar spine.[5,16,17] Moderate to severe vertebral fractures can often be seen well on plain films, particularly in the thoracolumbar area; the difficulty in diagnosis, however, lies in the determination of mild fractures and physiological variants.[17,18] Recognizing the need to identify and measure osteoporotic fracture in order to guide subsequent treatment strategies, visual semiquantitative assessment tools have been proposed since 1960.[19] Subsequently, many more assessment tools have been proposed,[20] but the semiquantitative visual and morphometric tool by Genant et al remains the most utilized in clinical practice and in research settings.[21,22,23] Severity assessment can be made

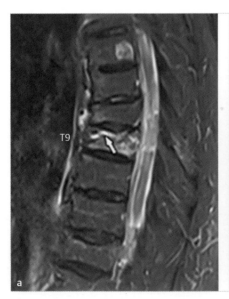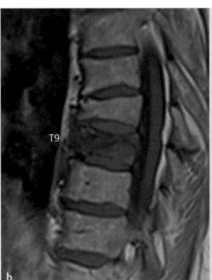

Fig. 16.1 Magnetic resonance (MR) study of the thoracolumbar spine. Sagittal T1-weighted (**a**) and short tau inversion recovery (STIR) (**b**) sequences of the thoracic spine demonstrated a wedge compression fracture with a linear high STIR signal fracture-cleft (white arrows) extending from the anterior aspect of the vertebral body to the posterosuperior end plate. There was no extension to the posterior elements. Courtesy: Dr. Danoob Dalili.

as Grade 1 (mild; fracture, defined as a fracture with 20 to 25% loss of vertebral height), Grade 2 (moderate fracture, defined as 25 to 40% loss of height), and Grade 3 (severe fracture, defined as > 40% loss of height). Mild vertebral compression fractures can be confused with physiological wedging (particularly in the mid-thoracic to upper lumbar region), short vertebral height,[24] Scheuermann's disease, degenerative scoliosis, Schmorl's nodes,[25] and Cupid's bow deformity.[26] When plain radiographs are not conclusive, neoplasm or ligamentous involvement is suspected, age of the fracture is unknown, or there is diagnostic doubt, MRI should be obtained, including a sagittal short tau inversion recovery (STIR) sequence to attain a more in-depth study.[5,27] Computed tomography (CT) is utilized if MRI is not available, in acute trauma settings, or if there is concern for bone fragments extending into the spinal canal as these could directly impinge upon the cord. A dual energy X-ray absorptiometry (DEXA) scan is also advocated to diagnose and quantify the extent of bone mineral density change, which may help in determining the risk of further fractures for the same patient.[8,17,20,28,29,30,31,32,33,34,35,36,37,38]

Vertebral fractures on radiographs are typically diagnosed and graded in two ways: the semi-quantitative method[21] and quantitative morphometric method.[32] The semi-quantitative morphometry defines a vertebral compression fracture as present if there is a 20% or greater reduction in height in the anterior, mid-, or posterior planes by visual estimation.[21] Quantitative morphometry compares vertebral body height with that of the adjacent vertebrae. Using this method, a vertebral fracture is diagnosed if there is a greater than three standard deviation difference in vertebral height between adjacent vertebrae.[39]

16.2.2 Treatment

Vertebral compression fractures are typically managed with pain medication and physiotherapy as first-line strategies.[40,41,42] In addition to spinal bracing, these regions typically consist of non-steroidal anti-inflammatory drugs, opioids, bisphosphonates, and calcium supplements.[43] Although many studies have shown good resolution of pain in 8 to 12 weeks,[5,44] the risks of progression of vertebral height loss, further kyphosis, and deformity of the spine in the future remain unaddressed.[13,45] As such, new methods such as VP and kyphoplasty (KP) have been implemented to improve vertebral fracture outcome. VP has proven not only to be highly effective in pain reduction (with up to 90% of patients describing long-term improvement),[46,47] but recent systematic reviews have highlighted the reduction in 12-month all-cause mortality in patients treated with VP or KP compared to conservative management.[48]

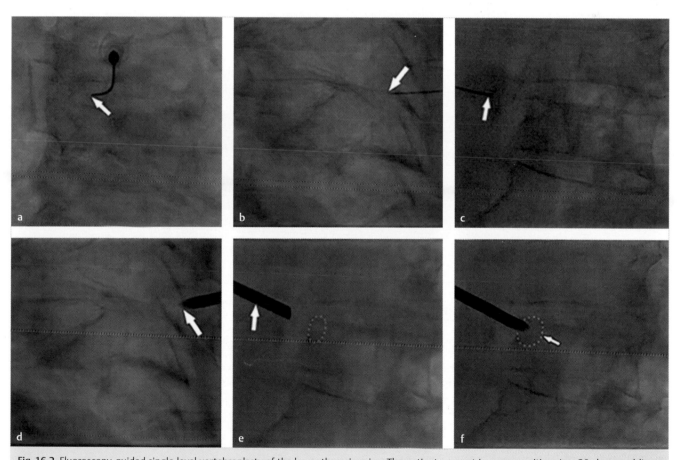

Fig. 16.2 Fluoroscopy-guided single level vertebroplasty of the lower thoracic spine. The patient was put in prone position. In a 20-degree oblique projection a standard spinal needle (**a**, white arrow) was advanced to the periosteum of the pedicle and confirmed on the lateral (**b**) and AP (**c**) projections. The bone trocar was positioned in the same trajectory (**d**) and advanced toward the upper outer margin of the pedicle (**e**), dotted white line).

(Continued)

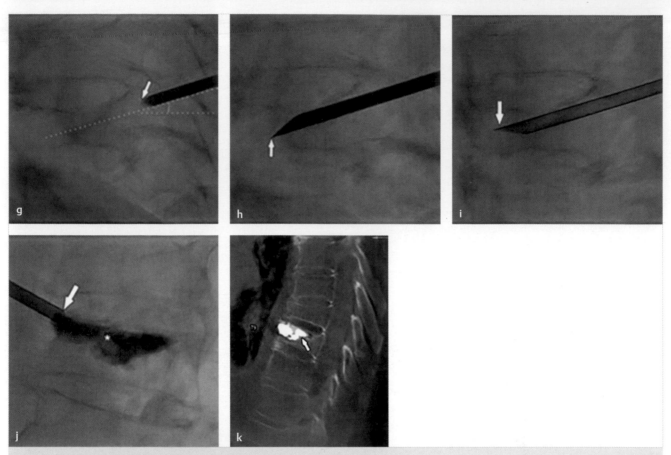

Fig. 16.2 (*Continued*) Once it pierced the cortex of the pedicle (**f**), it was advanced in a craniocaudal trajectory by approximately 25 to 30 degrees to reach the posterior aspect of the vertebral body (dashed line) (**g**). The trocar was then medialized and advanced to reach the antero-inferior one-third of the vertebral body (**h**) and the bevel was turned to face the caudal direction (**i**). About 2 to 4 mL of polymethyl methacrylate (PMMA) cement was injected under continuous fluoroscopic monitoring, ensuring an even spread across the midline (**j**, white arrow) from the superior to inferior end plate, encompassing the fracture line. Postprocedure sagittal computed tomography (CT) delineated the filling and indicated absence of cement leakage (**k**). Courtesy: Dr. Danoob Dalili.

VP is typically performed under local anesthesia and sedation.[5,49,50,51] The patient is placed in the prone position for thoracic and lumbar levels, and in the supine position for cervical vertebrae. Dual image-guidance of CT and C-arm fluoroscopy or biplanar fluoroscopy modalities are preferred. Initially CT is used to map out nerve roots, vascular structures, and visceral tissues. The needle sizes vary dependent on the radiologist's preference and anatomical target level and are between 10 G and 15 G with larger gauges typically being used in the cervical vertebrae.[51,52] Technical success is defined by appropriate cannulation of the pedicles and placement of the needle in the anteromedial portion of the vertebral body[53] in the transpedicular approach.

Transpedicular or extrapedicular approaches can be used depending on the fracture pattern and underlying anatomical remodeling. Multiple approaches have been described, with a bipedicular approach being used most commonly. Some authors have reported that a unipedicular approach may be as effective as a bipedicular approach when comparing cement filling across the midline of the vertebra and vertebral height restoration.[54,55]

The transpedicular (uni- and/or bipedicular) approaches are used most commonly and are viable if the pedicles are at least 4 to 5 mm wide. This approach targets the needle trajectory along the dorsal aspect of the vertebral posterior element into the vertebral body.[46,54,55,56,57,58,59] It allows easier compression of the overlying soft tissues following removal of the needle, thus promoting hemostasis at the insertion site. The extrapedicular (parapedicular and/or posteriolateral) approaches can be used if the pedicles are too small, as is typically noted above T8.[53] Using such approaches make it more difficult to achieve hemostasis.[58]

Once the needle is positioned in a satisfactory position, cement is injected under real-time fluoroscopy. Some clinicians opt to perform contrast venography prior to cement injection in order to reduce the risk of causing a venous thromboembolism; however, evidence for this is limited.[60] Cement should be injected while it is in a "pasty" phase to allow for better control. If a leak is identified, injection should cease until a plug is formed secondary to solidification of cement.[51] According to Belkoff et al and Gangi et al, typical cement injection volumes are 2.5 to 3 mL in the upper thoracic spine, 3 to 4 mL in the thoraco-lumbar junction, and 6 to 8 mL in the lumbar spine.[51,61] The cement should at least cross the midline on anteroposterior (AP) fluoroscopy. After injection the needle can be removed, and pressure applied to prevent hematoma formation.

The most common and serious complications of VP are cement leak, infection, and postprocedural pain.[2,4,53,62,63,64,65,66,67,68,69,70,71,72,73,74,75,76,77,78,79] Cement can leak into the epidural veins and neural foramina causing cement emboli and neuralgia or cord compression, respectively.[80,81,82,83,84] It is for this reason that constant fluoroscopic monitoring is paramount. Allergic reaction and hypertension are less commonly seen.[51]

Barriers to successful VP include osteolytic metastases, whereby the extent of bone destruction may lead to a higher chance of cement leak[85] into the canal or even displacement of the tumor into the canal with subsequent cord compression.[76] Severely compressed fractures with vertebral height loss greater than 75% can pose technical challenges with needle insertion; however, once this has been overcome appropriate cement filling can achieve good vertebral height.[86] Refracturing is another complication of VP that often occurs due to insufficient cement filling.[58]

16.3 Conclusion

Vertebroplasty has emerged as the most effective treatment of vertebral fractures, restoring function and height while reducing chronic pain. Although there are risks to this procedure, the incidence of adverse events remains relatively low. The advancement of VP and introduction of vertebral augmentation devices in this procedure may result in even better outcomes in the future.

References

[1] Galibert P, Deramond H, Rosat P, Le Gars D. Note préliminaire sur le traitement des angiomes vertébraux par vertébroplastie acrylique percutanée [Preliminary note on the treatment of vertebral angioma by percutaneous acrylic vertebroplasty]. Neurochirurgie. 1987; 33(2):166–168

[2] Garnon J, Doré B, Auloge P, et al. Efficacy of the vertebral body stenting system for the restoration of vertebral height in acute traumatic compression fractures in a non-osteoporotic population. Cardiovasc Intervent Radiol. 2019; 42(11):1579–1587

[3] Martikos K, Greggi T, Vommaro F, et al. Vertebroplasty in the treatment of osteoporotic vertebral compression fractures: patient selection and perspectives. Open Access Rheumatol. 2019; 11:157–161

[4] Burton AW, Rhines LD, Mendel E. Vertebroplasty and kyphoplasty: a comprehensive review. Neurosurg Focus. 2005; 18(3):e1

[5] McConnell CT , Jr, Wippold FJ , II, Ray CE , Jr, et al. ACR appropriateness criteria management of vertebral compression fractures. J Am Coll Radiol. 2014; 11(8):757–763

[6] Barzilai O, Boriani S, Fisher CG, et al. Essential concepts for the management of metastatic spine disease: what the surgeon should know and practice. Global Spine J. 2019; 9(1) Suppl:98S–107S

[7] Kendler DL, Bauer DC, Davison KS, et al. Vertebral fractures: clinical importance and management. Am J Med. 2016; 129(2):221.e1–221.e10

[8] Clynes MA, Harvey NC, Curtis EM, Fuggle NR, Dennison EM, Cooper C. The epidemiology of osteoporosis. Br Med Bull. 2020; 133(1):105–117

[9] Nevitt MC, Ettinger B, Black DM, et al. The association of radiographically detected vertebral fractures with back pain and function: a prospective study. Ann Intern Med. 1998; 128(10):793–800

[10] Ettinger B, Black DM, Nevitt MC, et al. The Study of Osteoporotic Fractures Research Group. Contribution of vertebral deformities to chronic back pain and disability. J Bone Miner Res. 1992; 7(4):449–456

[11] Sheon R, Rosen H. Clinical manifestations and treatment of osteoporotic thoracolumbar vertebral compression fractures. UpToDate. 2012. pp. 2–3

[12] Ong T, Sahota O, Gladman JRF. The Nottingham Spinal Health (NoSH) Study: a cohort study of patients hospitalised with vertebral fragility fractures. Osteoporos Int. 2020; 31(2):363–370

[13] Francis RM, Aspray TJ, Hide G, Sutcliffe AM, Wilkinson P. Back pain in osteoporotic vertebral fractures. Osteoporos Int. 2008; 19(7):895–903

[14] Schlaich C, Minne HW, Bruckner T, et al. Reduced pulmonary function in patients with spinal osteoporotic fractures. Osteoporos Int. 1998; 8(3):261–267

[15] Afrin N, Sund R, Honkanen R, et al. A fall in the previous 12 months predicts fracture in the subsequent 5 years in postmenopausal women. Osteoporos Int. 2020; 31(5):839–847

[16] Kaptoge S, Armbrecht G, Felsenberg D, et al. Whom to treat? The contribution of vertebral X-rays to risk-based algorithms for fracture prediction. Results from the European Prospective Osteoporosis Study. Osteoporos Int. 2006; 17(9):1369–1381

[17] Griffith JF. Identifying osteoporotic vertebral fracture. Quant Imaging Med Surg. 2015; 5(4):592–602

[18] The Royal College of Radiologists. Radiological guidance for the recognition and reporting of osteoporotic vertebral fragility fractures (VFFs). RCR guidelines. 2021. https://www.rcr.ac.uk/system/files/publication/field_publication_files/bfcr215_reporting_of_vff.pdf

[19] Smith RW, Jr, Eyler WR, Mellinger RC. On the incidence of senile osteoporosis. Ann Intern Med. 1960; 52:773–781

[20] Delmas PD, van de Langerijt L, Watts NB, et al. IMPACT Study Group. Underdiagnosis of vertebral fractures is a worldwide problem: the IMPACT study. J Bone Miner Res. 2005; 20(4):557–563

[21] Genant HK, Wu CY, van Kuijk C, Nevitt MC. Vertebral fracture assessment using a semiquantitative technique. J Bone Miner Res. 1993; 8(9):1137–1148

[22] Genant HK, Jergas M. Assessment of prevalent and incident vertebral fractures in osteoporosis research. Osteoporos Int. 2003; 14 Suppl 3:S43–S55

[23] Genant HK, Jergas M, Palermo L, et al. Comparison of semiquantitative visual and quantitative morphometric assessment of prevalent and incident vertebral fractures in osteoporosis The Study of Osteoporotic Fractures Research Group. J Bone Miner Res. 1996; 11(7):984–996

[24] Ferrar L, Jiang G, Armbrecht G, et al. Is short vertebral height always an osteoporotic fracture? The Osteoporosis and Ultrasound Study (OPUS). Bone. 2007; 41(1):5–12

[25] Abbas J, Hamoud K, Peled N, Hershkovitz I. Lumbar Schmorl's nodes and their correlation with spine configuration and degeneration. BioMed Res Int. 2018; 2018:1574020

[26] Jaremko JL, Siminoski K, Firth GB, et al. Canadian STOPP Consortium National Pediatric Bone Health Working Group. Common normal variants of pediatric vertebral development that mimic fractures: a pictorial review from a national longitudinal bone health study. Pediatr Radiol. 2015; 45(4):593–605

[27] Panda A, Das CJ, Baruah U. Imaging of vertebral fractures. Indian J Endocrinol Metab. 2014; 18(3):295–303

[28] Wilson DJ. Osteoporosis and sport. Eur J Radiol. 2019; 110:169–174

[29] Oei L, Koromani F, Rivadeneira F, Zillikens MC, Oei EHG. Quantitative imaging methods in osteoporosis. Quant Imaging Med Surg. 2016; 6(6):680–698

[30] Morgan SL, Prater GL. Quality in dual-energy X-ray absorptiometry scans. Bone. 2017; 104:13–28

[31] Lewiecki EM, Binkley N, Morgan SL, et al. International Society for Clinical Densitometry. Best practices for dual-energy X-ray absorptiometry measurement and reporting: International Society for Clinical Densitometry Guidance. J Clin Densitom. 2016; 19(2):127–140

[32] Diacinti D, Guglielmi G. Vertebral morphometry. Radiol Clin North Am. 2010; 48(3):561–575

[33] Cooper C, Atkinson EJ, O'Fallon WM, Melton LJ, III. Incidence of clinically diagnosed vertebral fractures: a population-based study in Rochester, Minnesota, 1985–1989. J Bone Miner Res. 1992; 7(2):221–227

[34] Shayganfar A, Ebrahimian S, Masjedi M, Daryaei S. A study on bone mass density using dual energy X-ray absorptiometry: does high body mass index have protective effect on bone density in obese patients? J Res Med Sci. 2020; 25:4

[35] Mazzoccoli G. Body composition: where and when. Eur J Radiol. 2016; 85(8):1456–1460

[36] Dalili D, Bazzocchi A, Dalili DE, Guglielmi G, Isaac A. The role of body composition assessment in obesity and eating disorders. Eur J Radiol. 2020; 131(August):109227

[37] Lewiecki EM, Binkley N. DXA: 30 years and counting: introduction to the 30th anniversary issue. Bone. 2017; 104:1–3

[38] Guerri S, Mercatelli D, Aparisi Gómez MP, et al. Quantitative imaging techniques for the assessment of osteoporosis and sarcopenia. Quant Imaging Med Surg. 2018; 8(1):60–85

[39] McCloskey EV, Spector TD, Eyres KS, et al. The assessment of vertebral deformity: a method for use in population studies and clinical trials. Osteoporos Int. 1993; 3(3):138–147

[40] NICE; The National Institute for Health and Care Excellence. NICE. Osteoporosis—prevention of fragility fractures, Management. 2016. [Accessed May 22, 2020]

[41] Hernlund E, Svedbom A, Ivergård M, et al. Osteoporosis in the European Union: medical management, epidemiology and economic burden. A report prepared in collaboration with the International Osteoporosis Foundation (IOF) and the European Federation of Pharmaceutical Industry Associations (EFPIA). Arch Osteoporos. 2013; 8(1–2):136

[42] Tarantino U, Iolascon G, Cianferotti L, et al. Clinical guidelines for the prevention and treatment of osteoporosis: summary statements and recommendations from the Italian Society for Orthopaedics and Traumatology. J Orthop Traumatol 2017;18(Suppl 1):3–36

[43] Ensrud KE, Schousboe JT. Clinical practice. Vertebral fractures. N Engl J Med. 2011; 364(17):1634–1642

[44] Mazanec DJ, Podichetty VK, Mompoint A, Potnis A. Vertebral compression fractures: manage aggressively to prevent sequelae. Cleve Clin J Med. 2003; 70(2):147–156

[45] Stadhouder A, Buskens E, Vergroesen DA, Fidler MW, de Nies F, Öner FC. Nonoperative treatment of thoracic and lumbar spine fractures: a prospective randomized study of different treatment options. J Orthop Trauma. 2009; 23(8):588–594

[46] Rapan S, Jovanović S, Gulan G. Vertebroplasty for vertebral compression fracture. Coll Antropol. 2009; 33(3):911–914

[47] Muijs SPJ, Nieuwenhuijse MJ, Van Erkel AR, Dijkstra PDS. Percutaneous vertebroplasty for the treatment of osteoporotic vertebral compression fractures: evaluation after 36 months. J Bone Joint Surg Br. 2009; 91(3):379–384

[48] Cazzato RL, Bellone T, Scardapane M, et al. Vertebral augmentation reduces the 12-month mortality and morbidity in patients with osteoporotic vertebral compression fractures. Eur Radiol. 2021; 31(11):8246–8255

[49] Wilhelm K. Vertebroplastie -"state of the art [Vertebroplasty—state of the art]. Radiologe. 2015; 55(10):847–852

[50] Laredo JD, Hamze B. Complications of percutaneous vertebroplasty and their prevention. Skeletal Radiol. 2004; 33(9):493–505

[51] Gangi A, Guth S, Imbert JP, Marin H, Dietemann JL. Percutaneous vertebroplasty: indications, technique, and results. Radiographics. 2003; 23(2):e10

[52] Mpotsaris A, Abdolvahabi R, Hoffleith B, et al. Perkutane vertebroplastie von wirbelkörperfrakturen benigner und maligner genese: Eine prospektive studie mit 1 188 patienten und einem follow-up von zwölf monaten. Dtsch Arztebl. 2011; 108(19):331–338

[53] McCall T, Cole C, Dailey A. Vertebroplasty and kyphoplasty: a comparative review of efficacy and adverse events. Curr Rev Musculoskelet Med. 2008; 1 (1):17–23

[54] Kim AK, Jensen ME, Dion JE, Schweickert PA, Kaufmann TJ, Kallmes DF. Unilateral transpedicular percutaneous vertebroplasty: initial experience. Radiology. 2002; 222(3):737–741

[55] Steinmann J, Tingey CT, Cruz G, Dai Q. Biomechanical comparison of unipedicular versus bipedicular kyphoplasty. Spine. 2005; 30(2):201–205

[56] Fritz J, U-Thainual P, Ungi T, et al. MR-guided vertebroplasty with augmented reality image overlay navigation. Cardiovasc Intervent Radiol. 2014; 37(6): 1589–1596

[57] Prabhuraj AR, Mishra A, Mishra RK, Pruthi N, Saini J, Arvinda HR. Per-operative glue embolization with surgical decompression: a multimodality treatment for aggressive vertebral haemangioma. Interv Neuroradiol. 2019; 25(5):570–578

[58] Hiwatashi A, Moritani T, Numaguchi Y, Westesson PL. Increase in vertebral body height after vertebroplasty. AJNR Am J Neuroradiol. 2003; 24(2):185–189

[59] Liu PY, Lin SC, Lai PL, Lin CL. Investigation into whether or not PMMA bone cement transpedicular screw augmentation stabilizes pedicle screw loosening. J Mech Med Biol. 2019; 19(2)

[60] Vasconcelos C, Gailloud P, Beauchamp NJ, Heck DV, Murphy KJ. Is percutaneous vertebroplasty without pretreatment venography safe? Evaluation of 205 consecutives procedures. AJNR Am J Neuroradiol. 2002; 23 (6):913–917

[61] Belkoff SM, Mathis JM, Jasper LE, Deramond H. The biomechanics of vertebroplasty. The effect of cement volume on mechanical behavior. Spine. 2001; 26(14):1537–1541

[62] Autrusseau P-A, Garnon J, Bertucci G, et al. Complications of percutaneous image-guided screw fixation: an analysis of 94 consecutive patients. Diagn Interv Imaging. 2021; 102(6):347–353

[63] Cazzato RL, De Marini P, Leonard-Lorant I, et al. Percutaneous thermal ablation of sacral metastases: assessment of pain relief and local tumor control. Diagn Interv Imaging. 2021; 102(6):355–361

[64] Cazzato RL, Auloge P, Dalili D, et al. Percutaneous image-guided cryoablation of osteoblastoma. AJR Am J Roentgenol. 2019; 213(5):1157–1162

[65] Autrusseau P-A, Heidelberg D, Stacoffe N, et al. Percutaneous image-guided anterior screw fixation of the odontoid process. Cardiovasc Intervent Radiol. 2021; 44(4):647–653

[66] De Marini P, Cazzato RL, Auloge P, et al. Percutaneous image-guided thermal ablation of bone metastases: a retrospective propensity study comparing the safety profile of radio-frequency ablation and cryo-ablation. Int J Hyperthermia. 2020; 37(1):1386–1394

[67] Cazzato RL, Auloge P, De Marini P, et al. Spinal tumor ablation: indications, techniques, and clinical management. Tech Vasc Interv Radiol. 2020; 23(2): 100677

[68] Dalili D, Isaac A, Bazzocchi A, et al. Interventional techniques for bone and musculoskeletal soft tissue tumors: current practices and future directions - Part I. Ablation. Semin Musculoskelet Radiol. 2020; 24(6):692–709

[69] Garnon J, Meylheuc L, Auloge P, et al. Continuous injection of large volumes of cement through a single 10G vertebroplasty needle in cases of large osteolytic lesions. Cardiovasc Intervent Radiol. 2020; 43(4):658–661

[70] Autrusseau P-A, Garnon J, Auloge P, Dalili D, Cazzato RL, Gangi A. Percutaneous C2-C3 screw fixation combined with cementoplasty to consolidate an impending fracture of C2. Diagn Interv Imaging. 2020; 101(9): 619–621

[71] Garnon J, Meylheuc L, De Marini P, et al. Subjective analysis of the filling of an acetabular osteolytic lesion following percutaneous cementoplasty: is it reliable? Cardiovasc Intervent Radiol. 2020; 43(3):445–452

[72] Katsanos K, Sabharwal T, Adam A. Percutaneous cementoplasty. Semin Intervent Radiol. 2010; 27(2):137–147

[73] Dalili D, Isaac A, Cazzato RL, et al. Interventional techniques for bone and musculoskeletal soft tissue tumors: current practices and future directions - Part II. Stabilization. Semin Musculoskelet Radiol. 2020; 24(6):710–725

[74] Noriega DC, Krüger A, Ramajo RH, Ardura F, Munoz M, Sahin S. Long-term benefits of percutaneous anatomical restoration of vertebral compression fractures linked to malignancy. Turk Neurosurg. 2016; 26(4):608–614

[75] Zhang HR, Xu MY, Yang XG, Qiao RQ, Li JK, Hu YC. Percutaneous vertebral augmentation procedures in the management of spinal metastases. Cancer Lett. 2020; 475:136–142

[76] Barr JD, Mathis JM. Extreme vertebroplasty: techniques for treating difficult lesions. In: Percutaneous Vertebroplasty and Kyphoplasty. Springer New York; 2006:185–196

[77] Liu HF, Wu CG, Tian QH, Wang T, Yi F. Application of percutaneous osteoplasty in treating pelvic bone metastases: efficacy and safety. Cardiovasc Intervent Radiol. 2019; 42(12):1738–1744

[78] Greif DN, Ghasem A, Butler A, Rivera S, Al Maaieh M, Conway SA. Multidisciplinary management of spinal metastasis and vertebral instability: a systematic review. World Neurosurg. 2019; 128:e944–e955

[79] Cazzato RL, Palussière J, Auloge P, et al. Complications following percutaneous image-guided radiofrequency ablation of bone tumors: a 10-year dual-center experience. Radiology. 2020; 296(1):227–235

[80] Harrington KD. Major neurological complications following percutaneous vertebroplasty with polymethylmethacrylate: a case report. J Bone Joint Surg Am. 2001; 83(7):1070–1073

[81] Jean SN, Chen YF, Chen JF, Chen SJ, Lo TC, Hwang SJ. Pulmonary embolism of polymethylmethacrylate after percutaneous vertebroplasty: a case report. Zhonghua Fang She Xue Za Zhi. 2006; 31(1):47–51

[82] Lee BJ, Lee SR, Yoo TY. Paraplegia as a complication of percutaneous vertebroplasty with polymethylmethacrylate: a case report. Spine. 2002; 27 (19):E419–E422

[83] Padovani B, Kasriel O, Brunner P, Peretti-Viton P. Pulmonary embolism caused by acrylic cement: a rare complication of percutaneous vertebroplasty. AJNR Am J Neuroradiol. 1999; 20(3):375–377

[84] Ratliff J, Nguyen T, Heiss J. Root and spinal cord compression from methylmethacrylate vertebroplasty. Spine. 2001; 26(13):E300–E302

[85] Cotten A, Dewatre F, Cortet B, et al. Percutaneous vertebroplasty for osteolytic metastases and myeloma: effects of the percentage of lesion filling and the leakage of methyl methacrylate at clinical follow-up. Radiology. 1996; 200(2):525–530

[86] Peh WCG, Gilula LA, Peck DD. Percutaneous vertebroplasty for severe osteoporotic vertebral body compression fractures. Radiology. 2002; 223(1): 121–126

17 Osteoporotic Fracture II

Jon Marshall

17.1 Case Presentation

An 83-year-old woman presented to the emergency room with 10/10 back pain. The patient had a history of rheumatoid arthritis for which she has intermittently taking oral steroids. There was no evidence of radiculopathy or lower extremity muscle weakness on physical examination. On deep palpation, the patient complained of point tenderness of her spinous process in the mid-thoracic spine.

Plain radiographs of the thoracic and lumbar spine demonstrated an age-indeterminant compression fracture of the T8 vertebral body. The patient was given 0.5 mg of intravenous (IV) Dilaudid and discharged with oral naproxen.

The patient returned to the emergency department 5 days later, again complaining of 10/10 back pain; the pain was refractory to her discharge medications. She also complained of decreased mobility, to the point where she could not get out of bed. In addition, the patient complained of right calf swelling. She was admitted to the hospital for pain control, and subsequently underwent magnetic resonance imaging (MRI) of the thoracic spine (▶ Fig. 17.1a, b). Imaging demonstrated an acute compression deformity of the T8 vertebral body. The patient also had a Doppler ultrasound of the lower extremity, which demonstrated a nonocclusive thrombus in the peroneal and popliteal veins of the right lower extremity.

While admitted for observation, the patient's pain was refractory to IV analgesics, and she was referred to interventional radiology for possible kyphoplasty. The patient underwent fluoroscopic-guided kyphoplasty in the interventional suite (▶ Fig. 17.1c–f). She was discharged home 4 hours after completion of the procedure. The patient rated her pain as 2/10 immediately following the procedure, which increased to 6/10 for 3 days following the procedure, and then eventually completely resolved.

17.2 Discussion

Vertebral compression fractures (VCFs) are exceedingly common and present a significant financial burden on the health care system, costing billions of dollars per year.[1] There is no shortage of controversy surrounding the clinical decision-making when deciding between operative and nonoperative therapies in the treatment of VCFs. Nonoperative therapies include bed rest, analgesia, and bracing operative treatment (referred to as vertebral augmentation [VA]).

As a result of the prevalence of nonspecific low back pain, a substantial number of VCFs are missed entirely, or there is a significant delay in diagnosis. Up to 34 to 52% of fractures are not visualized on initial plain radiographs, and as many as 23% are not even clinically recognized.[2,3,4,5]

The majority of patients who are evaluated either in the hospital, emergency department, or in their primary care clinics with painful VCF are treated conservatively with opioid analgesics. Adverse reactions to such medications were noted in one study to occur in up to 10% of cases, with a higher incidence of such reactions in patients of advanced age.[6]

For referring providers, "nonoperative management" may imply an absence of risk. This belief is, clearly, untrue. Nonoperative conservative management such as bed rest or other significant decreased mobility are proven to be associated with increased rates of institutional readmission, reduction in activities of daily living, and increased mortality.[7]

Prolonged bed rest leads to bone density diminution of 2% per week and can be even worse in the first 12 weeks.[8] Bed rest also decreases muscle strength by 10 to 15% per week[9] and leads to increased contractures. Furthermore, pressure sores occur most commonly in bedridden patients older than 70 years of age[10] and can lead to an increase in management costs by as much as 20%. The cardiovascular effects of prolonged immobility should also not be ignored, and include a decrease in cardiac output, stroke volume, coronary blood flow, cerebral perfusion, and left ventricular function.[9] The risk of deep venous thrombosis (DVT) and pulmonary embolism (PE) should also not be ignored with prolonged bed rest, with DVT occurring in up to 61% of patients and fatal PE occurring in the range of 0.5 to 10%.[8]

The morbidity of VCFs can lead to deconditioning of the respiratory muscles, which can result in a subsequent 25 to 50% decrease in respiratory function. This effect creates a favorable environment for the development of respiratory infections.[10] It has been reported that the use of VA can result in a significant improvement in pulmonary function in patients with VCFs.[11,12]

Balloon kyphoplasty (BKP), and the now less commonly performed vertebroplasty, are both VA procedures. Both procedures are performed by percutaneously inserting needles into the vertebral body by an intrapedicular or extrapedicular approach. Depending on the geometry of the vertebral body, and extent and location of the fracture, one (unilateral) or two (bilateral) needles can be used. BKP differs from vertebroplasty with the inflation of a durable balloon within the vertebral body, which is subsequently deflated and removed, and used to restore vertebral body height and create a cavity for the injection of polymethylmethacrylate (PMMA) bone cement.

Vertebral augmentation is typically performed using a fixed angiographic table in an interventional suite, a C-arm in an operating room, or in an office-based lab. In most cases, VA can be performed using local anesthetic and moderate sedation, with general anesthesia reserved for the most complicated patients. Many different percutaneous access needles and stabilization products exist; however, review of these is beyond the scope of this chapter.

Anecdotally, most patients experience improvement in their pain immediately following the procedure, with a return of pain within 24 hours. This return of symptoms is likely a result of a combination of inflammation and paraspinal muscle spasm. Most patients experience near-complete improvement by 10 to 14 days post procedure. Significant adverse events occur in 1.0 to 1.5% of cases.[13,14,15,16,17] The most commonly noted adverse events include: epidural cement leakage requiring decompression, dural injury, asymptomatic cement PE, hematoma, osteomyelitis, asthma attack, and urinary tract infection. Although it was initially believed that vertebra adjacent to a treated level

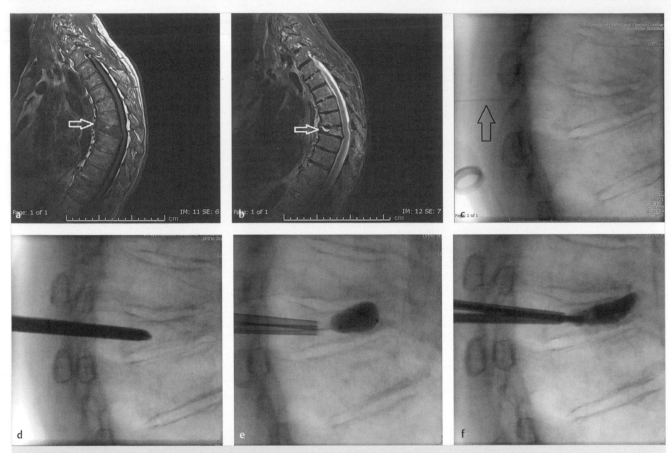

Fig. 17.1 (a, b) Sagittal tau-weighted image and sagittal short tau inversion recovery (STIR) image demonstrating moderate compression deformity of the T8 vertebral body (arrows), with T1 hypointensity and STIR hyperintensity consistent with edema. Prevertebral edema is also noted. (c) Lateral fluoroscopic view of the thoracic spine demonstrating a marking needle (arrow) confirming the correct level and trajectory of the pedicle. (d) An 8-gauge Jamshidi (Becton, Dickinson and Company; Franklin Lakes, NJ, USA) needle entering the vertebral body using an extrapedicular technique. (e) An inflated 10-gauge, 20-mm balloon used to create a cavity for cement fill. (f) Cement filling a large portion of the anterior vertebral cavity, without significant extravasation.

were susceptible to fracture, this has been disproven. Multiple studies have demonstrated frequency of fractures at adjacent levels is similar to the natural progression of VCFs in osteoporotic patients.

Absolute contraindications to VA include active infection (locally or systemically), particularly acute osteomyelitis of the vertebrae. Relative contraindications include an uncorrectable coagulopathy, allergy to PMMA, pregnancy, myelopathy or neurologic deficit, and spinal instability.

A decline in VA was noted in the Medicare population between 2004 and 2014. Many authors attribute this to two *New England Journal of Medicine* articles, by Kallmes et al and Buchbinder et al.[13,14,18,19] Both of these articles failed to demonstrate clinical improvement in patients undergoing vertebroplasty. Subsequent studies, however, have shown benefit conferred by VA. On such study, the Fracture Reduction Evaluation (FREE) study, evaluated 300 patients, 149 patients of whom underwent BKP while 151 had conservative management only.[20] Both the primary outcome measure of improvement in the physical component score (SF-36) and the secondary outcome measure of improved back pain disability were statistically improved in the BKP group.

Many of the major evaluations of VA use vertebroplasty exclusively as the operative procedure. Edidin et al performed a retrospective analysis of 858,978 Medicare patients diagnosed with a VCF over a 4-year period.[21] Of these patients, 13.9% were treated with BKP and another 7.4% were treated with vertebroplasty. The patients undergoing VA demonstrated a higher adjusted survival rate when compared with patients undergoing conservative management alone. Further analysis also demonstrated a higher adjusted survival rate for BKP over vertebroplasty.

References

[1] Hirsch JA, Beall DP, Chambers MR, et al. Management of vertebral fragility fractures: a clinical care pathway developed by a multispecialty panel using the RAND/UCLA Appropriateness Method. Spine J. 2018; 18(11):2152–2161

[2] Gehlbach SH, Bigelow C, Heimisdottir M, May S, Walker M, Kirkwood JR. Recognition of vertebral fracture in a clinical setting. Osteoporos Int. 2000; 11(7):577–582

[3] Delmas PD, van de Langerijt L, Watts NB, et al. IMPACT Study Group. Underdiagnosis of vertebral fractures is a worldwide problem: the IMPACT study. J Bone Miner Res. 2005; 20(4):557–563

[4] Fink HA, Milavetz DL, Palermo L, et al. Fracture Intervention Trial Research Group. What proportion of incident radiographic vertebral deformities is

clinically diagnosed and vice versa? J Bone Miner Res. 2005; 20(7):1216–1222

[5] Ensrud KE, Blackwell TL, Fink HA, et al. Osteoporotic Fractures in Men (MrOS) Research Group. What proportion of incident radiographic vertebral fractures in older men is clinically diagnosed and vice versa: a prospective study. J Bone Miner Res. 2016; 31(8):1500–1503

[6] Cherasse A, Muller G, Ornetti P, Piroth C, Tavernier C, Maillefert JF. Tolerability of opioids in patients with acute pain due to nonmalignant musculoskeletal disease. A hospital-based observational study. Joint Bone Spine. 2004; 71(6):572–576

[7] Brown CJ, Friedkin RJ, Inouye SK. Prevalence and outcomes of low mobility in hospitalized older patients. J Am Geriatr Soc. 2004; 52(8):1263–1270

[8] Babayev M, Lachmann E, Nagler W. The controversy surrounding sacral insufficiency fractures: to ambulate or not to ambulate? Am J Phys Med Rehabil. 2000; 79(4):404–409

[9] Dittmer DK, Teasell R. Complications of immobilization and bed rest. Part 1: Musculoskeletal and cardiovascular complications. Can Fam Physician. 1993; 39:1428–1432, 1435–1437

[10] Teasell R, Dittmer DK. Complications of immobilization and bed rest. Part 2: Other complications. Can Fam Physician. 1993; 39:1440–1442, 1445–1446

[11] Dong R, Chen L, Gu Y, et al. Improvement in respiratory function after vertebroplasty and kyphoplasty. Int Orthop. 2009; 33(6):1689–1694

[12] Tanigawa N, Kariya S, Kojima H, et al. Improvement in respiratory function by percutaneous vertebroplasty. Acta Radiol. 2008; 49(6):638–643

[13] Buchbinder R, Osborne RH, Ebeling PR, et al. A randomized trial of vertebroplasty for painful osteoporotic vertebral fractures. N Engl J Med. 2009; 361(6):557–568

[14] Kallmes DF, Comstock BA, Heagerty PJ, et al. A randomized trial of vertebroplasty for osteoporotic spinal fractures. N Engl J Med. 2009; 361(6): 569–579

[15] Rousing R, Hansen KL, Andersen MO, Jespersen SM, Thomsen K, Lauritsen JM. Twelve-months follow-up in forty-nine patients with acute/semiacute osteoporotic vertebral fractures treated conservatively or with percutaneous vertebroplasty: a clinical randomized study. Spine. 2010; 35(5):478–482

[16] Rousing R, Andersen MO, Jespersen SM, Thomsen K, Lauritsen J. Percutaneous vertebroplasty compared to conservative treatment in patients with painful acute or subacute osteoporotic vertebral fractures: three-months follow-up in a clinical randomized study. Spine. 2009; 34(13):1349–1354

[17] Wardlaw D, Cummings SR, Van Meirhaeghe J, et al. Efficacy and safety of balloon kyphoplasty compared with non-surgical care for vertebral compression fracture (FREE): a randomised controlled trial. Lancet. 2009; 373(9668):1016–1024

[18] Ong KL, Beall DP, Frohbergh M, Lau E, Hirsch JA. Were VCF patients at higher risk of mortality following the 2009 publication of the vertebroplasty "sham" trials? Osteoporos Int. 2018; 29(2):375–383

[19] Hirsch JA, Chandra RV, Pampati V, Barr JD, Brook AL, Manchikanti L. Analysis of vertebral augmentation practice patterns: a 2016 update. J Neurointerv Surg. 2016; 8(12):1299–1304

[20] Wardlaw D, Cummings SR, Van Meirhaeghe J, et al. Efficacy and safety of balloon kyphoplasty compared with non-surgical care for vertebral compression fracture (FREE): a randomised controlled trial. Lancet. 2009; 373(9668):1016–1024

[21] Edidin AA, Ong KL, Lau E, Kurtz SM. Mortality risk for operated and nonoperated vertebral fracture patients in the medicare population. J Bone Miner Res. 2011; 26(7):1617–1626

18 Osteoporotic Fracture III: Vertebral Augmentation Devices

Danoob Dalili, Nicolas Theumann, Nicolas Amoretti, Daniel E. Dalili, Amanda Isaac, and Jan Fritz

18.1 Case Presentation

A 65-year-old woman presented with a painful (6.5/10) osteoporotic impaction fracture of the L2 vertebra with 50% vertebral body collapse (Magerl type A3.1).[1] Percutaneous fluoroscopy-guided SpineJack® (Stryker Corp., Portage, MI, USA) vertebral augmentation was performed at this level (L2) (▶ Fig. 18.1).

Utilizing a percutaneous transpedicular/parapedicular approach, an implant-specific bone trocar (working cannula) was inserted until it reached the posterior third of the vertebral body as observed in a lateral/sagittal plane. At this point the inner part was replaced with a guidewire and a reamer (bone drill). The guidewire was removed, and drilling was performed until the desired position of the implant was reached. The drill should terminate just short of the anterior vertebral body cortex. The drill was replaced with a template device which "cleaned" the desired implant site. This process was repeated on the contralateral pedicle, and the implant expanders were inserted through the working cannulae on both sides. The devices were gradually expanded simultaneously. Intermittent fluoroscopic acquisition ensured the implants expanded safely and appropriately to achieve the desired fracture reduction, without

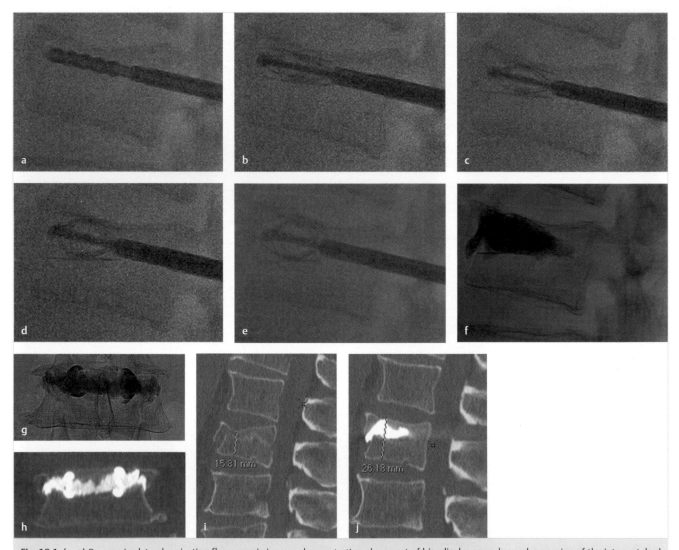

Fig. 18.1 **(a–e)** Progressive lateral projection fluoroscopic images demonstrating placement of bipedicular cannulae and expansion of the intravertebral spacing device. **(f, g)** Lateral and anteroposterior (AP) projections following instillation of polymethylmethacrylate. **(h)** Postprocedural coronal computed tomography (CT) demonstrating the satisfactory implant positioning and lack of cement leakage. **(i)** Preprocedural CT demonstrating the loss of central vertebral body height (15.81 mm). **(j)** Postprocedural CT demonstrating excellent near-normal anatomical height restoration (26.18 mm). Courtesy: Dr Nicolas Theumann.

breaching the superior end plate or changing direction. Once the desired vertebral height restoration was achieved, expansion was ceased and the expander device removed, leaving the implant and working cannula in place. Biomaterials in the form of implant-specific polymethylmethacrylate (PMMA) cement were injected simultaneously under continuous fluoroscopy on both sides until the desired quantity was injected. The final result was observed with an anteroposterior (AP) control projection.

On postprocedure day 1, the patient was able to ambulate and the visual analog pain scores reduced from 6.5 preprocedure to 1; there was a reduction in the kyphotic angle by 11 degrees.

18.2 Discussion

Vertebroplasty has become the primary method of definitive treatment for vertebral compression fractures over the last 10 to 20 years. This procedure is described in depth elsewhere in chapter 16. With the advancement of medical technology, new variants of routine vertebroplasty have emerged, namely, kyphoplasty and vertebral augmentation devices (VADs). These procedures have emerged as beneficial in cases of significant vertebral height loss of greater than 30%,[2] allowing better structural integrity and a closer return to normal bony anatomy. While kyphoplasty makes use of a balloon to restore vertebral height and create a cavity for subsequent cement injection,[3] VADs are new tools devised to achieve a similar effect.[4,5,6,7,8,9]

Kyphoplasty has historically been the treatment of choice for restoring vertebral body height.[3,6,10,11,12] Its mechanism involves using a percutaneous balloon that is inserted into the vertebral body via a transpedicular or an extrapedicular approach and inflated until the vertebral body achieves normal or near-normal height. This in turn creates a cavity that can then be filled with cement. In theory this should result in a rigid vertebral body with restored height; however, total or partial collapse following the procedure is not uncommon.[13] Failure to restore vertebral body height does not seem to interfere with the excellent pain management and good functional outcomes observed with kyphoplasty. However, in an attempt to improve the patient's overall outcomes and to indefinitely restore vertebral height, alternative techniques involving the use of VADs have emerged.[8,14]

Each VAD has its own procedures.[7,15,16,17,18] The most common devices are SpineJack®, Vertebral Body Stenting System (DePuy Synthes, West Chester, PA, USA), and OsseoFix Spinal Fracture Reduction System (Alphatec Spine, Inc., Carlsbad, CA, USA).

18.3 Specific Devices

18.3.1 SpineJack®

SpineJack® is a titanium implant used to restore vertebral body height in osteoporotic vertebral fractures, traumatic fractures, and primary or secondary bone tumors (▶ Fig. 18.2). This device is a mechanical system whereby longitudinal compression of the device causes inferior–superior expansion of the vertebral body with controlled restoration of height.[8,15] Similar to standard vertebroplasty and kyphoplasty practices, SpineJack® vertebral

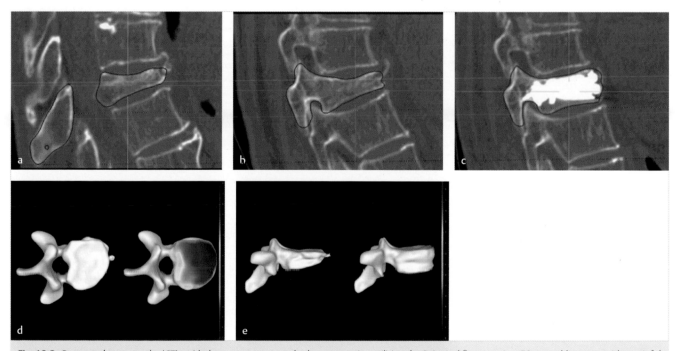

Fig. 18.2 Computed tomography (CT)-guided percutaneous vertebral augmentation utilizing the SpineJack® system in a 70-year-old woman with a painful (7.5/10) osteoporotic fracture of the L2 vertebra (Magerl type A3.3). **(a, b)** Sagittal reconstructed preprocedure CT demonstrates the degree of vertebral collapse and kyphotic deformity. **(c)** Following augmentation and vertebroplasty with the expansion device, there has been significant improvement in the degree of height restoration, which appears near-normal anatomical. On postprocedure day 3, at the time of discharge, the patient reported a significant pain reduction with a pain score of 2/10. There was a total reduction in kyphotic angle deformity by 24 degrees. **(d)** Color-coded axial and **(e)** sagittal view reconstructions illustrate the increase in anterior and central vertebral body height. Courtesy: Dr Nicolas Theumann.

cementing occurs under fluoroscopy. Patients are placed prone, and under fluoroscopic guidance a trocar containing the 5-mm device is inserted into the vertebral body using a bilateral transpedicular approach. Once in satisfactory position, a tool is used to expand the device using a mechanical (as opposed to hydraulic) mechanism. This inferior–superior expansion creates a cavity in the vertebral body within which SpineJack® resides. The device is then locked in place, creating space for cementing. As with vertebroplasty, PMMA is most commonly used as the cementing agent of choice. It is inserted through the already-placed trocar filling the cavity in the vertebral body and around the SpineJack® device. This is performed under constant fluoroscopic surveillance to assess for adequate filling and positioning of the implant and to ensure no cement leaks. A multicenter study by Noriega et al[8] demonstrated significant pain improvement post intervention, with 81.5% of patients stating pain relief 48 hours post procedure, with similar relief extending up to 12 months post procedure. Additionally, over 90% decrease in analgesia use was documented in the treated population.

18.3.2 Vertebral Body Stenting System (VBS)

The Vertebral Body Stenting System (VBS) is a fixation method suitable for compression fractures from T5 to L5.[11,19,20] This technique uses an expandable titanium device in the form of a stent to reduce pain and restore height to the fractured vertebra.[11] The stent is inserted using the same balloon as conventional kyphoplasty, and is placed under fluoroscopic guidance via a bipedicular approach. After balloon inflation, the stent remains expanded in place in the vertebra and the balloon is removed. Similar to the SpineJack system, PMMA is injected into the cavity created by the stent through the same cannula as device insertion. The viscous PMMA solidifies and helps to maintain that restored vertebral height created by the stent. Evidence has shown a greater reduction in vertebral height loss after balloon removal following VBS than standard kyphoplasty,[21] and VBS has been shown to significantly reduce pain and restore function as well as vertebral body height and kyphotic correction at 12 months post insertion.[7,12,22,23]

18.3.3 OsseoFix® Spine Reduction System

This method of fracture stabilization also utilizes an implantable titanium device. Its mechanism of action to reduce vertebral fractures and decrease kyphotic deformity is mechanical compression of trabecular bone.[15,24] OsseoFix® is recommended for use in stable traumatic and atraumatic compression fractures from T6 to L5. For this procedure, retropulsed fragments and dural sac or cord compression are absolute contraindications.[25] The OsseoFix® device is inserted under fluoroscopic guidance into the anterior third of the vertebral body.[15] The implant is placed in correct position by directing the insertion device tip to the anterior third of the vertebral body, after which the screw handle is used to expand the device. Expansion of the device causes compaction of surrounding bone and an increase in vertebral body height.[26] Similar to the vertebral body stenting system, the implant is left in the vertebral body after removal of the insertion device and

PMMA is injected through the cannula. Due to the nature of the implant, significantly less PMMA is required in comparison to standard kyphoplasty, and a more stable fixation is achieved due an interlocking effect being formed between the bone and the titanium mesh.[25] The system is reported to have reduced risk of cement leakage and provides good effectiveness in reducing pain and kyphotic deformity.[24,26]

18.4 Conclusion

VADs have emerged as new alternatives to balloon kyphoplasty with reported reduced complications and improved long-term outcomes. While OsseoFix® and SpineJack® use a mechanical method of implantation, VBS uses a hydraulic mechanism. Each method has a different mode of action with different techniques for implantation, and each offers inherent advantages and disadvantages that need to be considered prior to planning the intervention.[2] Multidisciplinary discussions are warranted to patient selection for the procedure and offer a patient-specific procedural plan to improve outcomes.[27,28,29,30]

References

[1] Magerl F, Aebi M, Gertzbein SD, Harms J, Nazarian S. A comprehensive classification of thoracic and lumbar injuries. Eur Spine J. 1994; 3(4):184–201

[2] Vanni D, Galzio R, Kazakova A, et al. Third-generation percutaneous vertebral augmentation systems. J Spine Surg. 2016; 2(1):13–20

[3] Shaibani A, Ali S, Bhatt H. Vertebroplasty and kyphoplasty for the palliation of pain. Semin Intervent Radiol 2007;24(4):409–418

[4] Dalili D, Isaac A, Cazzato RL, et al. Interventional techniques for bone and musculoskeletal soft tissue tumors: current practices and future directions - Part II. Stabilization. Semin Musculoskelet Radiol. 2020; 24(6):710–725

[5] Buy X, Catena V, Roubaud G, Crombe A, Kind M, Palussiere J. Image-guided bone consolidation in oncology. Semin Intervent Radiol. 2018; 35(4):221–228

[6] Noriega DC, Krüger A, Ramajo RH, Ardura F, Munoz M, Sahin S. Long-term benefits of percutaneous anatomical restoration of vertebral compression fractures linked to malignancy. Turk Neurosurg. 2016; 26(4):608–614

[7] Noriega D, Marcia S, Theumann N, et al. A prospective, international, randomized, noninferiority study comparing an implantable titanium vertebral augmentation device versus balloon kyphoplasty in the reduction of vertebral compression fractures (SAKOS study). Spine J. 2019; 19(11):1782–1795

[8] Noriega D, Maestretti G, Renaud C, et al. Clinical performance and safety of 108 SpineJack implantations: 1-year results of a prospective multicentre single-arm registry study. BioMed Res Int. 2015; 2015:173872

[9] Noriega D, Krüger A, Ardura F, et al. Clinical outcome after the use of a new craniocaudal expandable implant for vertebral compression fracture treatment: one year results from a prospective multicentric study. BioMed Res Int. 2015; 2015:927813

[10] McConnell CT, Jr, Wippold FJ, II, Ray CE, Jr, et al. ACR appropriateness criteria management of vertebral compression fractures. J Am Coll Radiol. 2014; 11(8):757–763

[11] Disch AC, Schmoelz W. Cement augmentation in a thoracolumbar fracture model: reduction and stability after balloon kyphoplasty versus vertebral body stenting. Spine. 2014; 39(19):E1147–E1153

[12] Werner CML, Osterhoff G, Schlickeiser J, et al. Vertebral body stenting versus kyphoplasty for the treatment of osteoporotic vertebral compression fractures: a randomized trial. J Bone Joint Surg Am. 2013; 95(7):577–584

[13] Feltes C, Fountas KN, Machinis T, et al. Immediate and early postoperative pain relief after kyphoplasty without significant restoration of vertebral body height in acute osteoporotic vertebral fractures. Neurosurg Focus. 2005; 18(3):e5

[14] Rotter R, Martin H, Fuerderer S, et al. Vertebral body stenting: a new method for vertebral augmentation versus kyphoplasty. Eur Spine J. 2010; 19(6):916–923

[15] Long Y, Yi W, Yang D. Advances in vertebral augmentation systems for osteoporotic vertebral compression fractures. Pain Res Manag. 2020; 2020: 3947368

[16] Chang M, Zhang C, Shi J, et al. Comparison between 7 osteoporotic vertebral compression fractures treatments: systematic review and network meta-analysis. World Neurosurg. 2021; 145:462–470.e1

[17] Cornelis FH, Joly Q, Nouri-Neuville M, et al. Innovative spine implants for improved augmentation and stability in neoplastic vertebral compression fracture. Medicina (Kaunas). 2019; 55(8):5–10

[18] Filippiadis DK, Marcia S, Ryan A, et al. New implant-based technologies in the spine. Cardiovasc Intervent Radiol. 2018; 41(10):1463–1473

[19] Klezl Z, Majeed H, Bommireddy R, John J. Early results after vertebral body stenting for fractures of the anterior column of the thoracolumbar spine. Injury. 2011; 42(10):1038–1042

[20] Fürderer S, Anders M, Schwindling B, et al. Vertebral body stenting. Eine methode zur reposition und augmentation von wirbelkörperkompressionsfrakturen. [Vertebral body stenting. A method for repositioning and augmenting vertebral compression fractures]. Orthopade. 2002; 31(4):356–361

[21] Garnon J, Doré B, Auloge P, et al. Efficacy of the vertebral body stenting system for the restoration of vertebral height in acute traumatic compression fractures in a non-osteoporotic population. Cardiovasc Intervent Radiol. 2019; 42(11):1579–1587

[22] Diel P, Röder C, Perler G, et al. Radiographic and safety details of vertebral body stenting: results from a multicenter chart review. BMC Musculoskelet Disord. 2013; 14:233

[23] Muto M, Greco B, Setola F, Vassallo P, Ambrosanio G, Guarnieri G. Vertebral body stenting system for the treatment of osteoporotic vertebral compression fracture: follow-up at 12 months in 20 cases. Neuroradiol J. 2011; 24(4):610–619

[24] Eschler A, Ender SA, Ulmar B, Herlyn P, Mittlmeier T, Gradl G. Cementless fixation of osteoporotic VCFs using titanium mesh implants (OsseoFix): preliminary results. Biomed Res Int. 2014; 2014:853897

[25] Ender SA, Gradl G, Ender M, Langner S, Merk HR, Kayser R. Osseofix® system for percutaneous stabilization of osteoporotic and tumorous vertebral compression fractures—clinical and radiological results after 12 months. Röfo Fortschr Geb Röntgenstr Nuklearmed. 2014; 186(4):380–387

[26] Ender SA, Wetterau E, Ender M, Kühn JP, Merk HR, Kayser R. Percutaneous stabilization system Osseofix® for treatment of osteoporotic vertebral compression fractures—clinical and radiological results after 12 months. PLoS One. 2013; 8(6):e65119

[27] Dalili D, Isaac A, Bazzocchi A, et al. Interventional techniques for bone and musculoskeletal soft tissue tumors: current practices and future directions—Part I. Ablation. Semin Musculoskelet Radiol. 2020; 24(6):692–709

[28] Dalili D, Isaac A, Rashidi A, Åström G, Fritz J. Image-guided sports medicine and musculoskeletal tumor interventions: a patient-centered model. Semin Musculoskelet Radiol. 2020; 24(3):290–309

[29] Cazzato RL, Garnon J, De Marini P, et al. French multidisciplinary approach for the treatment of MSK tumors. Semin Musculoskelet Radiol. 2020; 24 (3):310–322

[30] Sequeiros RB, Fritz J, Ojala R, Carrino JA. Percutaneous magnetic resonance imaging-guided bone tumor management and magnetic resonance imaging-guided bone therapy. Top Magn Reson Imaging. 2011; 22(4):171–177

19 Osteoporotic Fracture IV: Curved Balloon Kyphoplasty

J. Reed McGraw and J. Kevin McGraw

19.1 Case Presentation

A 76-year-old woman sustained a fall in her bathroom. She was admitted to the hospital via the emergency room for pain control secondary to an L2 vertebral body compression fracture (▶ Fig. 19.1a–c), and interventional radiology (IR) was consulted for consideration of vertebral augmentation. On examination, the patient was neurologically intact but had focal tenderness in the mid-lumbar spine. The patient underwent balloon kyphoplasty (BK) via a unipedicular approach utilizing a curved balloon (AVAflex balloon system, Stryker, Kalamazoo, MI).

Informed consent was obtained. The patient was placed in the prone position in a biplane IR suite. Intravenous (IV) moderate sedation was performed. The right pedicle of the L2 vertebral

body was entered with a 10-gauge needle that was advanced to the center of the vertebral body as seen on a lateral view (▶ Fig. 19.2a, b). An AVAflex nitinol stylet and introducer sheath (Stryker) was coaxially inserted into the 10-gauge cannula and advanced horizontally into the contralateral hemivertebrae (▶ Fig. 19.3a, b). The stylet was removed, leaving the introducer in place, and the AVAflex balloon was advanced through the introducer. The balloon was exposed by retracting the introducer (▶ Fig. 19.4a, b). The balloon was inflated with an insufflator, creating a cavity within the vertebral body (▶ Fig. 19.5a, b), after which the balloon was deflated. The deflated balloon and the introducer were removed simultaneously leaving the 10-gauge cannula. A curved nitinol AVAflex needle was inserted into the vertebral body via the 10-gauge cannula (▶ Fig. 19.6a, b). Vertaplex HV bone cement (Stryker) was delivered into the vertebral

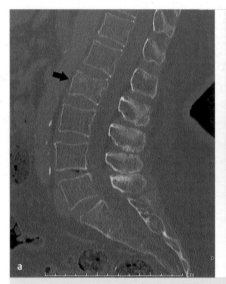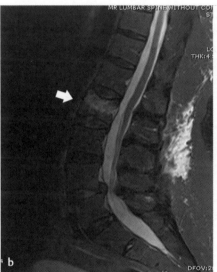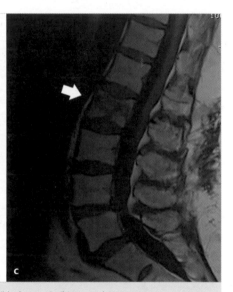

Fig. 19.1 (a) Sagittal reformatted computed tomography (CT) showing a compression fracture of L2 (black arrow). (b) Sagittal STIR magnetic resonance imaging (MRI) showing increased signal in the L2 vertebral body consistent with an acute compression fracture (white arrow). (c) Sagittal T1-weighted MRI showing decreased signal in the L2 vertebral body, also consistent with an acute compression fracture (white arrow).

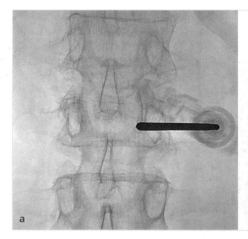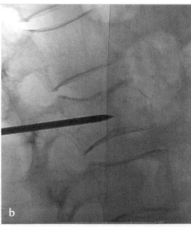

Fig. 19.2 (a, b) Frontal and lateral images showing a 10-gauge needle entering the right pedicle of the L2 vertebral body.

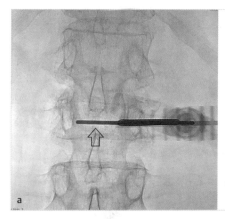
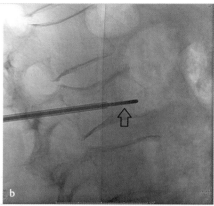

Fig. 19.3 (a, b) Frontal and lateral images showing the AVAflex nitinol stylet and introducer sheath (arrow) across the vertebral body.

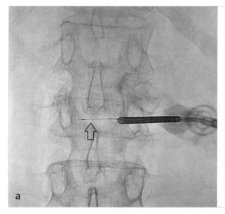
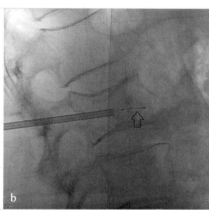

Fig. 19.4 (a, b) Frontal and lateral images showing the uninflated AVAflex balloon (arrow) in the vertebral body. The introducer sheath has been retracted.

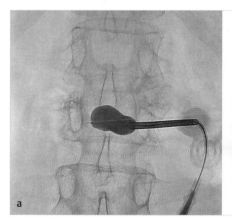
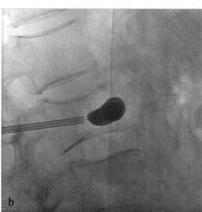

Fig. 19.5 (a, b) Frontal and lateral images showing balloon inflation. The balloon is compliant and in areas of hard bone it may not fully expand.

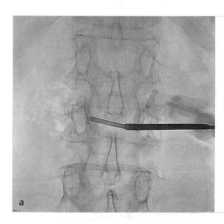
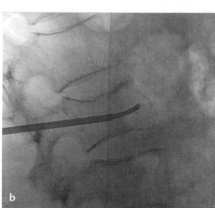

Fig. 19.6 (a, b) Frontal and lateral images showing the AVAflex needle (arrow) in the vertebral body prior to cement injection.

body (▶ Fig. 19.7a, b). The curved needle and cannula were removed, and a sterile dressing was applied.

On postprocedure day 1, the patient reported resolution of her pain for which the vertebral augmentation procedure was performed.

19.2 Discussion

Vertebral compression fractures (VCFs) are a significant and growing problem in the United States, with more than 700,000 new VCFs being diagnosed annually.[1] Treatment strategies for symptomatic VCFs revolve around pain management. Conservative approaches for VCF treatment include analgesics, bed rest, bracing, physical therapy, and nerve root blocks.[2] In patients in whom conservative therapy has failed or resulted in inadequate pain reduction, percutaneous vertebral augmentation can be considered.[2]

Vertebral augmentation was first described in the 1980s in France with the development of percutaneous vertebroplasty (VP).[3] Vertebroplasty was not performed in the United States until the mid-1990s.[4] It involves injection of bone cement, typically polymethylmethacrylate (PMMA), into the compressed vertebral body, typically utilizing a transpedicular approach under fluoroscopic guidance. Studies have reported VP to be associated with a significant reduction in pain due to VCFs and increased function.[4,5] The main drawbacks of VP include potential damage to the spinal cord and nerve roots due to cement leak.[4] This potential complication led to the development of BK in the late 1990s.

BK (which is effectively balloon-assisted VP) emerged as an attempt to enhance efficacy and reduce risk associated with VP.[4,5] Under fluoroscopic guidance, BK utilizes an inflatable balloon to create a cavity in the collapsed vertebral body prior to PMMA injection.[4,5] It has been associated with comparable pain reduction, height restoration, and kyphosis reduction to VP with the benefit of reduced risk of PMMA leakage. The major drawback to BK is cost.[4,5] Both VP and BK are widely used today in clinical practice.[6,7]

The AVAflex system received FDA approval in 2017.[8] BK with the AVAflex balloon system allows treatment via a unipedicular approach, saving time and decreasing potential risks related to a second transpedicular approach. The curved needle enables targeted cement placement, and depending upon the acuity of the fracture, the cavity created within the vertebral body can be quite substantial (▶ Fig. 19.5 and ▶ Fig. 19.6).[8]

Recently, new and innovative vertebral augmentation modalities such as the Kiva VCF treatment system (Benvenue Medical Inc., Santa Clara, CA), the SpineJack system (Stryker), and bone grafting have emerged. These techniques seek to not only relieve VCF-related pain but also to restore normal vertebral body height and to enhance fracture healing with minimal leakage of cement.[6,9,10,11,12] These new systems represent a move toward fixed, physician-controlled implantable devices.

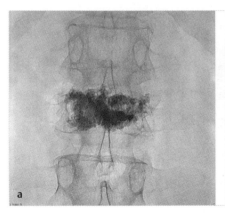
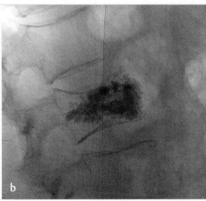

Fig. 19.7 (a, b) Frontal and lateral images showing vertebral body filling with the bone cement.

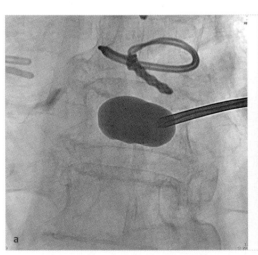
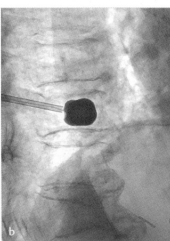

Fig. 19.8 (a, b) Frontal and lateral images of another patient demonstrating the balloon fully inflated in the T9 vertebral body.

The Kiva VCF treatment system utilizes a polyether ether ketone (PEEK) implant deployed over a nitinol coil via a transpedicular approach. Cement (PMMA) is injected and contained within the implant. Studies have found the Kiva system to be noninferior to BK, and effective at relieving pain and restoring height.[9] The SpineJack system relies on a titanium device, delivered via a transpedicular approach, that is expandable in the craniocaudal axis. Briefly, it relies on a titanium device, delivered via a transpedicular approach, that is expandable in the craniocaudal axis. The device is expanded to desired height, which is followed by injection of PMMA (▶ Fig. 19.7a–d). Preliminary studies have found the SpineJack system to be safe, effective at pain relief, and to have superior height restoration and kyphosis correction compared to BK.[10,11] Finally, early animal studies have found implantation of surface demineralized bone allograft to be effective at initiating osteoblastic response to promote bone healing in VCF.[12]

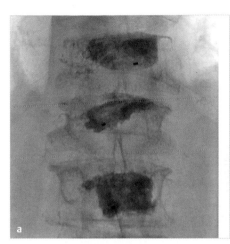
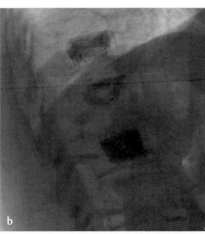

Fig. 19.9 (a, b) Frontal and lateral images following a three-level Kiva procedure.

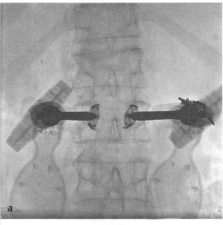
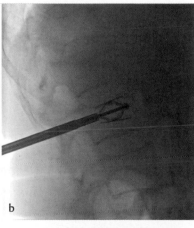
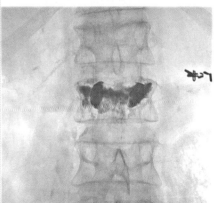
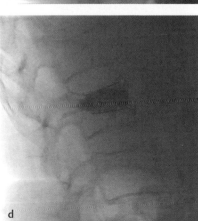

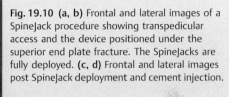

Fig. 19.10 (a, b) Frontal and lateral images of a SpineJack procedure showing transpedicular access and the device positioned under the superior end plate fracture. The SpineJacks are fully deployed. (c, d) Frontal and lateral images post SpineJack deployment and cement injection.

References

[1] Burge R, Dawson-Hughes B, Solomon DH, Wong JB, King A, Tosteson A. Incidence and economic burden of osteoporosis-related fractures in the United States, 2005–2025. J Bone Miner Res. 2007; 22(3):465–475

[2] Dewar C. Diagnosis and treatment of vertebral compression fractures. Radiol Technol. 2015; 86(3):301–320, quiz 321–323

[3] Galibert P, Deramond H, Rosat P, Le Gars D. [Preliminary note on the treatment of vertebral angioma by percutaneous acrylic vertebroplasty]. Neurochirurgie. 1987; 33(2):166–168

[4] Kushchayev SV, Wiener PC, Teytelboym OM, Arrington JA, Khan M, Preul MC. Percutaneous vertebroplasty: a history of procedure, technology, culture, specialty, and economics. Neuroimaging Clin N Am. 2019; 29(4):481–494

[5] Lieberman IH, Dudeney S, Reinhardt MK, Bell G. Initial outcome and efficacy of "kyphoplasty" in the treatment of painful osteoporotic vertebral compression fractures. Spine. 2001; 26(14):1631–1638

[6] Hargunani R, Le Corroller T, Khashoggi K, et al. An overview of vertebroplasty: current status, controversies, and future directions. Can Assoc Radiol J. 2012; 63(3) Suppl:S11–S17

[7] De Leacy R, Chandra RV, Barr JD, et al. The evidentiary basis of vertebral augmentation: a 2019 update. J Neurointerv Surg. 2020; 12(5):442–447

[8] Stryker AVAflex balloon system. https://strykerivs.com/products/families/avaflex#ref1. Published 2018. Accessed April 4, 2020

[9] Tutton SM, Pflugmacher R, Davidian M, Beall DP, Facchini FR, Garfin SR. KAST Study: The kiva system as a vertebral augmentation treatment—A safety and effectiveness trial: a randomized, noninferiority trial comparing the kiva system with balloon kyphoplasty in treatment of osteoporotic vertebral compression fractures. Spine. 2015; 40(12):865–875

[10] Premat K, Vande Perre S, Cormier É, et al. Vertebral augmentation with the SpineJack® in chronic vertebral compression fractures with major kyphosis. Eur Radiol. 2018; 28(12):4985–4991

[11] Noriega DC, Rodríguez-Monsalve F, Ramajo R, Sánchez-Lite I, Toribio B, Ardura F. Long-term safety and clinical performance of kyphoplasty and SpineJack® procedures in the treatment of osteoporotic vertebral compression fractures: a pilot, monocentric, investigator-initiated study. Osteoporos Int. 2019; 30(3):637–645

[12] Shetye SS, Lyons AS, Bhattacharjee AG, Abjornson C, Puttlitz CM. Radiographic and Histological Evaluation of a Surface Demineralized Flexible Allograft Chain in an Ovine Vertebra Body Model. 2019

20 Sacroplasty

Danoob Dalili, Nicolas Theumann, Nicolas Amoretti, Daniel E. Dalili, Amanda Isaac, and Jan Fritz

20.1 Case Presentation

A 65-year-old woman presented with persistent lower back and sacral pain in the absence of significant trauma. Magnetic resonance imaging (MRI) demonstrated left-sided sacral edema and fracture lines (▶ Fig. 20.1). Following failure of conservative measures for 2 months and outpatient clinical assessment, the patient was referred for a sacroplasty procedure (▶ Fig. 20.2, ▶ Fig. 20.3, and ▶ Fig. 20.4).

20.2 Discussion

The sacrum is the main stabilizer of the posterior pelvic wall and connects the lumbar vertebrae to the pelvis.[1] It serves to transmit axial loads from the trunk to the lower limbs and offers protection of the lumbosacral plexus and iliac vessels. There is an increased incidence in the diagnosis of sacral fractures with advanced age, with nonosteoporotic sacral fractures rising significantly to over 2.09 per 100,000 as reported by Bydon et al.[2] These fractures can typically be grouped into three categories according to the underlying mechanism, namely, traumatic, insufficiency, and pathological.

20.2.1 Fracture Types

Traumatic Fractures

Traumatic fractures of the sacrum commonly occur in a younger cohort and are typically secondary to high-impact or high-speed accidents. Only 5% of sacral fractures occur in isolation, with pelvic ring injuries, hip and lumbar spine fractures, abdominal or pelvic bleeding, open fractures, and soft tissue injuries being most commonly found in association.[3] Traumatic sacral fractures can have long-lasting neurological sequelae in up to 25% of patients.[2] Two methods have been used to categorize traumatic sacral fractures, namely, the Denis system and AO-Spine classification.

The Denis system[4] categorizes fractures into three zones based on location of fracture. Zone 1 is the most common (50%), and the fractures are confined to the sacral alar region, occasionally causing L5 nerve root injury. Zone 2 is the second most common type (34%) and involve the sacral foramina, with just under 28% resulting in a neurological deficit. Zone 3 fractures are confined to the spinal canal and sacral bodies. Although this is the least common type it holds the greatest potential (58%) for neurological injury, resulting in saddle anesthesia and potential for urinary or fecal incontinence.[4]

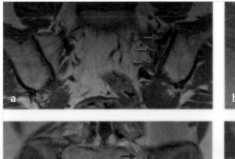
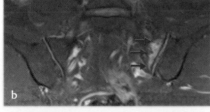
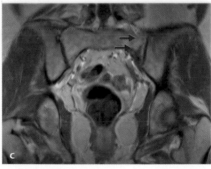
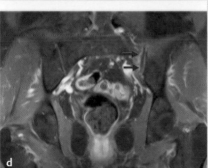

Fig. 20.1 Axial oblique (**a, b**) and coronal (**c, d**) magnetic resonance (MR) images of the sacrum demonstrating T1-weighted, low-signal, left-sided, longitudinal sacral alar fracture line (arrows in **a** and **c**) and Short tau inversion recovery (STIR) high signal fracture line with bone marrow edema (arrows in **b** and **d**).

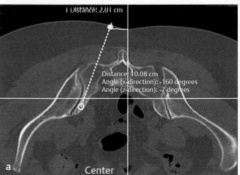
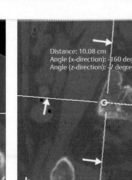

Fig. 20.2 Preprocedure planning computed tomography (CT) in the axial (**a**) and sagittal (**b**) planes for needle trajectory planning utilizing the long-axis approach. Note: As the patient is lying in prone position, the left sacral ala is now visible on the right.

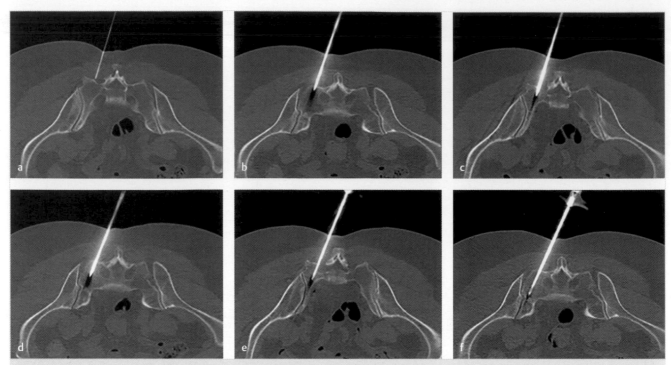

Fig. 20.3 Long-axis computed tomography (CT)-guided percutaneous sacroplasty. Standard spinal needle with anesthesia to the skin and needle tract, followed by elevation of the periosteum with 10 mL of 0.5% Marcaine (a). Thereafter, the 11-G vertebroplasty trocar is inserted in a medial–lateral, caudo-cranial trajectory (b–f).

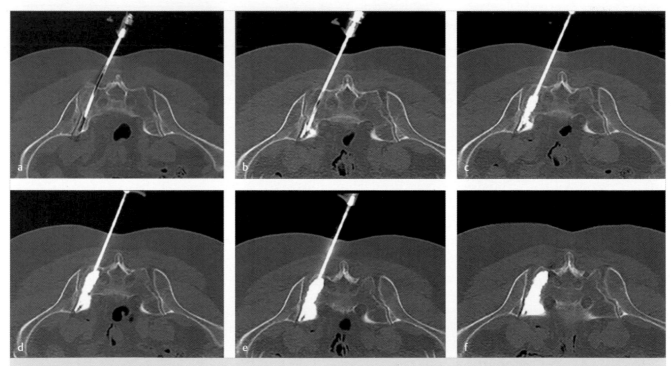

Fig. 20.4 The inner aspect of the trocar was removed and replaced with the cement injection needle (a). After the needle is directed according to the desired approach, the trocar is embedded into the fracture site, and eased half-way through the sacrum. Saline is then flushed down the tract that has been created to aid injecting air into the interosseous veins during the procedure. An iodine-based contrast is then injected through the trocar and continuous fluoroscopic images are acquired to depict an interosseous venogram. The contrast images can be analyzed to see if there is any extravasation from the vertebra, confirming a fracture at that site. When positioning of the trocar is deemed satisfactory in relation to images acquired it is flushed with sterile saline again in preparation for cementing.[1] High viscosity polymethylmethacrylate (PMMA) cement was injected distal to proximal (b–e), until consolidation was achieved across the fracture line (f). A contralateral, right-sided fracture was depicted during the procedure and the patient reported interval pain and limping following the original imaging. The steps were therefore repeated on the contralateral side.

Table 20.1 The AO-Spine classification scheme

Injury type	Subtype	Classification
A – Lower sacrococcygeal (normal spinopelvic stability)	1	Injury to the coccygeal region
	2	Nondisplaced transverse fractures below the level of the sacroiliac joint
	3	Displaced transverse fractures below the level of the sacroiliac joint
B – Posterior pelvic (unilateral and longitudinal in orientation; can affect pelvis stability)	1	Longitudinal fracture that is medial to the neural foramina and involves the spinal canal
	2	Longitudinal fracture that is lateral to the neural foramina and does not involve the spinal canal
	3	Longitudinal fracture that involves the foramen but not the spinal canal
C – Spinopelvic (spinopelvic instability)	0	Nondisplaced sacral U-type fracture
	1	Sacral U-type without posterior pelvic instability
	2	Bilateral complete B-type without transverse component
	3	Displaced sacral U-type

The AO-Spine[5] classification was developed in 2016 and categorizes fractures into three main types and three further subtypes. This classification scheme is outlined in ▶ Table 20.1.

Insufficiency Fractures

Sacral insufficiency fractures are a common cause of debilitating back pain in the elderly, and were first described as a unique entity by Lourie in 1982.[6] They typically occur in the elderly population with a predilection for postmenopausal women where low bone mineral density results in fractures of the weight-bearing (mechanical loading) areas. Low bone mineral density occurs secondary to malignancy, radiotherapy (with reported 21–34% prevalence),[7] metabolic bone disease, rheumatoid arthritis, and gynecological and gastrointestinal cancers among other causes. There is typically no precise mechanism of injury for these fractures and patients report very subtle but often repeated trauma, which would normally have no consequences in patients with normal bone metabolism.

Radiation-induced sacral insufficiency fractures have been increasingly identified with the increased use of radiotherapy. Depending on the location of the targeted organs, the sacrum can receive large radiation doses resulting in red to yellow marrow changes and loss of bone mineralization. A study by Park et al of 235 patients undergoing radiation therapy for nonmetastatic cervical cancer revealed an incidence of over 5% established sacral insufficiency fractures in the treated population.[8] Pathological fractures of the sacrum and pelvis can also occur secondary to benign tumors as well as primary malignancy and/or metastases disrupting bone architecture and compromising its mechanical integrity.[9] Tumor growth into the neural foramina or epidural space can further compress the exiting nerve roots, resulting in pain, and/or sensory and motor radiculopathy with secondary bladder and bowel incontinence.

20.2.2 Radiological Diagnosis

Plain radiographs are commonly performed initially; however, they suffer from low sensitivity (20–38%).[10] Radiograph interpretation is confounded by overlying bowel gas artefact and underlying osteopenia. In the presence of any diagnostic doubt, further imaging is warranted.[10] Often multiple plain film views are required (inlet, outlet, and lateral) to increase the cumulative sensitivity of the study and allow specific fracture patterns to become more apparent on certain views. For example, inlet and outlet views are optimal for identifying longitudinal fractures, while lateral views can better assess transverse fractures. Overall, this results in a considerable radiation dose to the patient, with relatively low yield.

Recent changes in evidence-based practices, particularly with imaging protocols for trauma, has led to computed tomography (CT) becoming the imaging modality of choice for suspected pelvic and sacral fractures. This is due to the fast acquisition of scans, cross-sectional display of structures, and high-resolution imaging with dedicated bone and soft tissue window reconstructions to optimize interrogation of any abnormalities present. Computed tomographic postprocessing algorithms also allow for three-dimensional reconstructions, which can enhance the display fractures and their extensions. This improves clinical decision-making for treatment. In addition to cortical breach, ancillary signs of fracture include perisacral hematoma and fat stranding denoting edema.

MRI is gaining popularity in guiding management strategies for sacral injuries. Fracture lines within the sacrum are T1[11] hypointense and surrounding marrow edema will appear hyperintense on short T1 inversion recovery images. T2 image can help determine the age of the fracture and assess lesions.[12] In acute cases, there will also be contrast enhancement of the fracture. MRI sensitivity has been reported to be as high as 100%.[10] Where MRI is contraindicated (pacemaker, implants, or claustrophobia) bone scintigraphy with Technetium-99 m has been found to be very useful in identifying sacral fractures, particularly insufficiency fractures, with a sensitivity of 96%.[10]

Fracture of one ala increases the risk of fracture of the contralateral ala, particularly in insufficiency fractures; this results in the classical appearance described as the H (Honda) sign on nuclear medicine studies (bone scan, single photon emission computed tomography [SPECT-CT] and positron emission tomography [PET-CT]),[13] as demonstrated in the case presented here. Active scrutiny for contralateral fractures is therefore advised. Patients with sacral insufficiency fractures should also have full spine assessment and imaging. Lateral plain radiographs of the entire spine and dual energy X-ray absorptiometry (DEXA) are the first-line investigative strategy in this cohort of patients.

Sacral factures can be managed conservatively or with a myriad of interventions. Conservative management of sacral fractures involves oral and topical analgesia, bed rest, and progressive weight-bearing alongside physiotherapy. This is only recommended in the case of stable fractures with minimal displacement (< 1 cm), in the absence of soft tissue compromise, neurological deficit, or unmanageable pain. The main drawback of conservative management is the potential for displacement of the fracture with weight-bearing, intractable pain, and confounding risks of decreased mobility such as deep vein thrombosis or pulmonary embolism as well as muscle atrophy. The latter is difficult to reverse in the elderly population.

Where intervention is required, sacral fractures have traditionally been managed by way of percutaneous screw fixation,[10] posterior tension band plating, and iliosacral and lumbopelvic fixation. All of these procedures are performed under fluoroscopy, and aside from the percutaneous screws are very invasive procedures with large incisions and prolonged hospital stays. Surgical fixation carries a high propensity for malunion, hardware loosening, and procedural failure when performed in osteoporotic bone (present in a large percentage of this patient cohort).[14] As a result, minimally invasive procedures such as sacroplasty have become more favorable.

20.2.3 Sacroplasty Procedure

First performed by Dehdashti et al in 2001, sacroplasty is a minimally invasive procedure used in the management of painful sacral metastases.[15,16,17,18] It is performed under fluoroscopic or CT guidance, and involves cementing of the sacral fracture to achieve mechanical stabilization.[19,20,21]

For the procedure, the patient is positioned prone and the procedure is performed under sedation. CT-guided procedures are carried out following similar steps to standard fluoroscopy, with the benefit of being able to initially have a reconstructed image to plan the optimal entry point.[22] In addition, during contrast injection extravasation around the sacral nerve roots can be better visualized under CT, which may prevent adverse effects. The steps of the procedure are illustrated in ▶ Fig. 20.1, ▶ Fig. 20.2, ▶ Fig. 20.3, ▶ Fig. 20.4, and ▶ Fig. 20.5.

Several needle approaches have been developed depending on user preference, site of fracture, and risk of cement leakage[23,24] (▶ Fig. 20.6). These approaches are the *long axis approach* where the needle is inserted in the cauda-cephalic direction; the *short axis approach* where the needle is inserted in the posterior–anterior direction; and the *transiliac approach* where the needle is positioned in the iliac bone to traverse the sacroiliac joint (▶ Fig. 20.1).

The most common approach is the long axis approach developed by Smith and Dix[25] in 2006, and has largely replaced the previously used short axis approach. The long axis approach is thought to be preferable to the short axis approach due to a variety of reasons. First, with the short axis approach it is difficult to ensure that the tip of the needle is located in the intramedullary space of the sacral ala before commencing cement injection. Injection of cement along the short axis can result in a collection at one aspect of the fracture but not along the entirety of the fracture line. There have also been reports of frequent cement extravasation in the injection process, resulting in premature cessation of cement injection and less than optimal filling of the fracture site. The long axis technique has therefore been adopted to address these technical issues and improve distribution of cement along the fracture line, reduce cement extravasation, and facilitate guidance of the needle into the optimal space.[26]

The cementing agent typically used in sacroplasty is a radiopaque polymethylmethacrylate (PMMA). Typical quantities of

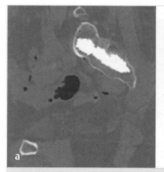
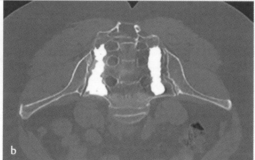
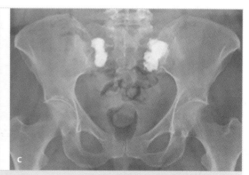

Fig. 20.5 Immediate postprocedure sagittal (**a**) and coronal-oblique (**b**) computed tomography (CT) multiplanar reformats demonstrating optimal osseous consolidation and cement filling of the sacrum from S1 to S5. Posteroanterior (PA) pelvic radiograph at 6 months follow-up (**c**) demonstrating satisfactory sacroplasty appearances, with significant reduction of visual analog scale (VAS) score to 1/10.

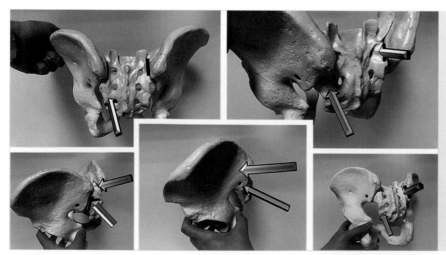

Fig. 20.6 Long axis (three-dimensional white arrow) and short axis (three-dimensional blue arrow) vertebroplasty technique trajectories demonstrated on a pelvic model.

cement vary from 2 to 8 mL[27] per fracture. In a proportion of cases, a second trocar may be inserted from a different entry point to target another segment of the fracture and allow for complete filling of the defect. This is performed in the same fashion as the first trocar. After satisfactory cementing of the fracture site, the trocar is removed, pressure is applied for hemostasis, and the patient is allowed to sit up. A vast majority of patients are allowed to ambulate the day after the procedure and will typically wear a protective brace for up to 3 months postoperatively.

Despite its percutaneous approach with proportionally decreased risk of infection when compared to open procedures, sacroplasty is not without risks. Although fairly uncommon,[27] the predominant adverse effects arising from sacroplasty are associated with cement issues or with the screw fixation.[28,29] Inadequate curing and thickening of the cement or inadequate use of imaging can result in intravascular or epidural injection.[30] Due to the innate exothermic[31] reaction of the PMMA, extravasation of cement into the sacral neural foramina can cause compression and damage of nerve roots. Intravascular injection of cement can result in cement emboli. The patient's underlying bone quality may also contribute to further fracturing of the sacrum at the injected site or elsewhere. These complications can result in further neurological symptoms.[32] These may require additional procedures such as decompression or fixation, albeit the need for decompression is quite rare with a reported incidence of 0.3%.[33]

A study by Yang et al has shown that inserting a balloon, which is expanded at the fracture site prior to cementing, can help to create a pre-sized cavity and compact the fracture chips, similar to balloon kyphoplasty.[34] Innovations in sacroplasty have been developed with the aim of reducing the amount of

cement leak. Studies have shown up to 55% cement leakage during a regular sacroplasty compared to 22% when using balloon assistance. This process could prevent untoward leak of cement outside of the fracture site, thereby reducing the chance of any adverse events.[35]

Sacroplasty has proven to be a consistently safe and effective method for alleviating pain[36] and improving functional outcomes in patients with sacral fractures. Frey et al[37] demonstrated a pain reduction in up to 90% of patients 1 year post sacroplasty. The results concur with subsequent studies which show significant ($P = 0.002$) reduction in pain, improved mobility, and decreased reliance on analgesia in a cohort of over 200 patients over a 10-year period.[38] A recent meta-analysis of 19 sacroplasty studies demonstrated statistically significant visual analog scale (VAS) score pain reductions in the short term (24–48 hours), and 6 and 12 months after the procedure.[33] Major complications were observed in up to 0.3% of patients, with three patients requiring surgical decompression for cement leakage. Random effects meta-analysis demonstrated statistically significant differences in the VAS pain level preprocedure, at 24 to 48 hours, 6 months, and 12 months, with cumulative pain scores of 8.32 ± 0.01, 3.55 ± 0.01, 1.48 ± 0.01, and 0.923 ± 0.01, respectively. Finally, multidisciplinary discussions are important to ensure rapid access to the service in the cohort of patients that would most benefit from this procedure.[21,39,40]

20.3 Companion Case

A companion case of a 60-year-old patient with osteoporosis and painful bilateral sacral insufficiency fractures is presented in ▶ Fig. 20.7, ▶ Fig. 20.8, ▶ Fig. 20.9, ▶ Fig. 20.10, ▶ Fig. 20.11, ▶ Fig. 20.12, and ▶ Fig. 20.13.

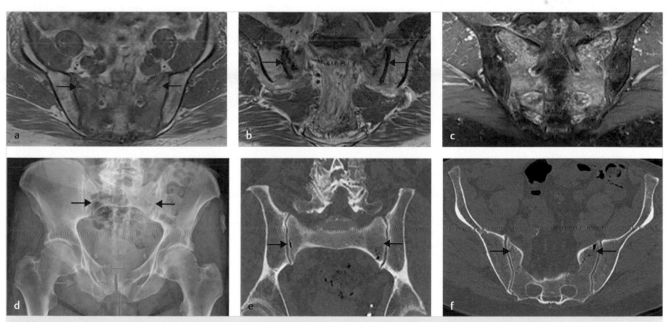

Fig. 20.7 A 60-year-old patient with osteoporosis and painful bilateral sacral insufficiency fractures seen as T1-weighted, low-signal linear lines on axial (**a**) and coronal-oblique (**b**) magnetic resonance imaging (MRI) images. Extensive sacral edema is seen bilaterally on STIRWI (**c**) sequences. Anteroposterior (AP) pelvic radiograph (**d**) demonstrates the fractures (red arrows) as well as further right superior and inferior pubic rami fractures (blue arrows). The sacral fractures are delineated on coronal (**e**) and axial (**f**) computed tomography (CT) with gas within the fracture margins (red arrows), consistent with ex-vacuo phenomenon compatible with fracture movement denoting instability.

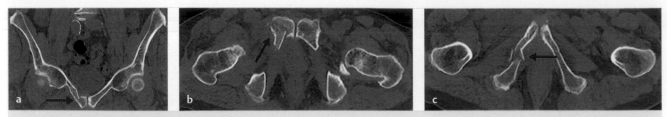

Fig. 20.8 Coronal (**a**) and axial (**b**) reformatted computed tomography (CT) images delineate the superior pubic rami fractures. A mildly displaced fracture of the inferior pubic ramus is also present (**c**).

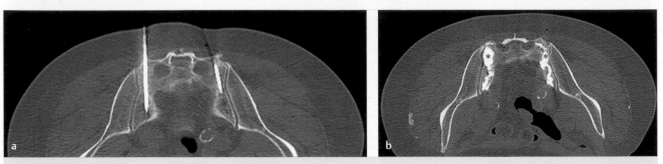

Fig. 20.9 Bilateral computed tomography (CT)-guided percutaneous sacroplasty was performed (**a**), with satisfactory fracture cement (*) filling (**b**).

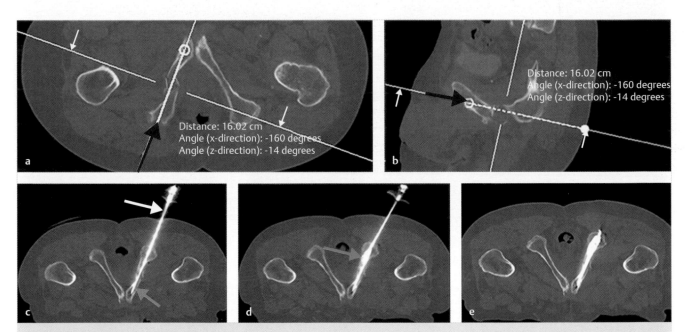

Fig. 20.10 Ischioplasty with cement-reinforced Kirschner (K) wire insertion in the same session to reduce the inferior pubic ramus fracture. Preplanning computed tomography (CT) with multiplanar reformatting (**a** and **b**) is performed with trajectory planning (red arrows). A K-wire (blue arrow) is fed through the vertebroplasty trocar (white arrow) across the fracture site (**c**). Thereafter, cementation (green arrow) is performed (**d**). Postprocedure CT demonstrates fracture reduction and cement reinforcement with K-wire (**e**).

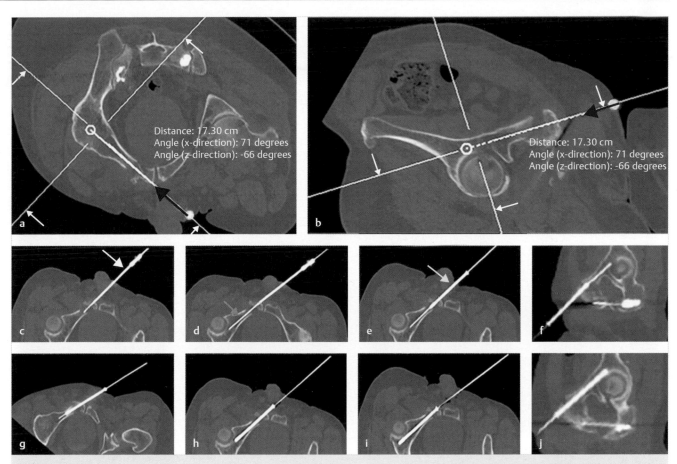

Fig. 20.11 Subsequently, ramoplasty was performed. Trajectory planning (red arrows) with preprocedure computed tomography (CT) (**a, b**). Once purchased into bone, the trocar (white arrow) allows K-wire (blue arrow) insertion and provides stability as it transgresses the superior pubic ramus fracture (**c, d**). A long, augmented screw (yellow arrow) replaces the trocar and is gradually passed along the wire (**e–j**) under intermittent low-dose CT, reducing the fracture.

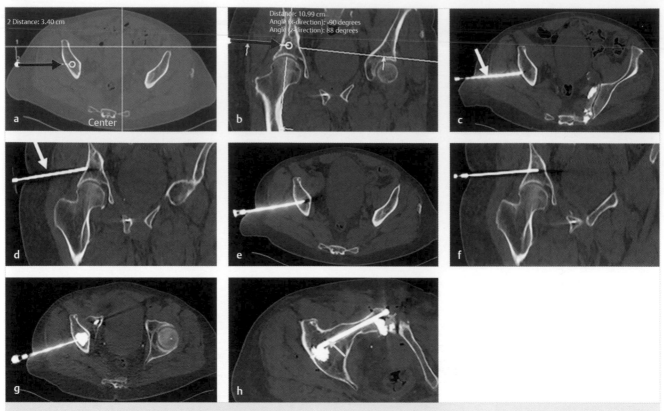

Fig. 20.12 Ilioplasty was performed to reinforce the distal aspect of the ramoplasty screw. Trajectory planning (red arrows) with preprocedure computed tomography (CT) (**a**, **b**). The trocar (white arrow) is advanced to the preplanned site (**c–f**). Cement is injected (**g**) to reinforce (**h**) the distal ramus screw (yellow arrow) as well as the proximal aspect of the screw concomitantly (blue arrow).

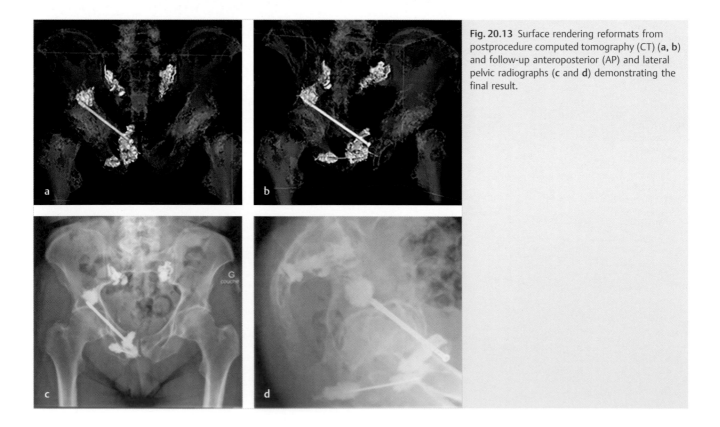

Fig. 20.13 Surface rendering reformats from postprocedure computed tomography (CT) (**a**, **b**) and follow-up anteroposterior (AP) and lateral pelvic radiographs (**c** and **d**) demonstrating the final result.

References

[1] Boortz-Marx RL. Atlas of interventional pain management. Mayo Clin Proc. 1999; 74(7):747

[2] Bydon M, De la Garza-Ramos R, Macki M, Desai A, Gokaslan AK, Bydon A. Incidence of sacral fractures and in-hospital postoperative complications in the United States: an analysis of 2002–2011 data. Spine. 2014; 39(18): E1103–E1109

[3] Rodrigues-Pinto R, Kurd MF, Schroeder GD, et al. Sacral fractures and associated injuries. Global Spine J. 2017; 7(7):609–616

[4] Denis F, Davis S, Comfort T. Sacral fractures: an important problem. Retrospective analysis of 236 cases. Clin Orthop Relat Res. 1988; 227(227): 67–81

[5] Bellabarba C, Schroeder GD, Kepler CK, et al. The AOSpine sacral fracture classification. Glob Spine J. 2017; 6 1_suppl:s-0036-1582696-s-0036-1582696

[6] Lourie H. Spontaneous osteoporotic fracture of the sacrum: an unrecognized syndrome of the elderly. JAMA. 1982; 248(6):715–717

[7] Peh WCG, Khong PL, Sham JST, Ho WY, Yeung HWD. Sacral and pubic insufficiency fractures after irradiation of gynaecological malignancies. Clin Oncol (R Coll Radiol). 1995; 7(2):117–122

[8] Park S-H, Kim J-C, Lee J-E, Park I-K. Pelvic insufficiency fracture after radiotherapy in patients with cervical cancer in the era of PET/CT. Radiat Oncol J. 2011; 29(4):269–276

[9] Agarwal MG, Nayak P. Management of skeletal metastases: an orthopaedic surgeon's guide. Indian J Orthop. 2015; 49(1):83–100

[10] Lyders EM, Whitlow CT, Baker MD, Morris PP. Imaging and treatment of sacral insufficiency fractures. AJNR Am J Neuroradiol. 2010; 31(2):201–210

[11] Cabarrus MC, Ambekar A, Lu Y, Link TM. MRI and CT of insufficiency fractures of the pelvis and the proximal femur. AJR Am J Roentgenol. 2008; 191(4): 995–1001

[12] Papakonstantinou O, Isaac A, Dalili D, Noebauer-Huhmann IM. T2-weighted hypointense tumors and tumor-like lesions. Semin Musculoskelet Radiol. 2019; 23(1):58–75

[13] Fujii M, Abe K, Hayashi K, et al. Honda sign and variants in patients suspected of having a sacral insufficiency fracture. Clin Nucl Med. 2005; 30(3):165–169

[14] Halawi MJ. Pelvic ring injuries: surgical management and long-term outcomes. J Clin Orthop Trauma. 2016; 7(1):1–6

[15] Dehdashti AR, Martin JB, Jean B, Rüfenacht DA. PMMA cementoplasty in symptomatic metastatic lesions of the S1 vertebral body. Cardiovasc Interv Radiol. 2000; 23(3):235–237

[16] Cazzato RL, De Marini P, Leonard-Lorant I, et al. Percutaneous thermal ablation of sacral metastases: assessment of pain relief and local tumor control. Diagn Interv Imaging. 2021; 102(6):355–361

[17] De Marini P, Cazzato RL, Auloge P, et al. Percutaneous image-guided thermal ablation of bone metastases: a retrospective propensity study comparing the safety profile of radio-frequency ablation and cryo-ablation. Int J Hyperthermia. 2020; 37(1):1386–1394

[18] Cazzato RL, Auloge P, De Marini P, et al. Spinal tumor ablation: indications, techniques, and clinical management. Tech Vasc Interv Radiol. 2020; 23(2): 100677

[19] Dalili D, Isaac A, Bazzocchi A, et al. Interventional techniques for bone and musculoskeletal soft tissue tumors: current practices and future directions - Part I. Ablation. Semin Musculoskelet Radiol. 2020; 24(6):692–709

[20] Dalili D, Isaac A, Cazzato RL, et al. Interventional techniques for bone and musculoskeletal soft tissue tumors: current practices and future directions - Part II. Stabilization. Semin Musculoskelet Radiol. 2020; 24(6): 710–725

[21] Cazzato RL, Garnon J, De Marini P, et al. French multidisciplinary approach for the treatment of MSK tumors. Semin Musculoskelet Radiol. 2020; 24(3):310–322

[22] Garnon J, Meylheuc L, Auloge P, et al. Continuous injection of large volumes of cement through a single 10G vertebroplasty needle in cases of large osteolytic lesions. Cardiovasc Intervent Radiol. 2020; 43(4):658–661

[23] Cazzato RL, de Marini P, Auloge P, et al. Percutaneous vertebroplasty of the cervical spine performed via a posterior trans-pedicular approach. Eur Radiol. 2021; 31(2):591–598

[24] Garnon J, Meylheuc L, De Marini P, et al. Subjective analysis of the filling of an acetabular osteolytic lesion following percutaneous cementoplasty: is it reliable? Cardiovasc Intervent Radiol. 2020; 43(3):445–452

[25] Smith DK, Dix JE. Percutaneous sacroplasty: long-axis injection technique. AJR Am J Roentgenol. 2006; 186(5):1252–1255

[26] Katsanos K, Sabharwal T, Adam A. Percutaneous cementoplasty. Semin Intervent Radiol. 2010; 27(2):137–147

[27] Bayley E, Srinivas S, Boszczyk BM. Clinical outcomes of sacroplasty in sacral insufficiency fractures: a review of the literature. Eur Spine J. 2009; 18(9): 1266–1271

[28] Autrusseau PA, Garnon J, Bertucci G, et al. Complications of percutaneous image-guided screw fixation: An analysis of 94 consecutive patients. Diagn Interv Imaging. 2021;102(6):347-353.

[29] Autrusseau P-A, Heidelberg D, Stacoffe N, et al. Percutaneous image-guided anterior screw fixation of the odontoid process. Cardiovasc Intervent Radiol. 2021; 44(4):647–653

[30] Garnon J, Auloge P, Dalili D, Koch G, Cazzato RL, Gangi A. Combined percutaneous screw fixation and cementoplasty of the odontoid process. J Vasc Interv Radiol. 2019; 30(10):1667–1669

[31] Khandaker M, Meng Z. The effect of nanoparticles and alternative monomer on the exothermic temperature of PMMA bone cement. Procedia Eng. 2015; 105:946–952

[32] Cazzato RL, Palussière J, Auloge P, et al. Complications following percutaneous image-guided radiofrequency ablation of bone tumors: a 10-year dual-center experience. Radiology. 2020; 296(1):227–235

[33] Chandra V, Wajswol E, Shukla P, Contractor S, Kumar A. Safety and efficacy of sacroplasty for sacral fractures: a systematic review and meta-analysis. J Vasc Interv Radiol. 2019; 30(11):1845–1854

[34] Andresen, R., Radmer, S., Lüdtke, C.W., Kamusella, P., Wissgott, C. and Schober, H.C. (2014) Balloon Sacroplasty as a Palliative Pain Treatment in Patients with Metastasis-Induced Bone Destruction and Pathological Fractures. Rofo, 186, 881–886.

[35] Garnon J, Doré B, Auloge P, et al. Efficacy of the vertebral body stenting system for the restoration of vertebral height in acute traumatic compression fractures in a non-osteoporotic population. Cardiovasc Intervent Radiol. 2019; 42(11):1579–1587

[36] Interventional Neuroradiology of the Spine: Clinical Features, Diagnosis and Therapy. Muto Mario. 2013. Muto Mario (Ed) Springer.

[37] Frey ME, Depalma MJ, Cifu DX, Bhagia SM, Carne W, Daitch JS. Percutaneous sacroplasty for osteoporotic sacral insufficiency fractures: a prospective, multicenter, observational pilot study. Spine J. 2008; 8(2):367–373

[38] Frey ME, Warner C, Thomas SM, et al. Sacroplasty: a ten-year analysis of prospective patients treated with percutaneous sacroplasty: literature review and technical considerations. Pain Physician. 2017; 20(7):E1063–E1072

[39] Dalili D, Isaac A, Rashidi A, Åström G, Fritz J. Image-guided sports medicine and musculoskeletal tumor interventions: a patient-centered model. Semin Musculoskelet Radiol. 2020; 24(3):290–309

[40] Cazzato RL, Garnon J, Koch G, et al. Musculoskeletal interventional oncology: current and future practices. Br J Radiol. 2020; 93(1115):20200465

21 Benign Lesions of the Spine I—Aneurysmal Bone Cysts

Danoob Dalili, Daniel E. Dalili, Amanda Isaac, and Jan Fritz

21.1 Case Presentation

A 9-year-old boy presented with significant back pain (visual analog scale [VAS] = 8/10), which was gradually increasing in severity. He also had lower leg weakness. Magnetic resonance imaging (MRI) study was performed which demonstrated an aneurysmal bone cyst (ABC) at T12 (▶ Fig. 21.1). Following discussion at the multidisciplinary tumor board, a computed tomography (CT)-guided biopsy of the lesion was performed.

21.2 Discussion

First described by Jaffe et al in 1942, ABCs are expansive benign osteolytic tumors with blood-filled cystic cavities.[1] Although occasionally aggressive in nature, causing bone disruption and impacting upon surrounding tissues, they very rarely transform into malignant tumors. They may occur as primary neoplasms or secondary lesions adjacent to osteoblastomas, chondroblastomas, chondromyxoid fibromas, nonossifying fibromas, and giant cell tumors.[2,3] They typically (80%) present in the first two decades of life, and have an incidence of 1.4/100,000, constituting 1% of all benign bone tumors.[4,5] ABCs have a predilection for long bone metaphysis[6] and the posterior elements of the spine, but they may also originate in the pelvis, sacrum, clavicle, feet, and fingers. Tumor diagnosis and decision on management strategies are based on clinical, radiological, and histological evaluations.[7,8,9,10]

21.3 Clinical Presentation

ABCs typically cause locoregional pain and swelling. They can disrupt the mechanical integrity of bone resulting in inherent bone weakness and pathological fractures.[11] Symptoms depend on the location of the tumor; and in the spine as demonstrated in the case presented above, the tumor can induce local mass effect with neurological deficit due to cord or nerve root compression.[12] When the tumor affects growth plates, ABCs may cause limb deformity and length discrepancies.[13,14,15]

21.4 Imaging Findings

Plain film radiographs are the preferred initial imaging modality.[16] ABCs will typically appear as expansile, well-circumscribed radiolucent cystic lesions with a thin layer of overlying cortical bone.[17] Due to distorted trabeculations within the lesion, they may have a multiloculated matrix dubbed as "soap bubble."[18] Although plain films can be used to identify the presence of a lesion, they may not fully characterize it, particularly its extent, cortical breach, or involvement of surrounding neurovascular structures. Therefore, further cross-sectional imaging (CT and MRI) is indicated. CT can

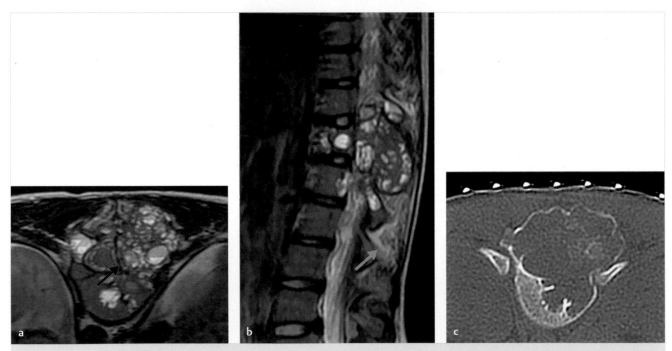

Fig. 21.1 (a–c) Axial and sagittal T2-weighted magnetic resonance (MR) sequences demonstrate a large expansile, multiloculated bone lesion centered on T12, predominantly demonstrating fluid-fluid levels throughout its matrix. The lesion is centered on the posterior elements, extending anteriorly into the vertebral body of T12 and L1 and in a craniocaudal direction from T11 to L1, while displacing and compressing the thoracic cord (**a**, red arrow). There is no radiological evidence of myelomalacia. The lesion is low signal on T1 with thinning of the cortices. There is extensive high T2 signal in the paraspinal muscles representing reactive edema (**b**, blue arrow). (**c**) Intraprocedural computed tomography (CT) confirmed cortical thinning, and disruption of the posterior cortex of the T12 vertebral body, delineating more accurately the extent of bone destruction and remodeling.

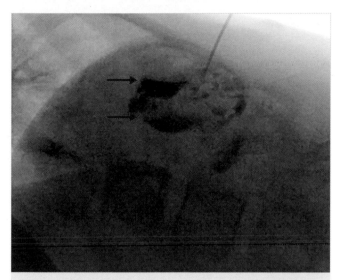

Fig. 21.2 Fluoroscopic-guided percutaneous injection of 4 mL of contrast agent (Omnipaque™ 270, GE Healthcare, USA) to exclude any communication with draining veins (particularly spinal) and the integrity of the thinned cortex displacing the thoracic cord. Note the fluid-fluid levels (red arrows). Once the absence of intradural leak was established, detergent sclerosant (STS) foam was created utilizing the Tessari method,[47] after which it was injected under continuous fluoroscopic monitoring.

demarcate the shape and size of the osseous borders of the lesion and may also identify fluid-fluid levels.[19] MRI will characterize the underlying soft tissue changes, identifying layering of blood of varying densities within the cyst, revealing internal septations and surrounding edema.[20] In addition, the mechanical impact on surrounding structures including the neurovascular structures, spinal cord, muscles, and epidural space can be elicited by MRI. The cystic components are classically demonstrated as hypointense on T1- and hyperintense on T2-weighted images.[21,22] A study by Mahnken et al demonstrated that, compared to each modality in isolation, using radiographs and MRI in combination improved the rate of accurate diagnosis.[23] Many of the characteristics of ABCs on imaging overlap with other lesions such as unicameral bone cysts, telangiectatic osteosarcoma (TOS), osteoblastomas, and giant cell tumors among others. For this reason, histological confirmation is paramount in the diagnosis of ABCs as with other tumors.

21.5 Histologic Findings

Macroscopically, ABCs are typically spongy, hemorrhagic masses encased in a thin shell of reactive bone. On microscopic analysis, red blood cells and brown hemosiderin are most commonly found. Within the cyst spaces, fibroblasts, mitotically active spindle cells, calcifications, and multinucleated giant cells can be visualized on histology.[24] While imaging modalities show overlap in conditions such as TOS and ABCs, high-power histological evaluation can show high-grade malignant sarcomatous cells along the periphery in TOS which are absent in ABCs.[25] The main method of obtaining these samples is incisional biopsy, which has been found to be preferable to fine-needle aspiration biopsy.[26,27]

21.6 Treatment Strategies

21.6.1 Surgical Treatments

Historically, ABCs were managed by surgical excision, curettage or resection, radiotherapy, and/or radionucleotide ablation.[28] En bloc excision was very common as it had low recurrence rates, but overall there were significant residual morbidities such as postoperative pain, limb length discrepancies, muscle weakness, and decreased function.[29] Resection of spinal ABCs can result in kyphoscoliosis, infection, and worsening of spinal cord compression.[30] As a result, despite reported success rates of 95 to 100% for localized control of the ABC,[31,32] surgical excision has become less commonly used and is typically reserved for recurrent lesions that are refractory to other treatments.

The current standard of care management of ABCs is open or endoscopic curettage with or without bone graft. With open procedures, there is a significant chance of excessive soft tissue damage[33] and growth disturbances when in close proximity to a physeal plate. Local control of ABCs has been reported to be up to 90% in high-speed burr augmented curettage, and endoscopic curettage has largely replaced open procedures.

21.6.2 Radiation Therapy

Although radiotherapy using external beam radiation to induce cellular death was used sparingly in the past due to risk of inducing sarcomatous transformation,[34] new advances in radiotherapeutic techniques have achieved successful treatment (100%) with no complications.[35]

21.6.3 Interventional Radiologic Treatments

Aneurysmal bone cysts may also be treated percutaneously with image-guided cryoablation. This procedure has been validated as a safe, effective, and viable management strategy for ABCs and other musculoskeletal tumors including low-flow vascular malformations and osteoblastomas.[36,37,38]

Due to wide variability in long-term results, a number of adjuvant treatments have been used to reduce recurrence rates after curettage. These include phenol sclerotherapy,[39] bone cement injection,[31] and argon beam cryotherapy.[40,41] Selective transarterial embolization is another technique that has been used both as a stand-alone treatment and combined with surgical resection to provide better outcomes.[42]

21.6.4 Sclerotherapy

Sclerotherapy Procedure

Over the last decade, sclerotherapy has emerged as one of the preferred techniques for treating ABCs. It is performed under fluoroscopic or CT guidance, whereby the lesion is punctured with a needle (16 to 22 G) and aspiration is performed to confirm correct needle positioning.[43] Instead of CT, which exposes the patient to ionizing radiation, MRI guidance can be especially valuable in pediatric patients.[36,44] After puncture, contrast is injected into the cystic cavity (► Fig. 21.2) to help identify the borders of the lesion and establish extension into other

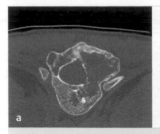
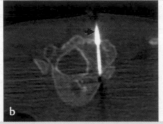
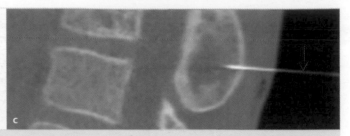

Fig. 21.3 Axial computed tomography (CT) at 3-month follow-up (**a**) demonstrates reduction of the cystic volume and progressive osseous consolidation with sclerosis and thickening of the cortex of the left pedicle (compare with ▶ Fig. 21.1c). Subsequent axial CT-guided sclerotherapy (**b**) utilizing a 14-gauge bone biopsy needle (red arrow) at 6 months follow-up. Note the further bony remodeling and reduction in the size of the lesion. Sagittal reformat of percutaneous CT-guided sclerotherapy of the residual spinous process component in the same patient at 9 months follow-up (**c**). Given the extent of the lesion in such a young patient, five total treatment cycles of sclerotherapy were performed over the course of 9 months.

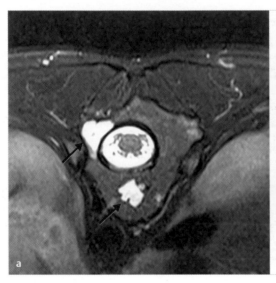
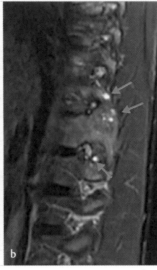

Fig. 21.4 Axial (**a**) and sagittal (**b**) Short tau inversion recovery (STIR) weighted magnetic resonance (MR) sequences at annual follow-up magnetic resonance imaging (MRI) of the aneurysmal bone cyst (ABC) 2 years post-procedure. (**a**) Two tiny residual "cystic" tumoral foci (**a**, red arrows) are seen. There was almost complete obliteration of the tumor, with minimal microcystic foci (**b**, blue arrows) in the remodeled enlarged left pedicle (**b**). The patient's pain largely resolved with occasional mechanical pain (VAS = 1) on exertion and playing sports.

structures, particularly large draining veins.[45] This is of particular importance in the spine, where it is crucial to confirm cortical integrity in order to prevent intradural or intravascular leakage of sclerosant into the spinal arteries (▶ Fig. 21.2). After exclusion of extraosseous leakage, the sclerosing agent is injected through the needle into the lesion. Often multiple injections are required at intervals of approximately 4 weeks to attain the desired effect while allowing time for bone remodeling (▶ Fig. 21.3).[46] In the authors' practice, a dedicated process for sclerotherapy utilizing sodium tetradecyl sulfate (STS) with repeat MRI at 3, 6, and 12 months postprocedure has been adopted. Long-term surveillance protocols depend on local practice and patient symptoms (▶ Fig. 21.4).

Alternative Sclerosants

There are a variety of available sclerosants, which have been increasing in number since their introduction in the 1920s. The prevailing detergent sclerosants that are used presently are doxycycline, hydroxy polyethoxydodecane (Polidocanol/POL), and STS. The mechanism of action of a sclerosant is determined by the coagulation cascade. Sclerosants cause endothelial damage by decreasing endothelial cell surface tension, interfering with cell surface lipids, disrupting intercellular adhesion, and extracting cell surface proteins.[48] Doxycycline has been reported to be successful in up to 94% of cases; this is due to its ability to inhibit matrix metalloproteinases and angiogenesis, resulting in healing of the ABC.[49] POL is a compound first used as an anesthetic in 1936. In the United Kingdom, it is currently the most commonly used sclerosant, mostly due to its ability to sclerose target areas without significant damage to surrounding tissues.[43] STS is a long chain fatty acid that has proven to be very useful as a sclerosing agent in ABCs and varicose veins alike.[50] Ethibloc is an alcohol-based fibrosing and sclerosing agent that has also shown favorable long-term outcomes in treating ABCs. Despite this, its use in sclerotherapy has diminished significantly due to high occurrence of inflammatory reactions (94%) and risk of pulmonary embolism, deep vein thrombosis, necrosis, and cerebellar infarction.[5,51] There has been at least one reported death of a 4-year-old child due to a vertebrobasilar system infarct after Ethibloc injection into a C2 ABC.[52]

Detergents often need to be administered in sufficient concentration to ensure adequate sclerosis; however, increasing concentrations may result in downstream effects and extravasation of sclerosing agents into undesirable nontargeted tissues.

Delivery of the sclerosants as foam reduces the rate of complications by delivering the chemical components in a more controlled physical form and allowing better coverage of the tumors from within, thereby targeting a larger area of the tumor in each session. Currently, doxycycline and STS can be reliably delivered as foam using the Tessari method.[47]

There is no unified consensus on a single sclerosant that would replace all others, and further studies are required. However, when performed safely in a high-volume center sclerotherapy has excellent short- and long-term outcomes with minimal side effects, thereby providing rapid and enduring relief of symptoms in young patients presenting with incapacitating manifestations of ABCs.

References

[1] Jaffe HL, Lichtenstein L. Solitary unicameral bone cyst: with emphasis on the roentgen picture, the pathologic appearance and the pathogenesis. Arch Surg. 1942; 44(6):1004–1025

[2] Bonakdarpour A, Levy WM, Aegerter E. Primary and secondary aneurysmal bone cyst: a radiological study of 75 cases. Radiology. 1978; 126(1):75–83

[3] Martinez V, Sissons HA. Aneurysmal bone cyst. A review of 123 cases including primary lesions and those secondary to other bone pathology. Cancer. 1988; 61(11):2291–2304

[4] Leithner A, Windhager R, Lang S, Haas OA, Kainberger F, Kotz R. Aneurysmal bone cyst. A population based epidemiologic study and literature review. Clin Orthop Relat Res. 1999(363):176–179

[5] Topouchian V, Mazda K, Hamze B, Laredo JD, Penneçot GF. Aneurysmal bone cysts in children: complications of fibrosing agent injection. Radiology. 2004; 232(2):522–526

[6] Dubois J, Chigot V, Grimard G, Isler M, Garel L. Sclerotherapy in aneurysmal bone cysts in children: a review of 17 cases. Pediatr Radiol. 2003; 33(6):365–372

[7] Dalili D, Isaac A, Bazzocchi A, et al. Interventional techniques for bone and musculoskeletal soft tissue tumors: current practices and future directions - Part I. Ablation. Semin Musculoskelet Radiol. 2020; 24(6):692–709

[8] Dalili D, Isaac A, Cazzato RL, et al. Interventional techniques for bone and musculoskeletal soft tissue tumors: current practices and future directions—Part II. Stabilization. Semin Musculoskelet Radiol. 2020; 24(6):710–725

[9] Cazzato RL, Garnon J, De Marini P, et al. French multidisciplinary approach for the treatment of MSK tumors. Semin Musculoskelet Radiol. 2020; 24(3):310–322

[10] Dalili D, Isaac A, Rashidi A, Åström G, Fritz J. Image-guided sports medicine and musculoskeletal tumor interventions: a patient-centered model. Semin Musculoskelet Radiol. 2020; 24(3):290–309

[11] Burch S, Hu S, Berven S. Aneurysmal bone cysts of the spine. Neurosurg Clin N Am. 2008; 19(1):41–47

[12] Novais EN, Rose PS, Yaszemski MJ, Sim FH. Aneurysmal bone cyst of the cervical spine in children. J Bone Joint Surg Am. 2011; 93(16):1534–1543

[13] Capanna R, Springfield DS, Biagini R, Ruggieri P, Giunti A. Juxtaepiphyseal aneurysmal bone cyst. Skeletal Radiol. 1985; 13(1):21–25

[14] McCarthy SM, Ogden JA. Epiphyseal extension of an aneurysmal bone cyst. J Pediatr Orthop. 1982; 2(2):171–175

[15] Rizzo M, Dellaero DT, Harrelson JM, Scully SP. Juxtaphyseal aneurysmal bone cysts. Clin Orthop Relat Res. 1999(364):205–212

[16] Lalam R, Bloem JL, Noebauer-Huhmann IM, et al. ESSR consensus document for detection, characterization, and referral pathway for tumors and tumorlike lesions of bone. Semin Musculoskelet Radiol. 2017; 21(5):630–647

[17] Boubbou M, Atarraf K, Chater L, Afifi A, Tizniti S. Aneurysmal bone cyst primary—about eight pediatric cases: radiological aspects and review of the literature. Pan Afr Med J. 2013; 15(Jul):111

[18] Kuna S, Gudena R. "Soap bubble" in the calcaneus. CMAJ. 2011; 183(10):1171

[19] Tsai JC, Dalinka MK, Fallon MD, Zlatkin MB, Kressel HY. Fluid-fluid level: a nonspecific finding in tumors of bone and soft tissue. Radiology. 1990; 175(3):779–782

[20] Revel MP, Vanel D, Sigal R, et al. Aneurysmal bone cysts of the jaws: CT and MR findings. J Comput Assist Tomogr. 1992; 16(1):84–86

[21] Beluffi G. Imaging in percutaneous musculoskeletal interventions. Radiol Med. 2010; 115:499–500

[22] Papakonstantinou O, Isaac A, Dalili D, Noebauer-Huhmann IM. T2-weighted hypointense tumors and tumor-like lesions. Semin Musculoskelet Radiol. 2019; 23(1):58–75

[23] Mahnken AH, Nolte-Ernsting CCA, Wildberger JE, et al. Aneurysmal bone cyst: value of MR imaging and conventional radiography. Eur Radiol. 2003; 13(5):1118–1124

[24] Hoda SA, Hoda RS. Robbins and Cotran pathologic basis of disease. Adv Anat Pathol. 2005; 12:103

[25] Murphey MD, wan Jaovisidha S, Temple HT, Gannon FH, Jelinek JS, Malawer MM. Telangiectatic osteosarcoma: radiologic-pathologic comparison. Radiology. 2003; 229(2):545–553

[26] Creager AJ, Madden CR, Bergman S, Geisinger KR. Aneurysmal bone cyst: fine-needle aspiration findings in 23 patients with clinical and radiologic correlation. Am J Clin Pathol. 2007; 128(5):740–745

[27] Layfield LJ, Armstrong K, Zaleski S, Eckardt J. Diagnostic accuracy and clinical utility of fine-needle aspiration cytology in the diagnosis of clinically primary bone lesions. Diagn Cytopathol. 1993; 9(2):168–173

[28] Park HY, Yang SK, Sheppard WL, et al. Current management of aneurysmal bone cysts. Curr Rev Musculoskelet Med. 2016; 9(4):435–444

[29] Flont P, Kolacinska-Flont M, Niedzielski K. A comparison of cyst wall curettage and en bloc excision in the treatment of aneurysmal bone cysts. World J Surg Oncol. 2013; 11:109

[30] Mesfin A, McCarthy EF, Kebaish KM. Surgical treatment of aneurysmal bone cysts of the spine. Iowa Orthop J. 2012; 32:40–45

[31] Mankin HJ, Hornicek FJ, Ortiz-Cruz E, Villafuerte J, Gebhardt MC. Aneurysmal bone cyst: a review of 150 patients. J Clin Oncol. 2005; 23(27):6756–6762

[32] Vergel De Dios AM, Bond JR, Shives TC, McLeod RA, Unni KK. Aneurysmal bone cyst. A clinicopathologic study of 238 cases. Cancer. 1992; 69(12):2921–2931

[33] Aiba H, Kobayashi M, Waguri-Nagaya Y, et al. Treatment of aneurysmal bone cysts using endoscopic curettage. BMC Musculoskelet Disord. 2018; 19(1):268

[34] Papagelopoulos PJ, Currier BL, Shaughnessy WJ, et al. Aneurysmal bone cyst of the spine. Management and outcome. Spine. 1998; 23(5):621–628

[35] Zhu S, Hitchcock KE, Mendenhall WM. Radiation therapy for aneurysmal bone cysts. Am J Clin Oncol. 2017; 40(6):621–624

[36] Fritz J, Sonnow L, Morris CD. Adjuvant MRI-guided percutaneous cryoablation treatment for aneurysmal bone cyst. Skeletal Radiol. 2019; 48(7):1149–1153

[37] Autrusseau P-A, Cazzato RL, De Marini P, et al. Percutaneous MR-guided cryoablation of low-flow vascular malformation: technical feasibility, safety and clinical efficacy. Cardiovasc Intervent Radiol. 2020; 43(6):858–865

[38] Cazzato RL, Auloge P, Dalili D, et al. Percutaneous image-guided cryoablation of osteoblastoma. AJR Am J Roentgenol. 2019; 213(5):1157–1162

[39] Capanna R, Sudanese A, Baldini N, Campanacci M. Phenol as an adjuvant in the control of local recurrence of benign neoplasms of bone treated by curettage. Ital J Orthop Traumatol. 1985; 11(3):381–388

[40] Cummings JE, Smith RA, Heck RK , Jr. Argon beam coagulation as adjuvant treatment after curettage of aneurysmal bone cysts: a preliminary study. Clin Orthop Relat Res. 2010; 468(1):231–237

[41] Schreuder HWB, Veth RPH, Pruszczynski M, Lemmens JAM, Koops HS, Molenaar WM. Aneurysmal bone cysts treated by curettage, cryotherapy and bone grafting. J Bone Joint Surg Br. 1997; 79(1):20–25

[42] Rossi G, Rimondi E, Bartalena T, et al. Selective arterial embolization of 36 aneurysmal bone cysts of the skeleton with N-2-butyl cyanoacrylate. Skeletal Radiol. 2010; 39(2):161–167

[43] Rastogi S, Varshney MK, Trikha V, Khan SA, Choudhury B, Safaya R. Treatment of aneurysmal bone cysts with percutaneous sclerotherapy using polidocanol. A review of 72 cases with long-term follow-up. J Bone Joint Surg Br. 2006; 88(9):1212–1216

[44] Sequeiros RB, Sinikumpu JJ, Ojala R, Järvinen J, Fritz J. Pediatric musculoskeletal interventional MRI. Top Magn Reson Imaging. 2018; 27(1):39–44

[45] Mascard E, Gomez-Brouchet A, Lambot K. Bone cysts: unicameral and aneurysmal bone cyst. Orthop Traumatol Surg Res. 2015; 101(1) Suppl:S119–S127

[46] Brosjö O, Pechon P, Hesla A, Tsagozis P, Bauer H. Sclerotherapy with polidocanol for treatment of aneurysmal bone cysts. Acta Orthop. 2013; 84(5):502–505

[47] Tessari L, Cavezzi A, Frullini A. Preliminary experience with a new sclerosing foam in the treatment of varicose veins. Dermatol Surg. 2001; 27(1):58–60

[48] Duffy DM. Sclerosants: a comparative review. Dermatol Surg. 2010; 36 Suppl 2:1010–1025

[49] Shiels WE , II, Beebe AC, Mayerson JL. Percutaneous doxycycline treatment of juxtaphyseal aneurysmal bone cysts. J Pediatr Orthop. 2016; 36(2):205–212

[50] Dalili D, Parker J, Mirzaian A, et al. Aneurysmal bone cysts in the spine, causing neurological compromise: safety and clinical efficacy of sclerotherapy utilizing sodium tetradecyl sulfate (STS) foam. Skeletal Radiol. 2021; 50(12):2433–2447

[51] Falappa P, Fassari FM, Fanelli A, et al. Aneurysmal bone cysts: treatment with direct percutaneous Ethibloc injection: long-term results. Cardiovasc Intervent Radiol. 2002; 25(4):282–290

[52] Peraud A, Drake JM, Armstrong D, Hedden D, Babyn P, Wilson G. Fatal ethibloc embolization of vertebrobasilar system following percutaneous injection into aneurysmal bone cyst of the second cervical vertebra. AJNR Am J Neuroradiol. 2004; 25(6):1116–1120

22 Benign Lesions of the Spine II: Hemangiomas

Alexis Kelekis and Dimitrios Filippiadis

22.1 Case Presentation

A 61-year-old woman arrived at the hospital reporting back pain and bilateral leg numbness. The patient was taking non-steroidal anti-inflammatory drugs (NSAIDs) for pain relief, but still reported a pain score of 9/10 numeric visual scale (NVS) units. Neurological examination demonstrated significant sensory and motor deficit affecting both legs. The level of neurological finding was estimated in the lower lumbar spinal levels. Furthermore, local pain and tenderness were noted upon palpation of the lower lumbar spinous processes.

Magnetic resonance imaging (MRI) with contrast injection to the lumbar spine was performed, revealing a high-intensity signal lesion in the L4 vertebral body, highly suspicious of an aggressive hemangioma of the vertebral body with an epidural component (▶ Fig. 22.1).

The patient was referred to our radiology department for percutaneous image-guided treatment. Direct sclerotherapy by means of intraosseous ethanol injection combined with vertebroplasty was decided as the first-choice therapy. Fluoroscopy-guided percutaneous vertebroplasty of L4 was performed through a bilateral transpedicular approach. Once the trocars were just beyond the posterior vertebral wall, digital subtraction venography (DSV) of bone (intraosseous injection of a small amount of contrast medium) was performed to assess for arteriovenous communications. When it was confirmed that there was no arteriovenous fistulae, injection of 1 mL of pure ethanol mixed with contrast medium was performed from each side. A second venography was performed post alcohol injection to assess for contrast stagnation. Vertebroplasty was completed with polymethylmethacrylate (PMMA) injection inside the vertebral body through each access cannula (starting from the anterior third) and both pedicles (▶ Fig. 22.2).

Computed tomography (CT) scan on the following morning demonstrated a good result and lack of immediate complications. There was also stagnation of contrast medium and presence of air bubbles (arrow) inside the epidural component of the hemangioma (▶ Fig. 22.3).

Clinical examination the morning after vertebroplasty revealed a pain score of 1/10 NVS units (significant pain reduction

of 8 NVS units), largely due to the minor discomfort on the skin entry sites. The recovery period remained uneventful, and following overnight observation the patient was discharged home the following day. Follow-up at 6 months following vertebroplasty demonstrated significant regression of paresthesia in both legs.

22.2 Discussion

Vertebral hemangiomas are benign, sometimes fat filled, usually asymptomatic, and commonly reported as incidental findings in spine CT or MRI examinations.[1,2] Rarely (in 0.9–1.2% of patients), active vertebral hemangiomas (with contrast uptake) can present as a symptomatic lesion, causing pain and/or neurologic compromise.[1,2] Pain is usually associated in the presence of a pathologic fracture, while extraosseous extension, collapse of the vertebral body, and neurologic compromise are usually associated with cord compression. These characteristics are more often encountered with aggressive hemangiomas with an epidural component.[1] The interventional approach for symptomatic vertebral hemangiomas includes transarterial embolization (typically performed with liquid agents), percutaneous vertebroplasty, and sclerotherapy. Other approaches include radiotherapy and surgery.[3]

In 1984, Galibert and Deramond introduced percutaneous vertebroplasty into clinical practice, initially reporting on the treatment of a painful and aggressive vertebral body hemangioma in the cervical spine.[4] As far as vertebral hemangiomas are concerned, percutaneous vertebroplasty (with or without sclerotherapy) is indicated in symptomatic lesions (aggressive or not) with or without neurologic compromise.[5] Additionally in the literature there are reports describing the use of kyphoplasty as an alternative to vertebroplasty in the percutaneous management of symptomatic vertebral hemangiomas.[6,7]

During percutaneous vertebroplasty, the hemangioma and main vascular bed are filled with the PMMA cement, stabilizing the vertebral body, solidifying the fracture, and thrombosing the perivertebral component.[1,8] Whenever hemangiomas extend to the vertebral pedicles, an alteration of standard vertebroplasty

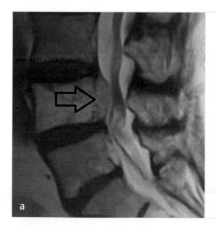
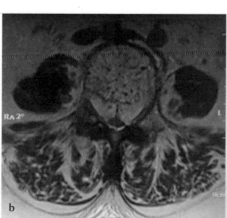

Fig. 22.1 T2-weighted sagittal (a) and axial (b) sequences revealing an L4 aggressive vertebral hemangioma with an epidural component (arrow). There is near-complete effacement of the thecal sac.

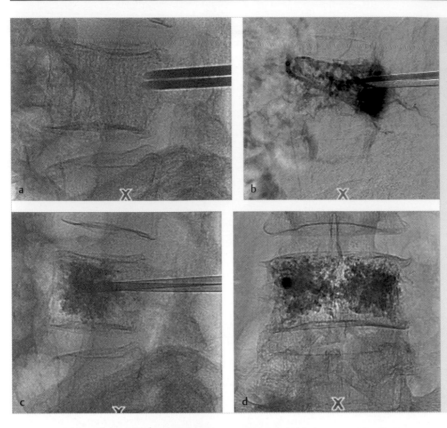

Fig. 22.2 (**a**) Lateral fluoroscopy view illustrating both trocars just beyond the posterior vertebral margin inside the vertebral body. (**b**) Lateral fluoroscopy view illustrating digital subtraction venography of bone at that level before alcohol injection. (**c**) Lateral fluoroscopy view during cement injection. (**d**) Posteroanterior (PA) fluoroscopy view illustrating satisfactory cement dispersion on both sides of the vertebral body extending from upper to lower end plate.

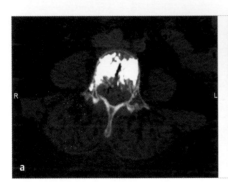
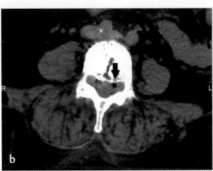

Fig. 22.3 Computed tomography axial scan evaluating osseous (**a**) and soft tissue (**b**) window cement dispersion inside the vertebral body and pedicles. There is a lack of extra-vertebral cement leakage, as well as stagnation of contrast medium and presence of air bubbles (arrow) inside the epidural component of the hemangioma.

may be necessary. Termed pediculoplasty, this technique involves injection of PMMA at the pedicular level and can be performed either with single- or double-needle technique.[9] Intralesional injection of ethanol results in devascularization and shrinkage of the lesion, with subsequent pressure reduction due to endothelial destruction and thrombosis of the vascular spaces.[1] Fluoroscopy with or without cone beam CT constitutes the ideal guidance method for this combination technique. In cases of intralesional sclerotherapy, direct contrast venography should be part of the protocol in order to exclude significant visualization of other systemic veins.

Combining percutaneous vertebroplasty and intralesional ethanol injection is a procedure that can be performed rapidly, within a total duration of less than 60 minutes. This procedure requires only a short hospital stay; patients are discharged the morning after the procedure, with a prophylactic short-course dose of oral cortisone for 6 days. Compared to surgery, the recovery from this percutaneous technique is faster and requires no rehabilitation.[8,9,10,11,12,13]

References

[1] Doppman JL, Oldfield EH, Heiss JD. Symptomatic vertebral hemangiomas: treatment by means of direct intralesional injection of ethanol. Radiology. 2000; 214(2):341–348

[2] Gabal AM. Percutaneous technique for sclerotherapy of vertebral hemangioma compressing spinal cord. Cardiovasc Intervent Radiol. 2002; 25 (6):494–500

[3] Kelekis A, Filippiadis DK, Martin JB, Kelekis NL. Aggressive vertebral hemangioma treated with combination of vertebroplasty and sclerotherapy through transpedicular and direct approach. Cardiovasc Intervent Radiol. 2014; 37(6):1638–1642

[4] Galibert P, Deramond H, Rosat P, Le Gars D. Note préliminaire sur le traitement des angiomes vertébraux par vertébroplastie acrylique percutanée [Preliminary note on the treatment of vertebral angioma by percutaneous acrylic vertebroplasty]. Neurochirurgie. 1987; 33(2):166–168

[5] Kelekis AD, Somon T, Yilmaz H, et al. Interventional spine procedures. Eur J Radiol. 2005; 55(3):362–383

[6] Moore JM, Poonnoose S, McDonald M. Kyphoplasty as a useful technique for complicated haemangiomas. J Clin Neurosci. 2012; 19(9):1291–1293

[7] Jones JO, Bruel BM, Vattam SR. Management of painful vertebral hemangiomas with kyphoplasty: a report of two cases and a literature review. Pain Physician. 2009; 12(4):E297–E303

[8] McAllister VL, Kendall BE, Bull JW. Symptomatic vertebral haemangiomas. Brain. 1975; 98(1):71–80

[9] Gailloud P, Beauchamp NJ, Martin JB, Murphy KJ. Percutaneous pediculoplasty: polymethylmethacrylate injection into lytic vertebral pedicle lesions. J Vasc Interv Radiol. 2002; 13(5):517–521

[10] Jian W. Symptomatic cervical vertebral hemangioma treated by percutaneous vertebroplasty. Pain Physician. 2013; 16(4):E419–E425

[11] Liu XW, Jin P, Wang LJ, Li M, Sun G. Vertebroplasty in the treatment of symptomatic vertebral haemangiomas without neurological deficit. Eur Radiol. 2013; 23(9):2575–2581

[12] Cianfoni A, Massari F, Dani G, et al. Percutaneous ethanol embolization and cement augmentation of aggressive vertebral hemangiomas at two adjacent vertebral levels. J Neuroradiol. 2014; 41(4):269–274

[13] Anselmetti GC, Bonaldi G, Carpeggiani P, Manfrè L, Masala S, Muto M. Vertebral augmentation: 7 years experience. Acta Neurochir Suppl (Wien). 2011; 108:147–161

23 Benign Lesions of the Spine III: Osteoblastoma

Nicholas Feinberg and Osman Ahmed

23.1 Case Presentation

A 17-year-old man with no significant past medical history presented with long-standing dull pain and aching in the lower neck. The pain was not relieved with nonsteroidal anti-inflammatory drugs (NSAIDs) or with rest at night. After radiographs demonstrated an abnormal finding, a noncontrast computed tomography (CT) of the cervical spine was obtained. This CT demonstrated a 1.9-cm mixed lucent and sclerotic lesion in the lateral body of C5 (▶ Fig. 23.1). The patient was evaluated by orthopedic oncology and offered both interventional and surgical approaches for treatment. The patient elected against surgery and interventional radiology (IR) consultation was obtained.

At consultation, the patient was offered concurrent CT-guided biopsy and radiofrequency ablation (RFA) for treatment. On the day of the procedure, general anesthesia was performed, and the patient was placed in the prone position. An 11-gauge introducer needle was placed into the target lesion and a coaxial bone biopsy was obtained. After biopsy, an RFA probe was placed, and three short burn cycles were performed (▶ Fig. 23.2). There were no immediate complications following the procedure; biopsy specimen revealed a diagnosis of osteoblastoma. The patient tolerated the procedure well, and at 1-month clinical follow-up reported resolution of symptoms.

23.2 Discussion

Osteoblastomas are rare, benign, bone-forming neoplasms with a predilection for the spine. They account for only 1 to 5% of all primary benign bone tumors, but account for 10% of primary osseous tumors of the spine.[1,2,3] Although first described in the English medical literature in 1932 by Jaffe and Mayer, they were likely originally characterized by Virchow in 1863.[4,5]

Osteoblastomas can occur at any point in a patient's life, but they primarily affect young males, with 80% of osteoblastomas occurring between the ages of 10 and 25 years.[6] They are two to three times more common in males than females.[6,7] Although they can affect any bone in the body, they are most frequently found (in 30 to 40% of cases) in the spine, particularly in the posterior elements of the spine.[1] Approximately 55% of osteoblastomas are entirely contained within the dorsal (posterior) elements, with approximately 40% extending from the dorsal elements into the adjacent vertebral body and fewer than 5%

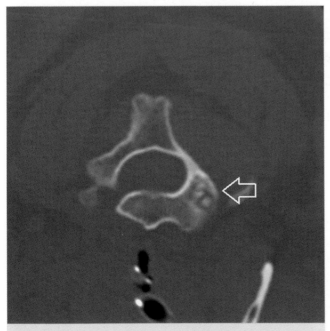

Fig. 23.1 Noncontrast computed tomography (CT) demonstrating a 1.9-cm lucent lesion mixed with matrix calcifications within the left lateral body of C5 (arrow). No cortical destruction or soft tissue extension was observed.

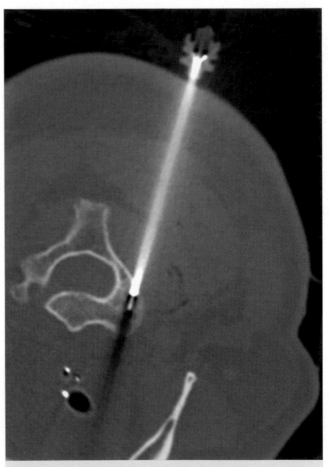

Fig. 23.2 Intraprocedural computed tomography (CT) image demonstrating the radiofrequency ablation (RFA) probe within the center of the lesion.

affecting the vertebral body alone.[1] Exclusive vertebral body involvement is more common in osteoblastomas originating within the cervical than thoracic or lumbar spine.[8]

Osteoblastomas share many histologic features with osteoid osteomas, but they are larger and are progressive while osteoid osteomas have self-limited growth. The average osteoblastoma measures 4 cm in diameter and by definition must be at least 1.5 cm to be classified as such.[1] In contrast, osteoid osteomas are smaller than 1.5 cm.[6]

23.2.1 Imaging

Osteoblastomas present with variable imaging findings. On plain radiographs, the most common pattern is an expansile lesion surrounded by a sclerotic rim containing a multitude of small calcifications.[1] They may also appear similar to osteoid osteomas, with a radiolucent nidus surrounded by sclerotic changes.[9] When particularly aggressive, osteoblastomas may present as expansile lesions with matrix calcifications, cortical destruction, and extension into the paravertebral and epidural spaces.[10] More aggressive osteoblastomas are frequently radiographically mistaken for aneurysmal bone cysts, osteosarcomas, or bone metastases.[11] It should be noted that the diagnostic accuracy for osteoblastomas of the spine by radiograph alone is fairly low at 66%; approximately 15% of radiographs are misinterpreted as malignant.[1]

CT is the imaging method of choice for osteoblastoma, as it provides the most detailed information on the location, size, extent, and composition of the tumor.[12,13] CT visualizes mineralization within the lesion as well as cortical destruction and soft-tissue extension.[14,15] On CT, osteoblastomas characteristically demonstrate areas of central mineralization, expansile bone remodeling, and peripheral reactive sclerosis with a thin marginal bone shell.[12]

Magnetic resonance imaging (MRI) of osteoblastoma must be interpreted carefully in order to avoid confusing the so-called "flare phenomenon"—a diffuse reactive inflammatory response within adjacent vertebrae, surrounding paraspinal soft tissues, and nearby ribs—with tumoral extension.[16,17] This phenomenon may lead the interpreting radiologist to mistake osteoblastoma with exuberant adjacent inflammation for Ewing's sarcoma or lymphoma.[17] Enhancement patterns on MRI are variable.[18] Osteoblastomas display an intermediate to low signal on T1-weighted sequences, and intermediate to high signal on T2-weighted sequences.[19] Bone remodeling at the level of the adjacent articular facets may present as facet hypertrophy, a result of the inflammatory reaction to the osteoblastoma.[7]

Bone scintigraphy is the most sensitive (but relatively nonspecific) imaging study for osteoblastomas, and Technetium-99 bone scans universally reveal avid uptake by the lesion.[9]

An osteoblastoma has neither malignant nor metastatic potential, and they have benign histological features even when they appear aggressive on imaging.[3] Any osteoblastoma reported to have malignant potential must be meticulously differentiated from other malignant bone tumors, in particular from the osteoblastoma-like variant of osteosarcoma.[20]

23.2.2 Clinical Presentation

Patients with osteoblastoma most commonly clinically present with complaints of dull, poorly localized, aching pain.[21] The pain is often progressive in nature. On average, patients present with symptoms for 16 to 24 months. In contrast to osteoid osteomas, osteoblastoma pain is not more severe at night and does not respond dramatically to NSAIDs.[22] Radicular symptoms may occur in up to 50% of patients, and neurological deficits such as paraparesis and paraplegia are seen in nearly one-third of cases.[19] Scoliosis is a common presentation of spinal osteoblastomas, especially in males, and painful scoliosis in a child should raise the index of suspicion for the possibility of an osteoblastoma.[19,23]

23.2.3 Treatment

An osteoblastoma must be treated because of its progressive nature, potential for bone destruction, and the risks associated with long-term NSAID therapy. Surgical intervention is the gold standard therapy, with either intralesional curettage or en bloc resection selected depending on the location and aggressiveness of the tumor. Resection of larger tumors or tumors in architecturally essential locations necessitates spinal stabilization in addition to resection. The decision to treat with curettage or en bloc resection is not standardized, but it is frequently based on the Enneking classification for benign musculoskeletal tumors.[7]

The surgical literature suggests that marginal resection should be undertaken for Enneking stage 1 and 2 lesions while stage 3 lesions generally require a more extensive resection to ensure that any soft-tissue involvement is excised.[24] Although this approach has guided therapy, it has not proven to reduce recurrence rates in spinal osteoblastomas.[25] Overall recurrence rates for spinal osteoblastomas following either curettage or en bloc resection is approximately 10%,[7] and recurrences have been reported as late as 9 years after resection.[26]

Although surgery has historically been the gold standard in the treatment of spinal osteoblastoma, interventional radiologists have published smaller series with promising results.[27,28,29,30] Using ablative techniques to treat smaller spinal osteoblastomas (1.5–2.8 cm nidus diameter), comparable or even superior rates of cure have been reported when compared to conventional surgery. In addition, ablation has been demonstrated to be cheaper and less morbid than spinal surgery.[30]

Proper patient selection is essential to ensure successful IR treatment of spinal osteoblastomas. Large and irregularly marginated osteoblastomas that cannot easily be ablated, destructive lesions that are at high risk for pathologic fracture, or lesions that cannot be separated (via hydrodissection or CO_2 insufflation) from at-risk neurovascular structures must be treated by alternative methods.

Prior to treatment, three-dimensional and multiplanar CT-guided access planning is recommended in all cases in order to define the optimal access trajectory and the number of needle positions needed to ablate the entire osteoblastoma nidus. RFA or cryoablation must take place using CT guidance to guarantee precise nidus penetration. As nidus penetration is very painful and may cause dangerous movement, general anesthesia is required. Delicate structures must be at least 5 mm from the ablation zone. If additional protection is required (e.g., the protection of a nerve root or the spinal cord itself), CO_2 insufflation into the epidural space or neuroforamina can be used to dissect and actively insulate the neural structures.[31,32,33,34] At the end of the procedure, 4 mg of corticosteroid (betamethasone 4 mg) can be administered directly into the ablated zone in order to reduce treatment-induced inflammation.[33] Such techniques have resulted in technical success rates of 95 to 100% and recurrence-free cure rates of 78 to 100%.

References

[1] Lucas DR, Unni KK, McLeod RA, O'Connor MI, Sim FH. Osteoblastoma: clinicopathologic study of 306 cases. Hum Pathol. 1994; 25(2):117–134

[2] Lucas DR. Osteoblastoma. Arch Pathol Lab Med. 2010; 134(10):1460–1466

[3] Berry M, Mankin H, Gebhardt M, Rosenberg A, Hornicek F. Osteoblastoma: a 30-year study of 99 cases. J Surg Oncol. 2008; 98(3):179–183

[4] Jaffe HL, Mayer L. An osteoblastic osteoid tissue-forming tumor of a metacarpal bone. Arch Surg. 1932; 24(4):550–564

[5] Virchow R. Die krankhaften Geschwülste. Berlin: A. Hirschwald; 1863;1:527

[6] Hochberg MC, Silman AJ, Smolen JS, Weinblatt ME, Weisman MH, eds. Rheumatology. 6th ed. Elsevier; 2015

[7] Galgano MA, Goulart CR, Iwenofu H, Chin LS, Lavelle W, Mendel E. Osteoblastomas of the spine: a comprehensive review. Neurosurg Focus. 2016; 41(2):E4

[8] Schwartz HS, Pinto M. Osteoblastomas of the cervical spine. J Spinal Disord. 1990; 3(2):179–182

[9] Boriani S, Weinstein JN. Oncologic classification of vertebral neoplasms. In: Dickman CA, Fehlings MG, Gokaslan ZL, eds. Spinal Cord and Spinal Column Tumors: Principles and Practice. New York: Thieme Medical Publishers; 2006

[10] Atesok KI, Alman BA, Schemitsch EH, Peyser A, Mankin H. Osteoid osteoma and osteoblastoma. J Am Acad Orthop Surg. 2011; 19(11):678–689

[11] Orguc S, Arkun R. Primary tumors of the spine. Semin Musculoskelet Radiol. 2014; 18(3):280–299

[12] Cerase A, Priolo F. Skeletal benign bone-forming lesions. Eur J Radiol. 1998; 27 Suppl 1:S91–S97

[13] Papaioannou G, Sebire NJ, McHugh K. Imaging of the unusual pediatric "blastomas.". Cancer Imaging. 2009; 9(1):1–11

[14] Arkader A, Dormans JP. Osteoblastoma in the skeletally immature. J Pediatr Orthop. 2008; 28(5):555–560

[15] Kroon HM, Schurmans J. Osteoblastoma: clinical and radiologic findings in 98 new cases. Radiology. 1990; 175(3):783–790

[16] Wu M, Xu K, Xie Y, et al. Diagnostic and management options of osteoblastoma in the spine. Med Sci Monit. 2019; 25:1362–1372

[17] Crim JR, Mirra JM, Eckardt JJ, Seeger LL. Widespread inflammatory response to osteoblastoma: the flare phenomenon. Radiology. 1990; 177 (3):835–836

[18] Jacobs WB, Fehlings MG. Primary vertebral column tumors. In: Dickman CA, Fehlings MG, Gokaslan ZL, eds. Spinal Cord and Spinal Column Tumors: Principles and Practice. New York: Thieme Medical Publishers; 2006

[19] Pobiel R, Pitt A. Radiologic Imaging of Tumors of the Spine, Spinal Cord, and Peripheral Nerves. New York: Thieme; 2006

[20] Bertoni F, Bacchini P, Donati D, Martini A, Picci P, Campanacci M. Osteoblastoma-like osteosarcoma. The Rizzoli Institute experience. Mod Pathol. 1993; 6(6):707–716

[21] Kafadar C, Incedayi M, Sildiroglu O, Ozturk E. Osteoblastoma of the thoracic spine presenting with back pain. Spine J. 2016; 16(7):e439–e440

[22] Hadgaonkar SR, Shyam AK, Shah KC, Khurjekar KS, Sancheti PK. Extraosseous thoracic foraminal osteoblastoma: diagnostic dilemma and management with 3 year follow-up. Asian Spine J. 2014; 8(5):689–694

[23] Akbarnia BA, Rooholamini SA. Scoliosis caused by benign osteoblastoma of the thoracic or lumbar spine. J Bone Joint Surg Am. 1981; 63(7):1146–1155

[24] Charles YP, Schuller S, Sfeir G, Steib J-P. Cervical osteoblastoma resection and posterior fusion. Eur Spine J. 2014; 23(3):711–712

[25] Versteeg AL, Dea N, Boriani S, et al. Surgical management of spinal osteoblastomas. J Neurosurg Spine. 2017; 27(3):321–327

[26] Jackson RP.. Recurrent osteoblastoma. Clin Orthop Relat Res. 1978(131):229–233

[27] Cazzato RL, Auloge P, Dalili D, et al. Percutaneous image-guided cryoablation of osteoblastomas. AJR Am J Roentgenol. 2019; 213(5):1157–1162

[28] Rehnitz C, Sprengel SD, Lehner B, et al. CT-guided radiofrequency ablation of osteoid osteoma and osteoblastoma: clinical success and long-term follow up in 77 patients. Eur J Radiol. 2012; 81(11):3426–3434

[29] Tomasian A, Wallace AN, Jennings JW. Benign spine lesions: advances in techniques for minimally invasive percutaneous treatment. AJNR Am J Neuroradiol. 2017; 38(5):852–861

[30] Weber M-A, Sprengel SD, Omlor GW, et al. Clinical long-term outcome, technical success, and cost analysis of radiofrequency ablation for the treatment of osteoblastomas and spinal osteoid osteomas in comparison to open surgical resection. Skeletal Radiol. 2015; 44(7):981–993

[31] Rybak LD, Gangi A, Buy X, La Rocca Vieira R, Wittig J. Thermal ablation of spinal osteoid osteomas close to neural elements: technical considerations. AJR Am J Roentgenol. 2010; 195(4):W293–8

[32] Tsoumakidou G, Koch G, Caudrelier J, et al. Image-guided spinal ablation: a review. Cardiovasc Intervent Radiol. 2016; 39(9):1229–1238

[33] Buy X, Tok C-H, Szwarc D, Bierry G, Gangi A. Thermal protection during percutaneous thermal ablation procedures: interest of carbon dioxide dissection and temperature monitoring. Cardiovasc Intervent Radiol. 2009; 32(3):529–534

[34] Tsoumakidou G, Garnon J, Ramamurthy N, Buy X, Gangi A. Interest of electrostimulation of peripheral motor nerves during percutaneous thermal ablation. Cardiovasc Intervent Radiol. 2013; 36(6):1624–1628

[35] Arrigoni F, Barile A, Zugaro L, et al. CT-guided radiofrequency ablation of spinal osteoblastoma: treatment and long-term follow-up. Int J Hyperthermia. 2018; 34(3):321–327

24 Axial Pain Related to Disk Disease (Epidurals vs. Biologics vs. Other)

Dimitrios Filippiadis and Alexis Kelekis

24.1 Case Presentation

A 35-year-old man arrived at the outpatient clinic reporting neck and left upper extremity pain at the distribution of C6 neurotome. The patient was taking nonsteroidal anti-inflammatory drugs (NSAIDs), and reported a pain score of 8/10 numeric visual scale (NVS) units. Neurological examination demonstrated mildly sensitive numbness in the left C6 territory, but no motor deficit affecting either upper extremity. Magnetic resonance imaging (MRI) of the cervical spine was performed, which revealed fusion of the C2 and C3 vertebral bodies (anatomic variation) as well as a C5–C6 left posterolateral intervertebral disk herniation causing pressure effect upon the spinal cord and the exiting nerve root (▶ Fig. 24.1).

After consultation and informed consent, the patient opted for image-guided percutaneous therapy by an interventional radiologist (IR) and an epidural infiltration was decided upon as the primary therapy. Computed tomography (CT) guidance with sequential scanning (120 kV peak, 240 mAs wavelength, and 1 mm slice thickness) was used for planning, targeting, and intraprocedural modification during the epidural session. After the initial CT scan, an appropriate skin entry point was selected. A 22-gauge spinal needle was inserted into the posterior epidural space at the C5–C6 level, and its approach was evaluated with intermittent CT scans. Contrast medium injection confirmed the correct extravascular needle location inside the epidural space. Following an uneventful medication injection, the procedure was terminated.

Clinical examination in the outpatient clinic 1 week after the epidural injection did not show changes in the pain score. Due to the lack of response, a percutaneous approach with chemical disk decompression was decided upon as a second-line treatment. With the patient in the supine position, under fluoroscopic guidance, the selected C5–C6 disk was recognized and aligned. Using an anterolateral right-sided approach (due to the presence of esophagus on the left side), an 18-gauge spinal needle was placed inside the C5–C6 intervertebral disk. To perform this, the larynx

was subluxed, and the trocar advanced between the larynx and jugular–carotid vessels until it reached the anterior longitudinal ligament. In the lateral projection, the trocar was advanced until it reached the middle of the disk. The final position of the needle inside the disk was toward the posterior third in the lateral projection and toward the midline in the anteroposterior (AP) projection, midway between the superior and inferior end plates of the adjacent vertebrae (▶ Fig. 24.2).

Once the needle was in its final location, under continuous fluoroscopy gelified ethanol with Tungsten for radio-opacity (DiscoGel, Hérouville-Saint-Clair, France) was slowly injected.[1] Cone-beam CT immediately after the injection showed stagnation of the gelified ethanol inside the disk and the herniated portion (▶ Fig. 24.3).

MRI at 6 months post-treatment demonstrated significant regression of the C5–C6 disk hernia (▶ Fig. 24.4).

24.2 Discussion

Intervertebral disk herniation accounts for approximately one-third of the neck and back pain cases with or without neuralgia. The most commonly affected disk levels are C5–C6 and C6–C7, as well as L4–L5 and L5–S1. Patients usually present between 30 and 40 years of age.[1,2,3,4] The therapeutic armamentarium for symptomatic intervertebral disk herniation includes conservative therapy, epidural infiltrations (interlaminar or transforaminal), advanced percutaneous therapeutic techniques, and surgical options.

Percutaneous therapeutic techniques are imaging-guided, minimally invasive treatments for intervertebral disk herniation that can be classified into four main groups: mechanical, thermal, chemical decompression, and biomaterials implantation.[5] Hijikata, Asher, and Choy provided the bio-mechanical proof of a theory stating that in the closed space of the intervertebral disk, removal of a small nuclear volume results in a significant drop in intradiskal pressure, creating the conditions for the herniation to regress inwards.[2,5,6]

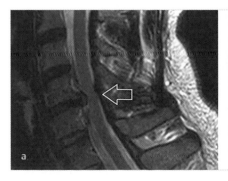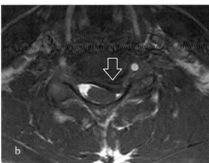

Fig. 24.1 Magnetic resonance imaging (MRI) T2-weighted sagittal (a) and axial (b) sequences illustrating a C5–C6 left posterolateral and foraminal intervertebral disk herniation (arrows) causing pressure effect upon the spinal cord and the exiting root.

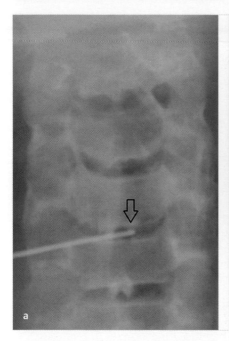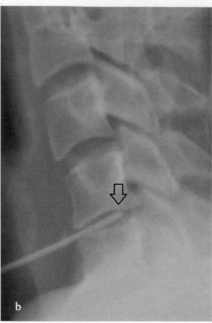

Fig. 24.2 Anteroposterior (AP) (a) and lateral (b) fluoroscopic views illustrating the final needle position. The intradiskal needle (arrow) is in the posterior third of the disk space in the lateral projection, and toward the midline in the AP projection. The needle should be at midway between the two end plates.

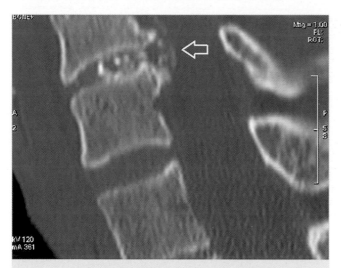

Fig. 24.3 Post-injection cone-beam computed tomography (CT) sagittal reconstruction immediately after intradiskal injection illustrates stagnation of the gelified ethanol inside the disk and the hernia (arrow).

Intradiskal biomaterials include implantation of hydrogel, platelet-rich plasma, and stem cell therapy aimed at regeneration of intervertebral disk material. This functions in a completely opposite way from the aforementioned decompression techniques.[7,8] To differentiate the two: the presence of a disk herniation that does not respond to conservative therapy, is symptomatic, and occupies less than one-third to half of the spinal canal's diameter is a clear indication for percutaneous decompression approaches. In contrast, the presence of a "black" disk on MRI that has lost its water content seems to be an indication for biomaterial implantation.[2,7,8,9] Contraindications to both procedure types include sequestration, infection, segmental instability (spondylolisthesis), uncorrected coagulopathy, or a patient unwilling to provide informed consent.[2,9]

Percutaneous decompression and biomaterial implantation techniques are performed as outpatient procedures. The patient is discharged within 34 hours following the procedure with instructions for bed rest, oral analgesics, avoidance of bending or rotatory movements for the first 2 weeks, and avoidance of heavy lifting and strenuous body activity for at least the same amount of time.[5]

The mean success rates for all decompression techniques range between 75 and 85%.[2,4,5,9] The complication rate is exceedingly low (approximately 0.5%), with the most common and fearsome complication being spondylodiskitis (with or without epidural abscess). This potentially devastating complication occurs in up to 0.24% of patients and 0.091% per disk.[1,3,4,8] When compared to conservative therapy or spinal infiltrations, in the correct patient population decompression techniques are favored due to better and longer lasting pain reduction.[10,11]

To date, there is no evidence favoring one percutaneous decompression technique over the other.[12,13] When compared to open diskectomy or microdiskectomy techniques, percutaneous decompression techniques show noninferiority in terms of efficacy and pain reduction.[14,15,16]

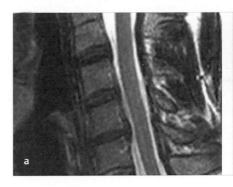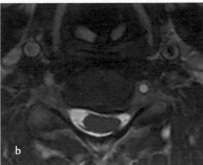

Fig. 24.4 Magnetic resonance imaging (MRI) T2-weighted sagittal (**a**) and axial (**b**) sequences illustrating significant size regression of C5–C6 left posterolateral intervertebral disk hernia (compare to ▶ Fig. 24.1).

References

[1] Théron J, Cuellar H, Sola T, Guimaraens L, Casasco A, Courtheoux P. Percutaneous treatment of cervical disk hernias using gelified ethanol. AJNR Am J Neuroradiol. 2010; 31(8):1454–1456

[2] Kelekis AD, Filippiadis DK, Martin JB, Brountzos E. Standards of practice: quality assurance guidelines for percutaneous treatments of intervertebral discs. Cardiovasc Intervent Radiol. 2010; 33(5):909–913

[3] Frymoyer JW. Lumbar disk disease: epidemiology. Instr Course Lect. 1992; 41:217–223

[4] Gangi A, Tsoumakidou G, Buy X, Cabral JF, Garnon J. Percutaneous techniques for cervical pain of discal origin. Semin Musculoskelet Radiol. 2011; 15(2): 172–180

[5] Kelekis A, Filippiadis DK. Percutaneous treatment of cervical and lumbar herniated disc. Eur J Radiol. 2015; 84(5):771–776

[6] Hijikata S. Percutaneous nucleotomy. A new concept technique and 12 years' experience. Clin Orthop Relat Res. 1989 Jan;(238):9-23.

[7] Nagae M, Ikeda T, Mikami Y, et al. Intervertebral disc regeneration using platelet-rich plasma and biodegradable gelatin hydrogel microspheres. Tissue Eng. 2007; 13(1):147–158

[8] Chan SC, Gantenbein-Ritter B. Intervertebral disc regeneration or repair with biomaterials and stem cell therapy—feasible or fiction? Swiss Med Wkly. 2012; 142:w13598

[9] Kelekis AD, Somon T, Yilmaz H, et al. Interventional spine procedures. Eur J Radiol. 2005; 55(3):362–383

[10] Erginousakis D, Filippiadis DK, Malagari A, et al. Comparative prospective randomized study comparing conservative treatment and percutaneous disk decompression for treatment of intervertebral disk herniation. Radiology. 2011; 260(2):487–493

[11] Gerszten PC, Smuck M, Rathmell JP, et al. SPINE Study Group. Plasma disc decompression compared with fluoroscopy-guided transforaminal epidural steroid injections for symptomatic contained lumbar disc herniation: a prospective, randomized, controlled trial. J Neurosurg Spine. 2010; 12(4): 357–371

[12] Lemcke J, Al-Zain F, Mutze S, Meier U. Minimally invasive spinal surgery using nucleoplasty and the Dekompressor tool: a comparison of two methods in a one year follow-up. Minim Invasive Neurosurg. 2010; 53(5–6):236–242

[13] Yan D, Li J, Zhu H, Zhang Z, Duan L. Percutaneous cervical nucleoplasty and percutaneous cervical discectomy treatments of the contained cervical disc herniation. Arch Orthop Trauma Surg. 2010; 130(11):1371–1376

[14] Adam D, Pevzner E, Gepstein R. Comparison of percutaneous nucleoplasty and open discectomy in patients with lumbar disc protrusions. Chirurgia (Bucur). 2013; 108(1):94–98

[15] Liu WG, Wu XT, Guo JH, Zhuang SY, Teng GJ. Long-term outcomes of patients with lumbar disc herniation treated with percutaneous discectomy: comparative study with microendoscopic discectomy. Cardiovasc Intervent Radiol. 2010; 33(4):780–786

[16] Tassi GP. Comparison of results of 500 microdiscectomies and 500 percutaneous laser disc decompression procedures for lumbar disc herniation. Photomed Laser Surg. 2006; 24(6):694–697

25 Axial Back Pain Related to Sacroiliac Disease

Danoob Dalili, Daniel E. Dalili, Amanda Isaac, and Jan Fritz

25.1 Case Presentation

A 26-year-old man presened with gradually worsening bilateral sacroiliac joint (SIJ) pain, which was greater on the right than the left. He had symptoms for 2 years, and conservative care had failed. Multimodality diagnostic imaging was performed, followed by therapeutic intervention (▶ Fig. 25.1).

25.2 Discussion

SIJ pain accounts for 10 to 25% of patients presenting with mechanical low back or leg pain.[1] SIJs are particularly prone to certain diseases,[2,3,4,5,6,7] including: inflammatory and erosive arthropathies, including ankylosing spondylitis; mechanical overuse injuries such as those seen in athletes, particularly joggers; insufficiency fractures (osteoporotic pathological fractures) involving the sacrum; and primary or metastatic bone disease affecting the pelvic bones and extending locally into the joint.

SIJ pain is confirmed by clinical examination, imaging, and response to analgesic intraarticular injections. Recently a diagnostic scoring system has been proposed and validated in differentiating SIJ pain from other causes of low back pain.[8]

Clinicians are recognizing sagittal imbalance more often and correlating it with the presenting symptoms.[6] As is the case in the abovementioned patient, sagittal imbalance probably also plays a role in SIJ pain. In sagittal imbalance, the posterior musculature must exert greater force to maintain an upright posture. With fascia and musculature originating from the ilium, this imbalance will exert a greater force on the posterior pelvis. If a patient has sagittal imbalance and SIJ pain is confirmed, correcting the sagittal imbalance surgically is probably the preferred treatment for improving alignment and posture[9] once conservative options are exhausted.

25.3 Therapeutic Approaches

The current therapeutic armamentarium is wide and includes oral nonsteroidal anti-inflammatory drugs (NSAIDs), sacral belting and/or orthotics,[10,11] activity modification and exercise,[10,12] manipulation and physiotherapy,[10,12] SIJ block,[13,14,15,16,17] acupuncture

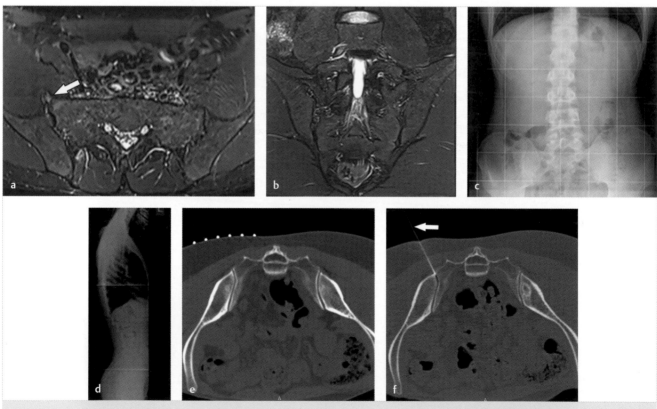

Fig. 25.1 (a) Axial and coronal oblique (b) short tau inversion recovery (STIR) magnetic resonance imaging (MRI) images demonstrate bilateral subtle subchondral sclerosis and subtle fatty metaplasia. In addition, the right sacroiliac joint demonstrates distal anterior bone bridging and marrow edema (arrow). Standing weight-bearing radiographs (c) and whole-spine radiographs (d) demonstrate scoliosis and sagittal imbalance, further contributing to symptoms. (e, f) Computed tomography (CT)-guided bilateral sacroiliac joint injections were performed. Arrow showing needle entering the right posterior sacroiliac joint. The numeral pain score improved from 8/10 preprocedure to 0/10 immediately after the procedure. After 6 weeks, the pain remained 0/10 on the left and 1/10 on the right.

prolotherapy, neuroaugmentation, viscosupplementation,[17] radiofrequency ablation,[16,18] and fusion.[19,20] Each technique has its own advantages and limitations. Treatments are often delivered in stages and escalated according to the patient's symptoms, associated comorbidies, and response to treatments provided. The escalation policy commonly followed is outlined below.

25.3.1 Conservative Therapies

Conservative therapies include medical treatments (analgesics, NSAIDs, oral steroids) and physiotherapy (including sacral belting and/or orthotics, activity modification and exercise, and manipulation and physiotherapy). These therapies are used for palliative control of symptoms rather than as curative, particularly in children and pregnant women. One drawback to these therapies is that they often fail to control progression of structural damage to the SIJ itself.[9,15,16,21,22]

25.3.2 Minimally Invasive Treatments

These treatments can be used in addition to or in combination with conservative therapies. They include acupuncture and percutaneous image-guided interventions, such as SIJ block, prolotherapy, neuroaugmentation, viscosupplementation, radiofrequency ablation, and fusion. Image-guided injections provide immediate and in some cases long-term pain relief that can improve mobility and allow a comfortable window of pain relief that facilitates complementary physiotherapy. In the USA, a study evaluating Medicare services between 2000 and 2015 showed an increase in facet and sacroiliac joint interventions by 313.3%, and a 316.9% increase in SIJ injections alone, calculated as an annual increase of 10.7%.[23,24,25] The overall accuracy and therapeutic effectiveness of SIJ interventions ranges between 70 and 90% in most level II and III studies, with further improved outcomes in patients undergoing multiple procedures.[17,26]

Procedures can be performed under ultrasound, fluoroscopy, computed tomography (CT), or magnetic resonance (MR) guidance.[13,27,28,29] SIJ injections are performed with the patient positioned prone on the procedural table, with adequate cushioning to ensure the patient is comfortable and in order to minimize motion. The SIJ space is also small (only 1–2 mm in width) and becomes narrower when inflicted by disease.[9,30] For this reason, CT- or MR-guided interventions are associated with more precise needle location and improved outcomes.[31,32,33,34,35] Cross-sectional imaging guidance improves visualization of the SIJs particularly when there is partial or complete ankylosis (e.g., in patients with ankylosing spondylitis). Fluoroscopy-guided corticosteroid injections of the joint have reported technical success rate in improving sacroiliac pain in only 50 to 64% of cases,[30,36,37] while CT-guided corticosteroid injections of the joint have reported high technical success rates and improved sacroiliac pain in up to 90% of patients. Similar to CT, MR-guided corticosteroid injections of the joint have reported high technical success rates and improved sacroiliac pain in about 90% of cases, with average pain intensity reduction by 62.5%.[34] The ability to visualize dissipation of fluid into the joint enhances the operator's confidence and can help radiologists adjust the administrated dose.[35]

25.3.3 Surgery

At least 17 different surgical techniques for SIJ fusion have been described. These invasive procedures are typically used only when more conservative treatments have failed.[38] Predictive outcome analysis reveals slightly inferior responses to these procedures in smokers and opioid users, and slightly greater improvements in those with longer pain durations and more advanced age.[20,38]

25.4 Anatomical Considerations

The SIJ is a true diarthrodial joint: matching articular surfaces separated by a joint space containing synovial fluid and enveloped by a thick fibrous capsule, with fibrocartilage and hyaline cartilage.[39] In addition, there is synovial lining in the lower two-thirds of the joints, rendering the joint susceptible to arthropathies that affect synovial joints (e.g., erosive and inflammatory arthropathies).[2] The articular surfaces have many ridges and depressions that minimize movement and enhance stability. Primary stability, however, is attributed to the many adjacent ligaments including the dorsal, ventral, and interosseous ligaments, the short and long dorsal sacroiliac ligaments, the dorsal and ventral transverse sacroiliac ligaments, and the iliolumbar ligaments.[9] There are also several myofascial structures that influence movement and stability, the most notable of which are the latissimus dorsi (via the thoracolumbar fascia), the gluteus maximus, and the piriformis.[39] The SIJs receive innervation from the L5 to S4 rami. The close proximity of the SIJs to the lumbosacral plexus and dorsal sacral rami as well as known defects in the anterior capsule of the SIJ explains why a response within the deep medial multifidis, gluteus maximus, piriformis, and quadratus lumborum is observed during some of the SIJ radiofrequency procedures.[9]

There are significant differences observed between men and women, with larger articular surfaces in men, as well as larger loading forces on standing and movement in men due to variation between genders in the gravitational axis of forces.[9]

Several studies have confirmed that the SIJs are mobile in pregnancy as a physiological phenomenon.[9,21,25] This may predispose to sacroiliac dysfunction during and after pregnancy.

25.5 Conclusion

A majority of diseases affecting the SIJs are chronic conditions that tend to progress with time, such as spondyloarthropathies, osteoporosis, and osteoarthritis. Treatment strategies therefore aim to offer medium- to long-term relief of symptoms, and to reduce the rate of progression of irreversible structural change within the SIJs such as erosions and ankylosis and/or mechanical remodeling associated with degenerative change. Image-guided interventions offer the fastest, least invasive, and most effective interventions that can achieve these goals with minimal complications. In addition, in select populations they can be offered in combination with conservative therapies to even further enhance patients' outcomes.

Although the current armamentarium of percutaneous image-guided interventions is broad, guidance with cross-sectional imaging modalities is preferred.[40,41] In the absence of contraindications to the procedure, MR-guided injections are considered quick, efficient, and safe procedures that incorporate the benefits of other imaging modalities and therefore promises to improve patients' outcomes.

References

[1] Thawrani DP, Agabegi SS, Asghar F. Diagnosing sacroiliac joint pain. J Am Acad Orthop Surg. 2019; 27(3):85–93

[2] Hemke R, Herregods N, Jaremko JL, et al. Imaging assessment of children presenting with suspected or known juvenile idiopathic arthritis: ESSR-ESPR points to consider. Eur Radiol. 2020; 30(10):5237–5249

[3] Afonso PD, Weber MA, Isaac A, Bloem JL. Hip and pelvis bone tumors: can you make it simple? Semin Musculoskelet Radiol. 2019; 23(3):e37–e57

[4] Isaac A, Dalili D, Dalili D, Weber M-A. State-of-the-art imaging for diagnosis of metastatic bone disease. Radiologe. 2020; 60 Suppl 1:1–16

[5] Plagou A, Teh J, Grainger AJ, et al. Recommendations of the ESSR Arthritis Subcommittee on Ultrasonography in Inflammatory Joint Disease. Semin Musculoskelet Radiol. 2016; 20(5):496–506

[6] Panchmatia JR, Isaac A, Muthukumar T, Gibson AJ, Lehovsky J. The 10 key steps for radiographic analysis of adolescent idiopathic scoliosis. Clin Radiol. 2015; 70(3):235–242

[7] Isaac A, Lecouvet F, Dalili D, et al. Detection and characterization of musculoskeletal cancer using whole-body magnetic resonance imaging. Semin Musculoskelet Radiol. 2020; 24(6):726–750

[8] Tonosu J, Oka H, Watanabe K, et al. Validation study of a diagnostic scoring system for sacroiliac joint-related pain. J Pain Res. 2018; 11:1659–1663

[9] Foley BS, Buschbacher RM. Sacroiliac joint pain: anatomy, biomechanics, diagnosis, and treatment. Am J Phys Med Rehabil. 2006; 85(12):997–1006

[10] Prather H, Bonnette M, Hunt D. Nonoperative treatment options for patients with sacroiliac joint pain. Int J Spine Surg. 2020; 14(Suppl 1):S35–S–40

[11] Hu H, Meijer OG, van Dieën JH, et al. Muscle activity during the active straight leg raise (ASLR), and the effects of a pelvic belt on the ASLR and on treadmill walking. J Biomech. 2010; 43(3):532–539

[12] Beales DJ, O'Sullivan PB, Briffa NK. The effects of manual pelvic compression on trunk motor control during an active straight leg raise in chronic pelvic girdle pain subjects. Man Ther. 2010; 15(2):190–199

[13] Fritz J, Sequeiros RB, Carrino JA. Magnetic resonance imaging-guided spine injections. Top Magn Reson Imaging. 2011; 22(4):143–151

[14] Gandhi Post S, Khuba S, Gandhi Post Graduate S, Agarwal A, Gautam S, Kumar S. Observational Study Fluoroscopic Sacroiliac Joint Injection: Is Oblique Angulation Really Necessary?

[15] Peebles R, Jonas CE. Sacroiliac joint dysfunction in the athlete: diagnosis and management. Curr Sports Med Rep. 2017; 16(5):336–342

[16] Soto Quijano DA, Otero Loperena E. Sacroiliac joint interventions. Phys Med Rehabil Clin N Am. 2018; 29(1):171–183

[17] Simopoulos TT, Manchikanti L, Gupta S, et al. Systematic review of the diagnostic accuracy and therapeutic effectiveness of sacroiliac joint interventions. Pain Physician. 2015; 18(5):E713–E756

[18] Huynh P, Hsu D. Comparison of Lateral Branched Pulsed Radiofrequency Denervation and Intraarticular Depot Methylprednisolone Injection for Sacroiliac Joint Pain: Inquiry for Additional Investigation. Pain Physician. 2019; 22(1):E53-E54.

[19] Polly DW , Jr. The sacroiliac joint. Neurosurg Clin N Am. 2017; 28(3):301–312

[20] Sachs D, Kovalsky D, Redmond A, et al. Durable intermediate-to long-term outcomes after minimally invasive transiliac sacroiliac joint fusion using triangular titanium implants. Med Devices (Auckl). 2016; 9:213–222

[21] Vincent R, Blackburn J, Wienecke G, Bautista A. Sacroiliac joint pain in pregnancy: a case report. A A Pract. 2019; 13(2):51–53

[22] Klauser AS, Sailer-Hoeck M, Abdellah MMH, et al. Feasibility of ultrasound-guided sacroiliac joint injections in children presenting with sacroiliitis. Ultraschall Med. 2016; 37(4):393–398

[23] Stelzer W, Stelzer D, Stelzer E, et al. Success rate of intra-articular sacroiliac joint injection: fluoroscopy vs ultrasound guidance—a cadaveric study. Pain Med. 2019; 20(10):1890–1897

[24] Schneider BJ, Huynh L, Levin J, Rinkaekan P, Kordi R, Kennedy DJ. Does immediate pain relief after an injection into the sacroiliac joint with anesthetic and corticosteroid predict subsequent pain relief? Pain Med. 2018; 19(2):244–251

[25] Cohen SP, Chen Y, Neufeld NJ. Sacroiliac joint pain: a comprehensive review of epidemiology, diagnosis and treatment. Expert Rev Neurother. 2013; 13 (1):99–116

[26] Zheng P, Schneider BJ, Yang A, McCormick ZL. Image-guided sacroiliac joint injections: an evidence-based review of best practices and clinical outcomes. PM R. 2019; 11 Suppl 1:S98–S104

[27] Dalili D, Isaac A, Rashidi A, Åström G, Fritz J. Image-guided sports medicine and musculoskeletal tumor interventions: a patient-centered model. Semin Musculoskelet Radiol. 2020; 24(3):290–309

[28] Fritz J, Niemeyer T, Clasen S, et al. Management of chronic low back pain: rationales, principles, and targets of imaging-guided spinal injections. Radiographics. 2007; 27(6):1751–1771

[29] Fritz J, U-Thainual P, Ungi T, et al. Augmented reality visualisation using an image overlay system for MR-guided interventions: technical performance of spine injection procedures in human cadavers at 1.5 Tesla. Eur Radiol. 2013; 23(1):235–245

[30] Kurosawa D, Murakami E, Aizawa T. Fluoroscopy-guided sacroiliac intraarticular injection via the middle portion of the joint. Pain Med. 2017; 18(9):1642–1648

[31] Fritz J, Henes JC, Thomas C, et al. Diagnostic and interventional MRI of the sacroiliac joints using a 1.5-T open-bore magnet: a one-stop-shopping approach. AJR Am J Roentgenol. 2008; 191(6):1717–1724

[32] Fritz J, Tzaribachev N, Thomas C, et al. Evaluation of MR imaging guided steroid injection of the sacroiliac joints for the treatment of children with refractory enthesitis-related arthritis. Eur Radiol. 2011; 21(5):1050–1057

[33] Fritz J, König CW, Günaydin I, et al. [Magnetic resonance imaging–guided corticosteroid-infiltration of the sacroiliac joints: pain therapy of sacroiliitis in patients with ankylosing spondylitis]. Röfo Fortschr Geb Röntgenstr Nuklearmed. 2005; 177(4):555–563

[34] Günaydin I, Pereira PL, Fritz J, König C, Kötter I. Magnetic resonance imaging guided corticosteroid injection of sacroiliac joints in patients with spondylarthropathy. Are multiple injections more beneficial? Rheumatol Int. 2006; 26(5):396–400

[35] Fritz J, Pereira PL. [MR-guided pain therapy: principles and clinical applications]. Röfo Fortschr Geb Röntgenstr Nuklearmed. 2007; 179(9):914–924

[36] Frey ME, Depalma MJ, Cifu DX, Bhagia SM, Carne W, Daitch JS. Percutaneous sacroplasty for osteoporotic sacral insufficiency fractures: a prospective, multicenter, observational pilot study. Spine J. 2008; 8(2):367–373

[37] Kasliwal PJ, Kasliwal S. Fluoroscopy-guided sacroiliac joint injection: description of a modified technique. Pain Physician. 2016; 19(2):E329–E338

[38] Yson SC, Sembrano JN, Polly DW , Jr. Sacroiliac joint fusion: approaches and recent outcomes. PM R. 2019; 11 Suppl 1:S114–S117

[39] Zou YC, Li YK, Yu CF, Yang XW, Chen RQ. A cadaveric study on sacroiliac joint injection. Int Surg. 2015; 100(2):320–327

[40] Dalili D, Isaac A, Bazzocchi A, et al. Interventional techniques for bone and musculoskeletal soft tissue tumors: current practices and future directions - Part I. Ablation. Semin Musculoskelet Radiol. 2020; 24(6):692–709

[41] Dalili D, Isaac A, Cazzato RL, et al. Interventional techniques for bone and musculoskeletal soft tissue tumors: current practices and future directions - Part II. Stabilization. Semin Musculoskelet Radiol. 2020; 24(6):710–725

26 Radicular Pain Related to Disk Disease I (Transforaminal Injections)

Jason W. Mitchell

26.1 Case Presentation

A 62-year-old woman self-referred to the interventional radiology (IR) clinic for back and hip pain. She described pain that started more than 5 years previously and had progressively worsened. The pain "shoots down her leg" and is worse with standing and walking, with only some recumbent positions able to partially relieve the pain. She stated that the worst it had been over the prior 24 hours is 10/10, and now she needed to use a cane to ambulate in order to not exacerbate the pain. Her balance without the cane was fine. Nonsteroidal anti-inflammatory drugs (NSAIDs) no longer seemed to alleviate the pain; she was opposed to taking opioids, even though the pain could bring her to tears. The pain extended across the left side of her back, across the front of her left leg, and over to the medial side of her left lower leg. The pain in her back was constant, sharp, and intense but not throbbing. The pain in her leg had changed from burning and electrical, to a steady dull pain, to periods of intense sharp pain. She had several "injections" by an orthopedist, which worked the first time several years ago but have failed to help since. Although she did not bring records of the procedures, she described the injections as being midline in location. She was evaluated for surgery by her orthopedist, who told her that she was too overweight to undergo surgery. She brought with her the most recent magnetic resonance imaging (MRI) exam performed during her surgical workup 2 months previously.

She had a history of hypertension and noninsulin-dependent diabetes, both of which appeared to be well controlled with multiple medications. She had never had any surgeries. Her only overnight hospital stays were the birth of her four children, all delivered naturally many years ago. She did not smoke, drink alcohol regularly, or take illicit drugs. She worked as an administrative assistant, which did not need much ambulating. She was active in her community and church and volunteers often. She was married with four living children and several grandchildren. Her medications were reviewed; it included 81 mg aspirin daily prescribed by her primary care physician as per preventative guidelines due to her cardiovascular risk.

On physical examination, she was found to be morbidly obese. Her pain mapped exactly to the left L4 dermatome, extending across her back, around her left hip, and down the left anterior thigh to the knee, and medially along her left lower leg to about the mid-tibia level. She had no loss of sensation along that or any other dermatome. She had good passive range of motion, fair active-assisted range of motion, and preserved strength except possibly a slight reduction (4+/5) in both knee extension and hip adduction.

Her outside MRI was reviewed which demonstrated loss of disk height with a broad-based circumferential disk bulge at L4–L5, causing mild central spinal canal stenosis and stenosis of the left L4–L5 neural foramen. There were mild disk hydration signal abnormalities at other levels. No other significant pathology was demonstrated (▶ Fig. 26.1).

After holding her aspirin for 5 days, she returned for a left L4 transforaminal injection with local anesthetic and steroid (▶ Fig. 26.2). She had near-immediate postprocedural relief, and ambulated without the need for her cane. She did not immediately report any alteration in sensation. She returned to the recovery area to prepare for discharge.

In the recovery area, the patient began to note decreased sensation across her thigh, and when standing to get dressed, her left leg "gave out" on her and she fell. Fortunately, her postprocedural nurse was supporting her, and she had no injuries from the controlled, supported fall. On examination, her strength on extension was reduced to 2+/5. She remained in recovery for 4 hours, after which she fully recovered her strength and her ability to safely and easily walk, and was able to be discharged home.

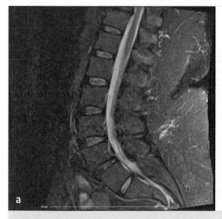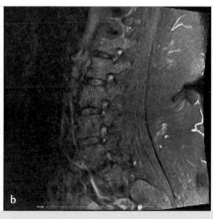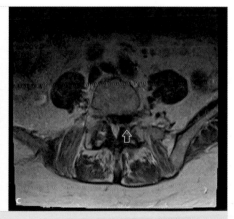

Fig. 26.1 Midline sagittal short tau inversion recovery (STIR) (a) and sagittal STIR (b) and axial fast-spin echo (FSE) T2 (c) through the left L4–L5 neural foramen demonstrate neural foraminal narrowing (arrow) secondary to disk bulge with no other significant pathology.

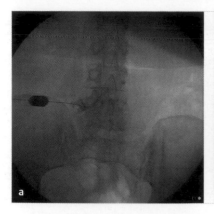
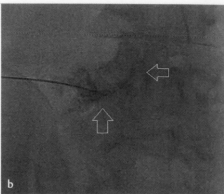

Fig. 26.2 Mildly obliqued fluoroscopic spot view (**a**) and digital magnification (**b**) after left L4–L5 transforaminal test injection of contrast. There is contrast extending superiorly and medially in the epidural space along the nerve root under the L4 pedicle, and out laterally (arrow).

On follow-up calls the following day and 2 weeks later, her pain over the preceding 24 hours had been reduced to 2/10, and she had returned to activities including comfortably increasing her level of activity. After 7 months, she still reported reasonable pain control.

26.2 Discussion

Transforaminal injections can be more specific than midline epidural injections in cases of radicular pain from disk disease or postlaminectomy pain.[1,2,3,4,5,6,7,8,9,10,11,12] Patient selection is critical for a successful transforaminal injection, and symptoms other than radiculopathy or postlaminectomy pain should cue the clinician that perhaps there are other sources of pain, limiting the effectiveness of transforaminal injection. In many patients, several nerve roots may be affected by disease, and therefore multiple injections in the same or successive settings may be necessary to achieve relief. The use of cross-sectional imaging may be helpful in complex cases, and review of imaging is recommended to correlate symptoms with anatomic pathology.

Recent consensus guidelines designate epidural injections as a high-risk procedure for bleeding, and therefore prothrombin time/international normalized ratio (PT/INR) and platelet count results should be obtained before the procedure and corrected appropriately. These guidelines set a suggested threshold for correction of INR to between 1.5 and 1.8, and transfusion of platelets up to 50×10^9/L. Also, the consensus guidelines recommend holding anticoagulation and antiplatelet medications prior to the procedure.[13]

Holding a patient *non per ora* (NPO) is not necessary, as sedation is not necessary; in fact, having a patient alert and able to communicate with the proceduralist is extremely helpful for determining immediate success. However, it is recommended that the patient bring a driver for after the procedure, as inadvertent motor blockade with local anesthetic is possible, as demonstrated in this case.

The procedure can be performed under fluoroscopic or computed tomography (CT) guidance; with readily identifiable landmarks, fluoroscopic guidance tends to be easy and quick. However, in postoperative patients, where surgical hardware can obscure landmarks on traditional views, CT guidance can be extremely useful.

Most injections are given in the so-called "safe triangle" as subpedicular approach through the "safe" triangle is easy to access and usually has little in the way of vascular structures.[2,3,11,12] This space is bordered superiorly by the pedicle, inferiorly (on the hypotenuse) by the dorsal root ganglion, and laterally by empty space. Another alternative approach, particularly when the "safe triangle" is inaccessible secondary to orthopedic hardware, is via Kambin's triangle, which is inferior to the dorsal root ganglion, and also relatively free of vascular structures. This approach is also commonly used during percutaneous diskectomy procedures. Kambin's triangle is bounded inferiorly by the pedicle, superiorly (on the hypotenuse) by the dorsal root ganglion, and medially by the articular process.[14] It should be noted that many of these borders, both for the "safe triangle" and for the alternative Kambin's triangle, are not clear on fluoroscopy, and therefore some of the borders are assumed (▶ Fig. 26.3a). The approach discussed herein is the fluoroscopically guided subpedicular or "safe triangle" approach, but the technique can be used by inference for Kambin's triangle injections and CT-guided injections.

For fluoroscopically guided transforaminal injections the patient is placed prone on the table, and the appropriate level is marked. An oblique view, showing the "Scotty dog" appearance of the facet joint, pars interarticularis, and pedicle, is used for needle entry. Local anesthesia at the needle entry site is a matter of operator preference, as the entire procedure can be performed with a single small-gauge needle access without much discomfort. A 21- to 25-gauge spinal or Quincke needle with stylet is used for access, and it is directed to the inferior edge of the pedicle visualized end-on in the oblique view. The needle is directed under the pedicle. Needle placement in the lumbar transforaminal space can be confirmed on an anteroposterior (AP) view, with the needle tip just under but not crossing medial to the pedicle (▶ Fig. 26.3b). On the lateral view, the needle tip should again be visualized just under the pedicle but in the posterior part of the neural foramen. Care should be taken to not advance too far forward (ventral) and inadvertently enter the dural space (▶ Fig. 26.3c).[2,3]

It is imperative to gently aspirate the needle prior to any injection to determine if the needle tip has been placed in a vascular structure.[2,3] The artery of Adamkiewicz is inconstant, and can be found in the lumbar range in a small minority of individuals,[15] and radicular arteries and venous plexuses are present in the neural foramina.[2,3,16] Although accessing the relatively safer triangles

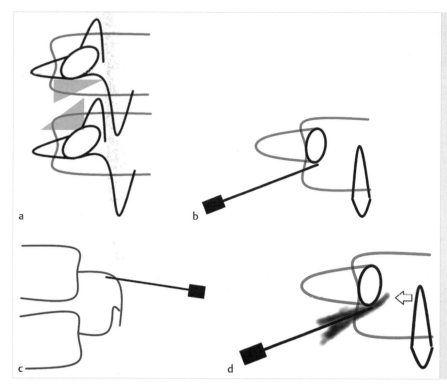

Fig. 26.3 Schematic representation of transforaminal injection. (**a**) An oblique "Scotty dog" view of a pair of typical lumbar vertebral bodies with visible fluoroscopic landmarks. The upper shaded triangle represents the subpedicular "safe triangle," and the lower shaded triangle represents Kambin's triangle. Anteroposterior (AP) (**b**) and lateral (**c**) views with visible fluoroscopic landmarks demonstrating needle position after accessing the "safe triangle." (**d**) A representation of an AP view, with a "blob" in the epidural space (arrow) after test injection of a small amount of contrast.

described above decreases the chance of puncture of these vascular structures, injecting material, particularly particulate steroid, into an artery can be catastrophic and result in paralysis; in cervical injections, even death has been reported.[2,3,16,17,18,19,20,21] After gentle aspiration yields no blood or cerebrospinal fluid, a small test injection of contrast material in the AP projection can confirm needle tip placement in the epidural space. There should be no flow of contrast in the spinal canal, with contrast limited to outlining the diagonally coursing nerve root (► Fig. 26.3d). The use of primed catheter tubing can help prevent needle motion on aspiration and injection, and prevent inadvertent dislodgement.

The use of particulate steroid has been linked to a higher rate of severe ischemic complications in case of occult or undetected vascular puncture, so nonparticulate dexamethasone or low-particulate betamethasone is preferred.[17,18,19,20,21,22,23,24,25] The use of local anesthetic, such as lidocaine or bupivacaine, can aid in immediate relief of symptoms; however, one should be prepared to advise the patient of sensory and motor deficits that may arise from partial or complete dorsal root blockade. Such deficits due to local anesthetic administration tend to be limited in scope and duration. A local anesthetic block can be used prior to steroid injection to determine the effect on symptoms. A total volume of 1 to 2 mL is injected after checking again for vascular placement of the needle tip by aspiration; more anesthetic can be injected (usually 5–6 mL) with visualization under fluoroscopy to further infiltrate the epidural space to the neighboring nerve roots. Care should be taken not to inject excessive doses of steroid, and any relative contraindications should be considered. Of particular concern is patients with diabetes, where blood glucose levels should be more closely monitored following steroid injection.[26]

26.3 Conclusion

Transforaminal injections are useful in patients with radiculopathies or postlaminectomy pain syndromes, and are better able to localize the effects of injections than central intralaminar epidural injection techniques. Patient selection is therefore critical, and a thorough understanding of the key anatomical landmarks makes the procedure quick, safe, relatively simple, and effective.

References

[1] Abdi S, Datta S, Trescot AM, et al. Epidural steroids in the management of chronic spinal pain: a systematic review. In: Database of Abstracts of Reviews of Effects (DARE): Quality-assessed Reviews [Internet]. York (UK): Centre for Reviews and Dissemination (UK); 1995. Review published: 2007. Available from: https://www.ncbi.nlm.nih.gov/books/NBK74551/

[2] Ranson MT, Deer TR. Epidural injections for the treatment of spine-related pain syndromes. In: Mathis JM, Golovac S, eds. Image-Guided Spine Interventions. New York, NY: Springer; 2011:157–174

[3] Suchy T, Diep J, Cheng J. Epidural steroid injections. In: Mao J, ed. Spine Pain Care. Cham: Springer International; 2020:281–290

[4] Lutz GE, Vad VB, Wisneski RJ. Fluoroscopic transforaminal lumbar epidural steroids: an outcome study. Arch Phys Med Rehabil. 1998; 79(11):1362–1366

[5] Ackerman WE, III, Ahmad M. The efficacy of lumbar epidural steroid injections in patients with lumbar disc herniations. Anesth Analg. 2007; 104 (5):1217–1222

[6] Vad VB, Bhat AL, Lutz GE, Cammisa F. Transforaminal epidural steroid injections in lumbosacral radiculopathy: a prospective randomized study. Spine. 2002; 27(1):11–16

[7] Manchikanti L, Buenaventura RM, Manchikanti KN, et al. Effectiveness of therapeutic lumbar transforaminal epidural steroid injections in managing lumbar spinal pain. In: Database of Abstracts of Reviews of Effects (DARE): Quality-assessed Reviews [Internet]. York (UK): Centre for Reviews and Dissemination (UK); 1995. Review published: 2012. Available from: https://www.ncbi.nlm.nih.gov/books/NBK116301/

[8] Schaufele MK, Hatch L, Jones W. Interlaminar versus transforaminal epidural injections for the treatment of symptomatic lumbar intervertebral disc herniations. Pain Physician. 2006; 9(4):361–366

[9] Rathmell JP, Aprill C, Bogduk N. Cervical transforaminal injection of steroids. Anesthesiology. 2004; 100(6):1595–1600

[10] Costandi SJ, Azer G, Eshraghi Y, et al. Cervical transforaminal epidural steroid injections: diagnostic and therapeutic value. Reg Anesth Pain Med. 2015; 40 (6):674–680

[11] Roberts ST, Willick SE, Rho ME, Rittenberg JD. Efficacy of lumbosacral transforaminal epidural steroid injections: a systematic review. PM R. 2009; 1(7):657–668

[12] Benny B, Azari P. The efficacy of lumbosacral transforaminal epidural steroid injections: a comprehensive literature review. J Back Musculoskeletal Rehabil. 2011; 24(2):67–76

[13] Patel IJ, Rahim S, Davidson JC, et al. Society of Interventional Radiology consensus guidelines for the periprocedural management of thrombotic and bleeding risk in patients undergoing percutaneous image-guided interventions—Part II: Recommendations: Endorsed by the Canadian Association for Interventional Radiology and the Cardiovascular and Interventional Radiological Society of Europe. J Vasc Interv Radiol. 2019; 30(8):1168–1184.e1

[14] Park JW, Nam HS, Cho SK, Jung HJ, Lee BJ, Park Y. Kambin's triangle approach of lumbar transforaminal epidural injection with spinal stenosis. Ann Rehabil Med. 2011; 35(6):833–843

[15] Alleyne CH , Jr, Cawley CM, Shengelaia GG, Barrow DL. Microsurgical anatomy of the artery of Adamkiewicz and its segmental artery. J Neurosurg. 1998; 89 (5):791–795

[16] Huntoon MA. Anatomy of the cervical intervertebral foramina: vulnerable arteries and ischemic neurologic injuries after transforaminal epidural injections. Pain. 2005; 117(1–2):104–111

[17] Scanlon GC, Moeller-Bertram T, Romanowsky SM, Wallace MS. Cervical transforaminal epidural steroid injections: more dangerous than we think? Spine. 2007; 32(11):1249–1256

[18] Baker R, Dreyfuss P, Mercer S, Bogduk N. Cervical transforaminal injection of corticosteroids into a radicular artery: a possible mechanism for spinal cord injury. Pain. 2003; 103(1–2):211–215

[19] Furman MB, Giovanniello MT, O'Brien EM. Incidence of intravascular penetration in transforaminal cervical epidural steroid injections. Spine. 2003; 28(1):21–25

[20] Huntoon MA, Martin DP. Paralysis after transforaminal epidural injection and previous spinal surgery. Reg Anesth Pain Med. 2004; 29(5):494–495

[21] Rathmell JP, Benzon HT. Transforaminal injection of steroids: should we continue? Reg Anesth Pain Med. 2004; 29(5):397–399

[22] Dreyfuss P, Baker R, Bogduk N. Comparative effectiveness of cervical transforaminal injections with particulate and nonparticulate corticosteroid preparations for cervical radicular pain. Pain Med. 2006; 7(3):237–242

[23] Gharibo C, Koo C, Chung J, Moroz A. Epidural steroid injections: an update on mechanisms of injury and safety. Tech Reg Anesth Pain Manage. 2009; 13: 266–271

[24] Benzon HT, Chew TL, McCarthy RJ, Benzon HA, Walega DR. Comparison of the particle sizes of different steroids and the effect of dilution: a review of the relative neurotoxicities of the steroids. Anesthesiology. 2007; 106(2): 331–338

[25] Zheng P, Schneider BJ, Kennedy DJ, McCormick ZL. Safe injectate choice, visualization, and delivery for lumbar transforaminal epidural steroid injections: evolving literature and considerations. Curr Phys Med Rehabil Rep. 2019; 7:414–421

[26] Younes M, Neffati F, Touzi M, et al. Systemic effects of epidural and intra-articular glucocorticoid injections in diabetic and non-diabetic patients. Joint Bone Spine. 2007; 74(5):472–476

27 Radicular Pain Related to Synovial Cysts

Danoob Dalili, Daniel E. Dalili, Amanda Isaac, and Jan Fritz

27.1 Case Presentation

An 86-year-old woman presented with low back pain that radiated down the left leg. On clinical examination, the pain was described as mainly "electric shock"-like but occasionally dull, scoring 7 to 9 on a 10 point visual analog pain scale (VAS score). Clinically, a diagnosis of sciatica was suspected. Her past medical history was significant for breast cancer. Laboratory evaluation demonstrated nonspecific increased inflammatory markers (erythrocyte sedimentation rate and C-reactive protein). Given her cancer history, magnetic resonance imaging (MRI) of the lumbosacral spine was performed to exclude a neoplastic or infectious etiology of her symptoms (▶ Fig. 27.1).

Following clinical review and discussion at a spinal multidisciplinary board meeting, and since the patient was deemed unfit for surgical intervention due to comorbidities, percutaneous left L3–L4 facet joint cyst rupture was requested to reduce the degree of spinal canal narrowing.

27.2 Companion Case Presentation

A 54-year-old woman presented with long-standing right-sided leg pain, which worsened following a fall from standing height. Her pain was incapacitating without relief despite analgesics. On clinical examination, she reported a 10/10 VAS score in a predominantly right L4 dermatomal distribution. Following discussion at the regional multidisciplinary spinal board meeting, a decision was made to perform computed tomography (CT)-guided indirect synovial cyst rupture.

27.3 Companion Case Presentation

A 77-year-old woman presented with 8/10 low back pain that radiated into the left thigh region. Conservative treatment consisting of physical therapy and analgesic oral medication were unsuccessful in providing meaningful pain relief. An MRI examination of the lumbar spine demonstrated multilevel disk degeneration, ligamentum flavum thickening, and facet joint arthrosis. At the L2–L3 level, an asymmetric disk bulge and left intracanalicular facet joint cyst contributed to high-grade central canal stenosis, with near-complete effacement of the cerebrospinal fluid (CSF) signal. In order to reduce the degree of central canal narrowing, the patient was subsequently referred for CT-guided percutaneous facet joint rupture.

27.4 Discussion

The first case of a spinal synovial cyst causing radiculopathy in a patient was described by Vossschulte and Borger in 1950.[1] Lumbar synovial cysts, also known as juxta-facet cysts, are intraspinal, foraminal, or paravertebral cysts first described by Kao et al in 1968.[2] They are most commonly located posteriorly within the spinal canal. In a prevalence MRI study, synovial facet cysts occurred in 6.5% of all patients, with 46% of the cases being discovered incidentally.[3] Synovial cysts are dilatations of the joint capsule that originate from the facet joints and protrude into the spinal canal.[3] Such cysts can contain serous, viscous, or hemorrhagic fluid.[4] The lumbar region at L3–L4 is the most common, followed by L4–L5 and L5–S1[5]; the thoracic and cervical spine are uncommon locations.[6,7,8] On CT and MRI, the cysts present as well-circumscribed, extradural, space-occupying lesions, often with visible communication with the facet joint, contributing to various degrees of central canal stenosis.[9] MRI remains the modality of choice for diagnosis, as it can confirm an extradural location as well as characterize the matrix of the cyst (fluid, proteinaceous content, presence of calcifications, or blood in case of hemorrhagic cysts). On MRI, a simple cyst is typically hyperintense on both T1- and T2-weighted images, and is likely easier to rupture than more complex cysts. On contrast-enhanced T1-weighted MR images, there is usually mild peripheral wall enhancement without enhancement of cyst contents.[10,11] Due

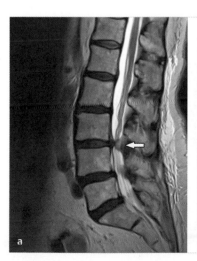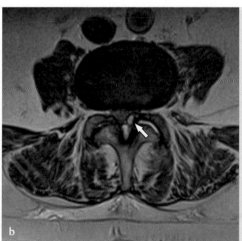

Fig. 27.1 Routine magnetic resonance imaging (MRI) of the lumbosacral spine. Sagittal (**a**) and axial (**b**) T2-weighted sequences demonstrating multilevel lumbar degeneration with degenerative grade 1 L4–L5 spondylolisthesis. At L3–L4, a right central disk extrusion, ligamentum flavum thickening, facet joint arthrosis, and a 7-mm left intracanalicular facet joint synovial cyst (arrow) resulted in moderate to severe central spinal canal stenosis, with near-complete effacement of the cerebrospinal fluid signal and nerve root redundancy above this level.

to hemosiderin deposition, hemorrhage presents as high signal on T1-weighted and low signal on gradient echo sequences. Owing to advances in MRI and improved access to MR scanners, symptomatic synovial cysts are being increasingly reported and referred for treatment.[12,13,14]

27.4.1 Risk Factors and Presentation

Common risk factors for synovial cysts are spinal degeneration, instability, and trauma. The incidence increases with age.[14] Although asymptomatic and found incidentally in nearly half of all cases, common symptoms of synovial cysts are back pain, radiculopathy, and sensory and motor deficits.[15] The initial presentation is cauda equina syndrome in up to 13% of patients.[16] Symptoms usually occur when the size of the cyst is large enough to cause higher grade central canal stenosis with compression of neural elements. The symptoms are often nonspecific and compounded by disk degeneration, facet joint arthrosis, and ligamentum flavum thickening.[17]

27.4.2 Diagnosis

Symptoms of synovial cysts may initially be attributed to neural compression caused mechanically by the cysts. Owing to the lack of specific symptoms, the diagnosis of an intracanalicular synovial cyst is difficult to make based on clinical presentation, history, and radiography alone.[14,18] Radiographs can diagnose osseous abnormalities but are not reliable in detecting synovial cysts due to their soft tissue nature. MRI is the most accurate imaging technique to diagnose facet joints cysts based on their typical T2 hyperintense cystic nature. Proteinaceous materials within the cyst may be depicted with higher signal intensity than the surrounding CSF on both T1- and T2-weighted imaging[10,19] (▶ Fig. 27.2). Synovial cysts can also be detected with CT when low tube voltages are used to allow sufficient soft tissue contrast. In addition, facet joints cysts are more conspicuous on CT images when there is mineralization of the cyst wall and when the cyst contains high attenuating blood products and low attenuating gas.[20,21] Given its high spatial and contrast resolution, MRI is the standard of reference for the imaging diagnosis of synovial cysts.[22]

27.4.3 Treatment

Multidisciplinary discussions are warranted to assess the threshold for intervention and the treatment options available in a patient-centered model.[23,24,25,26,27] Facet synovial cysts can either be managed conservatively, treated surgically, or treated with minimally invasive techniques. Typical conservative treatments include bed rest, oral and topical analgesic drugs, and physiotherapy.[4] Some studies have demonstrated complete resolution of symptoms with conservative management only.[28] However, in the majority of patients an intervention is more likely to lead to a successful outcome.[4]

In the past, surgical management was used in treating synovial cysts that were refractory to conservative management. The most common surgical procedures used to manage this condition are hemi-laminectomy and bilateral laminectomy. Endoscopic or open resection of the cyst, and optional instrumentation for stabilization, has also been used. The average clinical success rate of surgery is 80 to 90%.[29] Despite this high success rate, adverse effects are associated with surgery, particularly in the setting of laminectomy without instrumentation, resulting in spinal instability in approximately 20% of cases; in these patients, further surgery is required. Risks of open spinal surgery to treat synovial cysts also include epidural hematoma and diskitis, as well as risks of anesthesia.[30] There has been a reported incidence of dural tears in 4% of cases (and 17% of revision cases) while attempting to remove cysts that have adhered to the dura, resulting in CSF leaks and associated complications.[31]

Minimally invasive image-guided percutaneous interventions for synovial cysts include simple facet joint steroid injections and percutaneous cyst rupture. First reported by Casselman in 1985, steroid injections for treating synovial cysts have long become one of the initial management options prior to considering surgery.[32]

Facet joint injections are traditionally performed with fluoroscopy guidance with reported good effect in the early stages; 66% of such patients report initial resolution of pain. New approaches include CT- and MRI-guided facet joint injections.[27,33,34,35]

Recurrence of pain and adverse symptoms may occur over time following simple steroid injections.[36] Advancements in

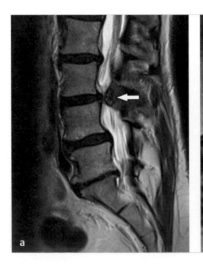
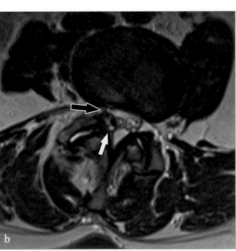

Fig. 27.2 Sagittal (**a**) and axial (**b**) T2-weighted (T2W) magnetic resonance (MR) images of the lumbar and sacral spine. Routine magnetic resonance imaging (MRI) of the lumbar and sacral spine demonstrating degenerative lumbar scoliosis with multilevel facet and disk degeneration. At the L3–L4 level, a 10-mm right intracanalicular facet joint cyst protrudes into the right lateral recess, indenting the thecal sac and compressing the traversing right L4 nerve root in the subarticular zone (black arrow). MRI demonstrates a thickened cyst wall with low T2 signal intensity (white arrow) suggestive of calcification.

imaging technology and the increasing popularity of percutaneous minimally invasive techniques have resulted in the establishment of percutaneous facet joint synovial cyst rupture as a first-line method for treating this condition, particularly if causing mechanical neural compromise. This procedure can be performed either fluoroscopically or under CT guidance, with the latter found to be more successful at follow-up.[37] Using either imaging modality, synovial cyst rupture utilizes a similar technique as facet joint injections. Typically, a 90-mm 22-G standard spinal needle is placed into the facet joint space and a small volume of radiopaque contrast (1–3 mL) is injected to confirm intra-articular positioning. Thereafter, continuous injection of contrast is performed to confirm the presence of a cyst by observing pooling of the contrast into one location anterior to the facet joint.

Then two established methods are used to rupture the cyst—indirect and direct. The indirect method involves injecting a combination of 2 mL of a nonparticulate steroid (dexamethasone 3.3 mg/mL), 4 mL of 0.25% Marcaine, and 1 mL of contrast into the facet joint. This injected volume causes the cyst to rupture, which is confirmed through perception of loss of resistance by the operator as well as extravasation of dye into the epidural space on continuous fluoroscopic or intermittent CT acquisition (▶ Fig. 27.3 and ▶ Fig. 27.4).

The direct method is more commonly confined to CT guidance, and involves direct puncture and aspiration of the cyst using a needle inserted in the interlaminar space[37] (▶ Fig. 27.5). For this method, an extrapedicular transforaminal approach is used. Better anatomical correlation augmented by reality navigation and freehand MRI-guided interventions may be helpful in increasing the safety of the procedure and improving the confidence of the interventional radiologist performing the procedure.[38,39]

This method of treating synovial cysts is reported to have an efficacy rate of 46% in a retrospective study of 101 cases in 2009.[40] Improved efficacy (over 82%) was reported in a more recent case study in 2018.[37] Similar to the latter study, in a recent population-based study, 79% of the patients reported short-term pain relief and almost a third of the patients had sustained relief and were able to avoid spinal surgery during long-term follow-up (median 11 years).[31] Percutaneous intervention for treating this condition inevitably carries a lower risk of adverse events compared to open procedures such as laminectomy and surgical fusion.

T2 signal on MRI can serve as a predictive tool in order to determine successful outcomes following percutaneous rupture procedures.[33] T2 hyperintense and intermediate signal intensity Lumbar facet joint synovial cysts (LFSCs) are easier to rupture, perhaps because the cysts contain a higher proportion of fluid and are less gelatinous or calcified than T2 hypointense cysts. Partly for this reason, patients with T2 hyperintense LFSCs are less likely to need surgery.[33]

27.4.4 Complications

The main adverse effect of attempted synovial cyst rupture is the possibility of cyst expansion with failure to rupture, resulting in further neuronal compression which could potentially lead to cauda equina syndrome. Other complications include a dural leak if the procedure injures the dura which could be adherent to the cyst wall in long-standing infection as noted with any invasive procedure or following repeat procedures and surgery.[32]

27.5 Conclusion

Symptomatic lumbar facet joint synovial cysts are fairly uncommon but when present can cause back pain and lower limb radiculopathy by direct mechanical compression on nerve roots. Accessibility to MRI and improvements in MR resolution have

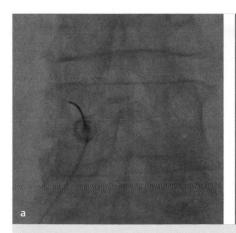
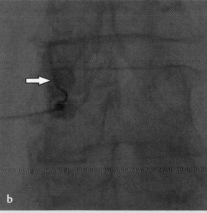
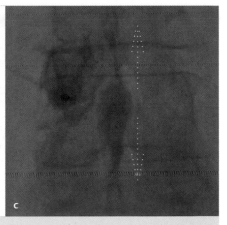

Fig. 27.3 Fluoroscopic images (**a**) demonstrating targeting of the left L3–L4 facet joint with a standard 90-mm-long 22-G spinal needle. A 10 degrees obliquity (mediolateral) of the fluoroscopy X-ray beam is used for optimal visualization of the inferomedial margin of the facet joint. Contrast is injected (**b**) to confirm intra-articular positioning of the needle tip and filling of the synovial cyst (arrow). Finally, a 6 mL mixture of 2 mL dexamethasone (3.3 mg/mL) and 4 mL Marcaine (0.25%) is injected with a Luer-lock syringe under high pressure until successful rupture of the synovial cyst occurrs (**c**), which is denoted by a sudden loss of resistance and fluoroscopic confirmation of contrast extravasation (dotted arrows) into the epidural space. Informed consent should include the likelihood of "crescendo"-like pain during the procedure due to the increasing size of the cyst immediately before rupture, which is then followed by decompression and subsiding pain/radiculopathy symptoms. The epidural leakage of steroid and anesthetic may have a prolonged epidural effect, which could be sensory, motor, or mixed.

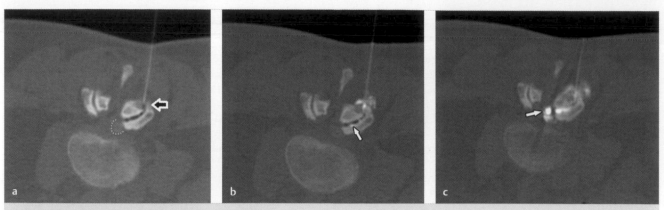

Fig. 27.4 Axial computed tomography (CT) slices through the L3–L4 level demonstrating technique for indirect CT-guided synovial cyst rupture. A 90-mm 22-G spinal needle (arrow) is utilized to puncture the right L3–L4 facet joint (**a**). CT images demonstrated calcifications within the wall of the cyst (dotted line). Iodine-based contrast injection (**b**) confirmed the intra-articular positioning of the needle tip within the facet joint (arrow). (**c**) The admixture of dexamethasone, bupivacaine, and iodine contrast agent is injected under high pressure until the cyst ruptures (arrow), which is accompanied by epidural spread of the injectate (arrow).

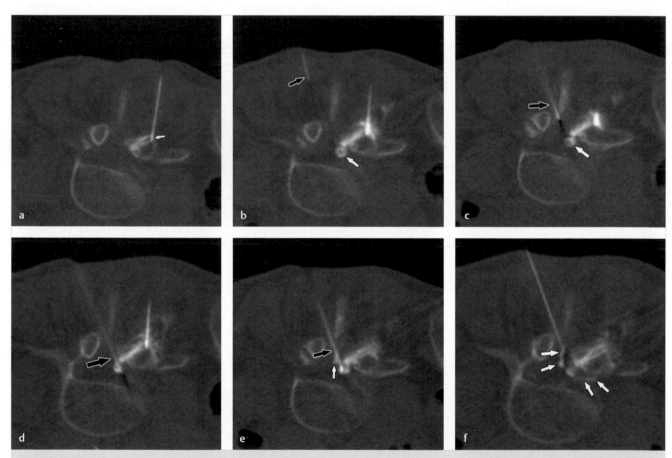

Fig. 27.5 Axial computed tomography (CT) slices through the L2–L3 level demonstrating technique for direct CT-guided synovial cyst rupture. (**a**) The left L2–L3 facet joint is punctured with a 20-gauge spinal needle (arrow). (**b**) The intra-articular needle tip position is confirmed with the injection of 0.5 mL of iodine contrast material. The intra-articular contrast material outlines the intracanalicular facet joint cyst (white arrow), which was distensible. Several attempts of cyst rupture were unsuccessful because of high pain levels before cyst rupture could occur. (**c, d**) Using a second 20-gauge needle (open arrow), the intracanalicular contrast-opacified cyst is targeted via a contralateral oblique interlaminar approach. (**e, f**) Using intermittent needle advancement and imaging control, the cyst was successfully punctured and fenestrated with multiple careful needle excursions. Subsequent injection of a mixture of 1% ropivacaine local anesthetic, dexamethasone, and iodine contrast demonstrated cyst rupture with epidural spread (white arrows).

led to increased reporting of symptomatic synovial cysts and referrals for management.[12,13,14]

Although surgical management is very successful in treating this condition, image-guided percutaneous interventions have shown comparable efficacies with a lower risk of adverse events.

Radiologically guided procedures offer safe and effective first-line treatment strategies for this condition once conservative therapies have failed to control the symptoms. Discussion in a multidisciplinary board with an interventional radiologist should be considered prior to referral for surgery. MRI is the modality of choice for diagnosis and characterization of the cysts, and their location as well as their effect on the surrounding neurological structures. T2 signal can serve as a predictive tool to determine successful outcomes following percutaneous rupture procedures.[41]

References

[1] Vossschulte K, Borger G. [Anatomic and functional studies of intervertebral disk hernia]. Langenbecks Arch Klin Chir Ver Dtsch Z Chir. 1950; 265(3–4):329–355

[2] Kao CC, Uihlein A, Bickel WH, Soule EH. Lumbar intraspinal extradural ganglion cyst. J Neurosurg. 1968; 29(2):168–172

[3] Epstein NE, Baisden J. The diagnosis and management of synovial cysts: efficacy of surgery versus cyst aspiration. Surg Neurol Int. 2012; 3(4) Suppl 3:S157–S166

[4] Shah RV, Lutz GE. Lumbar intraspinal synovial cysts: conservative management and review of the world's literature. Spine J. 2003; 3(6):479–488

[5] Sauvage P, Grimault L, Ben Salem D, Roussin I, Huguenin M, Falconnet M. [Lumbar intraspinal synovial cysts: imaging and treatment by percutaneous injection. Report of thirteen cases]. J Radiol. 2000; 81(1):33–38

[6] Epstein NE. Lumbar synovial cysts: a review of diagnosis, surgical management, and outcome assessment. J Spinal Disord Tech. 2004; 17(4):321–325

[7] Almefty R, Arnautović KI, Webber BL. Multilevel bilateral calcified thoracic spinal synovial cysts. J Neurosurg Spine. 2008; 8(5):473–477

[8] Costa F, Menghetti C, Cardia A, Fornari M, Ortolina A. Cervical synovial cyst: case report and review of literature. Eur Spine J. 2010; 19(2) Suppl 2:S100–S102

[9] Khan AM, Girardi F. Spinal lumbar synovial cysts. Diagnosis and management challenge. Eur Spine J. 2006; 15(8):1176–1182

[10] Jackson DE, Jr, Atlas SW, Mani JR, Norman D. Intraspinal synovial cysts: MR imaging. Radiology. 1989; 170(2):527–530

[11] Knox AM, Fon GT. The appearances of lumbar intraspinal synovial cysts. Clin Radiol. 1991; 44(6):397–401

[12] Kaneko K, Inoue Y. Haemorrhagic lumbar synovial cyst. A cause of acute radiculopathy. J Bone Joint Surg Br. 2000; 82(4):583–584

[13] Kao CC, Winkler SS, Turner JH. Synovial cyst of spinal facet. Case report. J Neurosurg. 1974; 41(3):372–376

[14] Boviatsis EJ, Stavrinou LC, Kouyialis AT, et al. Spinal synovial cysts: pathogenesis, diagnosis and surgical treatment in a series of seven cases and literature review. Eur Spine J. 2008; 17(6):831–837

[15] Bjorkengren AG, Kurz LT, Resnick D, Sartoris DJ, Garfin SR. Symptomatic intraspinal synovial cysts: opacification and treatment by percutaneous injection. AJR Am J Roentgenol. 1987; 149(1):105–107

[16] Baum JA, Hanley EN, Jr. Intraspinal synovial cyst simulating spinal stenosis. A case report. Spine. 1986; 11(5):487–489

[17] Sabo RA, Tracy PT, Weinger JM. A series of 60 juxtafacet cysts: clinical presentation, the role of spinal instability, and treatment. J Neurosurg. 1996; 85(4):560–565

[18] Reddy P, Satyanarayana S, Nanda A. Synovial cyst of lumbar spine presenting as disc disease: a case report and review of literature. J La State Med Soc. 2000; 152(11):563–566

[19] Papakonstantinou O, Isaac A, Dalili D, Noebauer-Huhmann IM. T2-weighted hypointense tumors and tumor-like lesions. Semin Musculoskelet Radiol. 2019; 23(1):58–75

[20] Liu SS, Williams KD, Drayer BP, Spetzler RF, Sonntag VKH. Synovial cysts of the lumbosacral spine: diagnosis by MR imaging. AJR Am J Roentgenol. 1990; 154(1):163–166

[21] Fardon DF, Simmons JD. Gas-filled intraspinal synovial cyst. A case report. Spine. 1989; 14(1):127–129

[22] Bermejo A, De Bustamante TD, Martinez A, Carrera R, Zabía E, Manjón P. MR imaging in the evaluation of cystic-appearing soft-tissue masses of the extremities. Radiographics. 2013; 33(3):833–855

[23] Dalili D, Isaac A, Rashidi A, Åström G, Fritz J. Image-guided sports medicine and musculoskeletal tumor interventions: a patient-centered model. Semin Musculoskelet Radiol. 2020; 24(3):290–309

[24] Dalili D, Isaac A, Bazzocchi A, et al. Interventional techniques for bone and musculoskeletal soft tissue tumors: current practices and future directions—part I. Ablation. Semin Musculoskelet Radiol. 2020; 24(6):692–709

[25] Dalili D, Isaac A, Cazzato RL, et al. Interventional techniques for bone and musculoskeletal soft tissue tumors: current practices and future directions—part II. Stabilization. Semin Musculoskelet Radiol. 2020; 24(6):710–725

[26] Cazzato RL, Garnon J, De Marini P, et al. French multidisciplinary approach for the treatment of MSK tumors. Semin Musculoskelet Radiol. 2020; 24(3):310–322

[27] Fritz J, Niemeyer T, Clasen S, et al. Management of chronic low back pain: rationales, principles, and targets of imaging-guided spinal injections. Radiographics. 2007; 27(6):1751–1771

[28] Métellus P, Fuentes S, Adetchessi T, et al. Retrospective study of 77 patients harbouring lumbar synovial cysts: functional and neurological outcome. Acta Neurochir (Wien). 2006; 148(1):47–54, discussion 54

[29] Bydon A, Xu R, Parker SL, et al. Recurrent back and leg pain and cyst reformation after surgical resection of spinal synovial cysts: systematic review of reported postoperative outcomes. Spine J. 2010; 10(9):820–826

[30] Lyons MK, Atkinson JLD, Wharen RE, Deen HG, Zimmerman RS, Lemens SM. Surgical evaluation and management of lumbar synovial cysts: the Mayo Clinic experience. J Neurosurg. 2000; 93(1) Suppl:53–57

[31] Epstein NE. Lumbar laminectomy for the resection of synovial cysts and coexisting lumbar spinal stenosis or degenerative spondylolisthesis: an outcome study. Spine. 2004; 29(9):1049–1055, discussion 1056

[32] Casselman ES. Radiologic recognition of symptomatic spinal synovial cysts. AJNR Am J Neuroradiol. 1985; 6(6):971–973

[33] Fritz J, Clasen S, Boss A, et al. Real-time MR fluoroscopy-navigated lumbar facet joint injections: feasibility and technical properties. Eur Radiol. 2008; 18(7):1513–1518

[34] Fritz J, Pereira PL. [MR-guided pain therapy: principles and clinical applications]. Röfo Fortschr Geb Röntgenstr Nuklearmed. 2007; 179(9):914–924

[35] Fritz J, Sequeiros RB, Carrino JA. Magnetic resonance imaging-guided spine injections. Top Magn Reson Imaging. 2011; 22(4):143–151

[36] Parlier-Cuau C, Wybier M, Nizard R, Champsaur P, Le Hir P, Laredo JD. Symptomatic lumbar facet joint synovial cysts: clinical assessment of facet joint steroid injection after 1 and 6 months and long-term follow-up in 30 patients. Radiology. 1999; 210(2):509–513

[37] Chazen JL, Leeman K, Singh JR, Schweitzer A. Percutaneous CT-guided facet joint synovial cyst rupture: success with refractory cases and technical considerations. Clin Imaging. 2018; 49:7–11

[38] Fritz J, U-Thainual P, Ungi T, et al. Augmented reality visualisation using an image overlay system for MR-guided interventions: technical performance of spine injection procedures in human cadavers at 1.5 Tesla. Eur Radiol. 2013; 23(1):235–245

[39] Fritz J, Thomas C, Clasen S, Claussen CD, Lewin JS, Pereira PL. Freehand real-time MRI-guided lumbar spinal injection procedures at 1.5 T: feasibility, accuracy, and safety. AJR Am J Roentgenol. 2009; 192(4):W161–7

[40] Martha JF, Swaim B, Wang DA, et al. Outcome of percutaneous rupture of lumbar synovial cysts: a case series of 101 patients. Spine J. 2009; 9(11):899–904

[41] Cambron SC, McIntyre JJ, Guerin SJ, Li Z, Pastel DA. Lumbar facet joint synovial cysts: does T2 signal intensity predict outcomes after percutaneous rupture? AJNR Am J Neuroradiol. 2013; 34(8):1661–1664

28 Percutaneous Spinal Decompression

Junjian Huang and Joshua A. Hirsch

28.1 Case Presentation

An 81-year-old man with prostate cancer, hypertension, and longstanding back pain that had been managed with epidural spine injections was referred for management of lower back pain. Specifically, he complained of lower back and leg pain with claudication that was relieved when hunched over. There was no evidence of saddle anesthesia or bowel dysfunction.

On physical examination, he was able to move all extremities, and demonstrated 5/5 strength in bilateral lower extremities

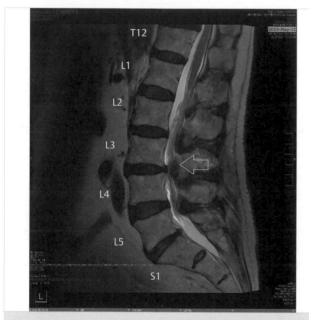

Fig. 28.1 Sagittal T2-weighted magnetic resonance imaging (MRI) of the lumbar spine demonstrating central stenosis at L3–L4 (arrow).

with intact sensation. Mild tenderness to palpation in the lower lumbar spinous process was noted. He was able to walk 50 feet (approximately 15 m) before noting bilateral leg cramping that was relieved by sitting and forward leaning. His visual analog scale pain score was reported as 8–9/10. His magnetic resonance imaging (MRI) evaluation of the lumbar spine demonstrated multilevel degenerative changes with spinal canal narrowing worst at L3–L4 (▶ Fig. 28.1).

Given that his conservative therapy options were exhausted, and he desired to avoid surgery, the Superion device (VertiFlex, Inc. San Clemente, CA, USA) procedure was offered to him as a nonsurgical option to alleviate his neurogenic claudication (NIC). The purposes, alternatives, risks (bleeding, infection, spinous process fracture, device migration, nerve damage including paralysis), and benefits were explained and discussed. The patient understood all the risks and demonstrated willingness to proceed.

28.2 Procedure

The L3–L4 interspinous space was marked under fluoroscopic guidance (▶ Fig. 28.2a, b). The needle insertion site was anesthetized with lidocaine injection. A 3-cm incision was made using a scalpel. The posterior spinal ligament was incised using a scalpel. The Vertiflex Instrument Platform Kit (Vertiflex, Inc. San Clemente, CA, USA) was opened, and the cannula assembly was inserted under fluoroscopic guidance into the L3–L4 interspinous space (▶ Fig. 28.2c). This was advanced to the level of the lamina after which the dilator assembly was placed (▶ Fig. 28.2d). The cannula assembly was removed (▶ Fig. 28.2e). Subsequently, the interspinous gauge was inserted which measured a distance of approximately 12 mm (▶ Fig. 28.3a). The assembly was retracted into better position. The driver and inserter were then used to place the 12-mm implant under fluoroscopic guidance (▶ Fig. 28.3b).

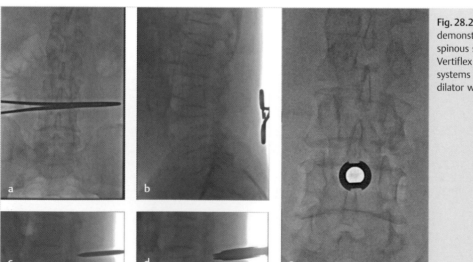

Fig. 28.2 Intraoperative fluoroscopic images demonstrating localization of the L3–L4 interspinous space (**a** and **b**) with placement of Vertiflex platform cannula (**c**) and dilator (**d**) systems with posteroanterior (PA) view of the dilator with cannula assembly removed (**e**).

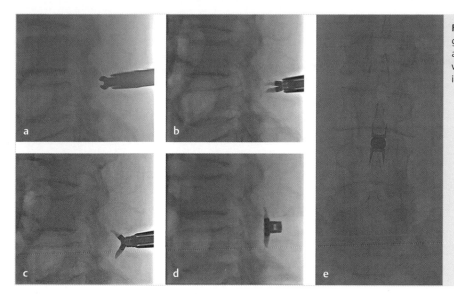

Fig. 28.3 Intraoperative fluoroscopic interspinous gauge (**a**) was inserted to measure the distance and then replaced by the driver and inserter, which were then used to place the 12-mm implant under fluoroscopic guidance (**b–e**).

The driver and inserter were then removed, which demonstrated appropriate positioning of the implant (▶ Fig. 28.3c). The incision was closed with deep 3–0 resorbable braided suture layer and superficial 4–0 nonresorbable monofilament suture, followed by Syvek patch (Marine Polymer Technologies, Inc.; Burlington, MA). Good hemostasis was achieved.

The patient tolerated the procedure well and was discharged the same day with relief of symptoms. Of note, now 5 months out from the procedure, the patient does not have any plans to have surgery performed.

28.3 Discussion

Interspinous process devices (IPDs) have been available for decades with numerous devices including: the Device for Intervertebral Assisted Motion (DIAM) (Medtronic Sofamor Danek, Memphis, TN), Wallis Stabilization System (Zimmer, Bordeaux, France), and COFLEX (Paradigm Spine, New York, NY). These devices have traditionally been marketed to surgeons aiming to perform "minimally" invasive surgery.[1] Studies performed on cadavers have demonstrated increased neural foraminal area and spinal canal area by 26 and 18%, respectively, following placement of IPD, as well as increased foraminal width and subarticular diameter by 41 and 50%.[2] Typically, IPDs are indicated in patients who have failed a 6-month trial of conservative therapy and are without posterior element instability greater than Meyerding Grade 1 spondylolisthesis.

The X STOP trial randomized 191 patients with neurogenic intermittent claudication (NIC) into treatment (100) and control (91) groups.[3] Quantitative improvement was measured based on the Zurich Claudication Questionnaire, and demonstrated significantly better outcomes 48 months in patients who underwent X STOP IPD placement compared to conservative therapy group.[3] Subsequent studies assessing inter-IPD differences demonstrated no significant differences in efficacy between the two groups.[4] Recently, a new second-generation percutaneous IPD was introduced named the SUPERION device. The PRESS trial is a randomized control trial comparing the efficacy of X STOP versus the SUPERION consisting of 391 patients with NIC to either group (190 SUPERION vs. 201 X STOP).

Results have demonstrated significantly improved back pain and leg symptoms in the SUPERION group at 2 years.[5] A literature comparison of SUPERION versus laminectomy demonstrates no significant difference for back pain or leg symptoms at 1 or 2 years.[6] Recent data for SUPERION as stand-alone therapy have demonstrated that at 5 years, 84% of patients have demonstrated durable results and 75% are free of surgery, reoperation, or revision.[7]

The main complications with all IPDs are spinous process fracture (3.3%) and prosthesis dislocation (rare).

In summary, IPDs can be helpful in patients with NIC and currently act as a bridge between conservative therapy and surgery. Currently, the American Pain Society guidelines give IPDs a "B" recommendation as there is moderate net benefit at 2 years.[8]

References

[1] Gazzeri R, Galarza M, Alfieri A. Controversies about interspinous process devices in the treatment of degenerative lumbar spine diseases: past, present, and future. BioMed Res Int. 2014; 2014:975052

[2] Richards JC, Majumdar S, Lindsey DP, Beaupré GS, Yerby SA. The treatment mechanism of an interspinous process implant for lumbar neurogenic intermittent claudication. Spine. 2005; 30(7):744–749

[3] Zucherman JF, Hsu KY, Hartjen CA, et al. A multicenter, prospective, randomized trial evaluating the X STOP interspinous process decompression system for the treatment of neurogenic intermittent claudication: two-year follow-up results. Spine. 2005; 30(12):1351–1358

[4] Sobottke R, Schlüter-Brust K, Kaulhausen T, et al. Interspinous implants (X Stop, Wallis, Diam) for the treatment of LSS: is there a correlation between radiological parameters and clinical outcome? Eur Spine J. 2009; 18(10):1494–1503

[5] Patel VV, Whang PG, Haley TR, et al. Two-year clinical outcomes of a multicenter randomized controlled trial comparing two interspinous spacers for treatment of moderate lumbar spinal stenosis. BMC Musculoskelet Disord. 2014; 15:221

[6] Lauryssen C, Jackson RJ, Baron JM, et al. Stand-alone interspinous spacer versus decompressive laminectomy for treatment of lumbar spinal stenosis. Expert Rev Med Devices. 2015; 12(6):763–769

[7] Nunley PD, Patel VV, Orndorff DG, Lavelle WF, Block JE, Geisler FH. Five-year durability of stand-alone interspinous process decompression for lumbar spinal stenosis. Clin Interv Aging. 2017; 12:1409–1417

[8] Chou R, Loeser JD, Owens DK, et al. American Pain Society Low Back Pain Guideline Panel. Interventional therapies, surgery, and interdisciplinary rehabilitation for low back pain: an evidence-based clinical practice guideline from the American Pain Society. Spine. 2009; 34(10):1066–1077

29 Neurostimulators

Vinita Singh and Jerry P. Kalangara

29.1 Case Presentation

A 44-year-old man with a history of metastatic renal cell carcinoma (▶ Fig. 29.1) presented with constant axial low back pain (left greater than right) located near the lumbosacral junction. He described his pain as burning, throbbing, and sharp. He also had bilateral anterior thigh pain, but his back pain was his predominant symptom. His medical history was significant for osseous metastasis throughout the entire spine including multiple vertebral bodies, sacrum, and ilium. He had a pathologic fracture of the L2 vertebral body with 50% height loss. Retropulsed bone and tumor resulted in severe spinal canal narrowing and cauda equina compression. Extraosseous metastasis included ventral epidural extension of the tumor effacing cerebrospinal fluid (CSF) at various levels in the thoracolumbar region (▶ Fig. 29.2), retroperitoneal lymphadenopathy, and direct tumoral extension into the left iliacus muscle.

His pain was refractory to medical management (opioids, adjuvants, and cannabinoids). The differential diagnosis for his pain included neuropathic pain from spinal stenosis, nociceptive pain from L2 vertebral body fracture, or referred visceral pain from the renal mass, and retroperitoneal lymphadenopathy.

The patient underwent various targeted radiation therapies and different interventional procedures without much benefit. Interventions included: transpedicular L2 radiofrequency ablation (RFA) and kyphoplasty; lumbar L3–L5 medial branch block and RFA; interlaminar L5–S1 and caudal epidural steroid injections; celiac plexus neurolysis; and intrathecal pump trial with a continuous epidural catheter.

Due to suboptimal pain relief, the decision was made for a conventional spinal cord stimulator (SCS) trial. Trial leads were placed at T8 and T9, which resulted in greater than 60% pain relief and improved function. An SCS with an external pulse generator was chosen for implant due to concern for delayed wound healing from previous lumbar radiation therapy and malnutrition. Following permanent implant, his pain was controlled with SCS therapy. He began gaining weight back, was able to work part time, and enjoyed spending time with his family for 6 months before he died.

29.2 Discussion

Spinal cord stimulation therapy was originally developed in 1967 by Dr. Norman Shealy, a neurosurgeon, for the treatment of neoplasm-related pain.[1,2] This therapy was originally based on the Melzack–Wall "gate-control" theory, which postulated that stimulation of large myelinated fibers could modulate pain perception by "closing the gate" to the dorsal horn neurons and thus preventing input from small pain fibers.[3] Based on this concept, conventional SCS therapy started becoming commercially available in the 1980s; presently, an estimated 50,000 SCS implants are performed every year.[4]

The mechanism of pain relief in SCS was initially attributed solely to dorsal column stimulation. Now, it is postulated that the mechanism behind SCS analgesia is more complex and nuanced than a straightforward spinoff of the gate-control therapy. Current theories include alteration of wide dynamic range (WDR) neuron excitability, modulation of the descending inhibitory

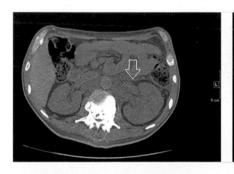
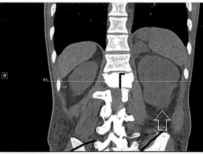

Fig. 29.1 Left renal cell carcinoma. Axial and coronal computed tomographic images demonstrate an infiltrative mass replacing the entirety of the left kidney (arrows). The mass is inseparable from adjacent retroperitoneal lymphadenopathy.

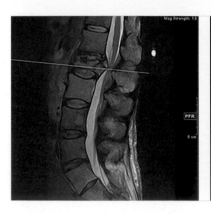
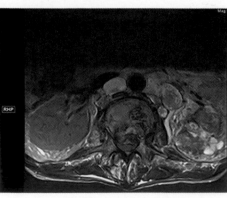

Fig. 29.2 Sagittal and axial magnetic resonance images demonstrating pathologic fracture of L2 vertebral body with severe spinal canal stenosis (level of the line).

pathway, changes among neurotransmitter activity, and even endogenous opioid receptor activation.[5]

The growth of SCS implantation has been driven by the increasing prevalence of neuropathic pain conditions such as diabetic neuropathy,[3] as well as the upsurge in failed back surgery syndrome (FBSS).[6] Other common indications for SCS therapy include combined trunk and limb pain (radiculopathies), complex regional pain syndrome, and angina pectoris. Yet

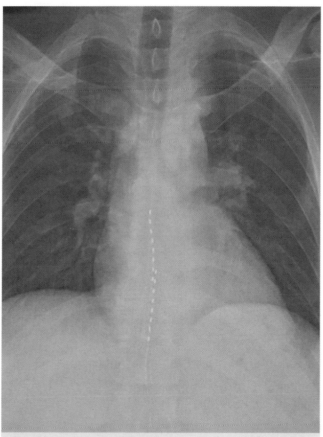

Fig. 29.3 Single frontal radiograph demonstrating spinal cord stimulator leads in the midline (arrow).

another factor for growth of the procedure has been the impetus for multimodal and steroid-sparing therapies in the treatment of chronic pain.

Although neoplasm-related pain is not traditionally seen as an indication for SCS therapy, SCS should still be considered in refractory situations. Cancer pain can often have multiple heterogeneous underlying mechanisms, including somatic-nociceptive and neuropathic components.[7] As in the case presented here, neuropathic pain from neoplasm may derive notable benefit from SCS therapy. Further, due to the multitude of adverse effects related to opioids often used in the treatment of pain caused by cancer, SCS therapy can be a useful adjunct in the appropriate patient and setting to prevent opioid dose escalation.

Following patient selection for SCS therapy, the patient initially undergoes an SCS trial of about 5 to 7 days prior to permanent neurostimulator implantation, with the aim of increasing the chances of successful treatment. During a trial, one to two percutaneous SCS lead(s) are advanced into the epidural space with a needle (usually a 14-gauge Tuohy) using a paramedian interlaminar approach under fluoroscopic guidance.[8] The specific level at which the leads are positioned is determined based on paresthesia mapping. With conventional SCS, the device elicits local paresthesia (tingling sensation), and the electrodes are adjusted until the patient experiences this paresthesia at the sites of his or her pain. Once the lead location is thus identified, the leads are secured in place to the patient's back and connected to an external generator until the end of the trial, at which point everything is completely removed.

Although the definition of a successful SCS trial varies among providers, significant pain relief (greater than 50%) and subjective improvements in functionality are generally accepted as indications to pursue a permanent SCS implant.[9] For this procedure, a pulse generator or battery is typically surgically placed in a small pocket in the posterior back and the SCS leads are secured in the fascial layer via a midline incision (► Fig. 29.3 and ► Fig. 29.4). These surgeries are usually performed in an ambulatory surgery center; patients are counseled regarding a typical recovery time of 1 to 2 weeks. In the patient presented here, an external pulse generator was used due to concerns of poor wound healing. Once the patient recovers from surgery, the SCS device programmer then modifies multiple parameters—amplitude,

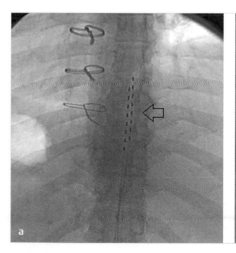
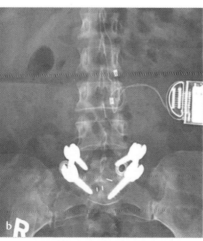

Fig. 29.4 Spinal cord stimulator (SCS) leads and internal pulse generator (IPG)/battery placement. (a) Fluoroscopic image demonstrating leads in the midline. (b) Postprocedure radiograph illustrating battery placement in the subcutaneous tissues laterally.

pulse width, frequency, and duty cycle—to optimize the patient's pain relief.[10]

SCS implantation is in general considered a safe procedure; however, standard perioperative safeguards should be in place to minimize infection risk. More commonly reported complications are hardware-related, and include migration and failure or fracture of the leads.[11]

29.3 Companion Case Presentation

A 49-year-old woman with a history of multiple back surgeries presented with chronic low back pain that radiated down the posterior aspect of her bilateral lower extremities. She initially underwent an L5–S1 partial diskectomy, which later was revised to L5–S1 laminectomy. Due to her continued pain, she eventually underwent an L5–S1 spinal fusion procedure. Despite these surgeries, she continued to have significant pain and poor functionality.

The patient described a constant, burning, aching pain that she localized 50% to her axial back and 50% to her lower extremities. Symptoms were unresponsive to multimodality therapy that included multiple medications (opioids, neuropathic medications, NSAIDs) and interventional procedures (epidural injections, RFA treatments).

Due to her poor response to prior treatments, she underwent an SCS trial with high frequency stimulation and staggered lead placement at the T8 level. This trial afforded about 70% pain relief and allowed her to be more active. Following the successful trial, the patient underwent a permanent SCS implant with an internal pulse generator. After recovery from surgery, the patient had excellent pain relief and significantly improved functionality. She was able to wean herself off opioid medications completely, and was able to start an exercise regimen that allowed her to lose weight. At 2 years following the implant, the patient continues to have her pain well controlled and is living a more active lifestyle.

29.4 Discussion

This second case illustrates the more typical SCS candidate. FBSS presents in 10 to 40% of patients who have undergone lumbar spine surgery, and although poorly understood, it is believed to be secondary to neuropathic leg and back pain. This entity is associated with decreased function, high pain scores, and significant socioeconomic burden.[6] An accumulating body of literature supports the use of SCS in this population.[12]

With advancements in technology, several new SCS modalities have emerged on the horizon in an attempt to circumvent limitations such as paresthesia and inadequate coverage of conventional SCS (cSCS) therapy. These developments in SCS include high frequency stimulation (HFS), unique waveforms, and even wireless receiver technology. These innovations have afforded greater versatility in patient selection and show promise for treating an even more extensive list of chronic pain conditions.

HFS generates a very high frequency of 10,000 Hz to provide pain relief as opposed to cSCS which typically has frequency parameters set between 60 and 100 Hz.[10] In general, patients do not feel any paresthesia with HFS therapy. Studies suggest that HFS is equivalent in safety and may be more effective than cSCS and, in particular, provides enhanced coverage for axial low back pain.[2,13] Clinical trials are underway for the application of HFS for various neuropathic pain conditions, and this modality is now considered a validated alternative SCS mode.

SCS energy delivery in terms of waveforms is also being extensively studied. For cSCS, the tonic waveform is used, which entails an action potential spike followed by immediate repolarization.[10] There are now alternative waveforms available for programming such as burst, which is a waveform consisting of a series of five pulses followed by a single repolarization pulse.[10] This waveform has similarities to thalamo-cortical firing patterns, and there is some evidence that suggests burst SCS may improve the emotional and affective components of pain.[14]

Another SCS treatment option includes a wireless system. In this system, the stimulator lead has a receiver that communicates with a wearable transmitter, which acts as a power source.[15] This technique is advantageous in that it allows the patient to avoid an invasive surgery for the implantation of an internal battery; the lead can be placed in a minimally invasive fashion via a percutaneous approach.

29.5 Summary

An accumulating body of literature supports an overwhelmingly positive response to SCS in subjects with chronic neuropathic pain diagnoses. With the advent of more recently developed stimulation paradigms, patients now have more choices than ever. SCS research and clinical applications will likely continue to grow exponentially as technology advances, allowing for better treatment of chronic pain conditions. Larger, nonindustry funded clinical trials remain an unmet need and could be used to compare the efficacy of available therapies in various pain phenotypes.

References

[1] Shealy CN, Mortimer JT, Reswick JB. Electrical inhibition of pain by stimulation of the dorsal columns: preliminary clinical report. Anesth Analg. 1967; 46(4):489–491

[2] Mekhail N, Visnjevac O, Azer G, Mehanny DS, Agrawal P, Foorsov V. Spinal cord stimulation 50 years later: clinical outcomes of spinal cord stimulation based on randomized clinical trials—a systematic review. Reg Anesth Pain Med. 2018; 43(4):391–406

[3] Geurts JW, Joosten EA, van Kleef M. Current status and future perspectives of spinal cord stimulation in treatment of chronic pain. Pain. 2017; 158(5): 771–774

[4] Sdrulla AD, Guan Y, Raja SN. Spinal cord stimulation: clinical efficacy and potential mechanisms. Pain Pract. 2018; 18(8):1048–1067

[5] Caylor J, Reddy R, Yin S, et al. Spinal cord stimulation in chronic pain: evidence and theory for mechanisms of action. Bioelectron Med. 2019; 5:12

[6] Thomson S. Failed back surgery syndrome—definition, epidemiology and demographics. Br J Pain. 2013; 7(1):56–59

[7] Peng L, Min S, Zejun Z, Wei K, Bennett MI. Spinal cord stimulation for cancer-related pain in adults. Cochrane Database Syst Rev. 2015(6):CD009389

[8] Zhu J, Falco F, Onyewu CO, Joesphson Y, Vesga R, Jari R. Alternative approach to needle placement in spinal cord stimulator trial/implantation. Pain Physician. 2011; 14(1):45–53

[9] Sitzman BT, Provenzano DA. Best practices in spinal cord stimulation. Spine. 2017; 42 Suppl 14:S67–S71

[10] Miller JP, Eldabe S, Buchser E, Johanek LM, Guan Y, Linderoth B. Parameters of spinal cord stimulation and their role in electrical charge delivery: a review. Neuromodulation. 2016; 19(4):373–384

[11] Eldabe S, Buchser E, Duarte RV. Complications of spinal cord stimulation and peripheral nerve stimulation techniques: a review of the literature. Pain Med. 2016; 17(2):325–336

[12] Cho JH, Lee JH, Song KS, et al. Treatment outcomes for patients with failed back surgery. Pain Physician. 2017; 20(1):E29–E43

[13] Kapural L, Yu C, Doust MW, et al. Comparison of 10-kHz high-frequency and traditional low-frequency spinal cord stimulation for the treatment of chronic back and leg pain: 24-month results from a multicenter, randomized, controlled pivotal trial. Neurosurgery. 2016; 79(5):667–677

[14] Kirketeig T, Schultheis C, Zuidema X, Hunter CW, Deer T. Burst spinal cord stimulation: a clinical review. Pain Med. 2019; 20 Suppl 1;S31–S40

[15] Bolash R, Creamer M, Rauck R, et al. Wireless high-frequency spinal cord stimulation (10 kHz) compared with multiwaveform low-frequency spinal cord stimulation in the management of chronic pain in failed back surgery syndrome subjects: preliminary results of a multicenter, prospective randomized controlled study. Pain Med. 2019; 20(10):1971–1979

30 Basivertebral Nerve Ablation

Ashley M. L. Nguyen and Dan T. D. Nguyen

30.1 Case Presentation

A 68-year-old man with a history of osteoarthritis and remote lumbar laminectomy presented with chronic low back pain. He has had trials of conservative management including nonsteroidal anti-inflammatory drugs (NSAIDs), physical therapy, injections to facet joints and sacroiliac joints, and lumbar diskography without improvement. He also had a lumbar medial branch radiofrequency ablation performed by an outside physician without pain relief and with a minor complication of right calf numbness afterward. On presentation he was taking tramadol pain medication without pain relief.

Upon presentation, it was noted that his back pain worsened with lumbar flexion and extension. His neurological examination showed normal motor, sensory, and deep tendon reflexes. Review of his outside lumbar magnetic resonance imaging (MRI) study revealed Modic end plate Type 2 changes at L3–L4, L4–L5, and L5–S1 levels (▶ Fig. 30.1). Given his historic presentation, basivertebral nerve ablation was discussed. After a detailed discussion with the patient about the procedure, risks, benefits, and clinical trial results, informed consent was obtained.

The patient underwent the basivertebral nerve ablation at L3, L4, L5, and S1 levels under general anesthesia (▶ Fig. 30.2). Following the procedure he had minor left hip pain that was deemed to be unrelated to the procedure and which resolved with a left hip injection. His chronic low back pain continued to improve, and he had a follow-up lumbar MRI at 6 weeks post procedure (▶ Fig. 30.3). At his 3-month postprocedure follow-up appointment, his chronic low back pain had improved to a steady 2/10 on the visual analog scale, and his daily activities were significantly improved compared to his preoperative state. At the time of follow-up he was only taking intermittent NSAIDs for his diffuse arthritic pain.

30.2 Discussion

Chronic low back pain is a common medical problem with a large societal impact. It occurs in all socioeconomic populations and affects individuals covered in both governmental sponsored[1] and private insurance plans. This medical condition is associated with increased age and obesity, and results in increased disability, lost workdays, depression, and sleep disturbances. Patients typically present to their primary care physicians for initial evaluation, and after trials of conservative management, a portion of this population gets forwarded to spine specialists. Treatment options include trials of NSAIDs, with some patients undergoing surgical interventions such as spinal arthroplasty or instrumental fusion. Despite radiographical success, instrumental fusion only results in 60 to 70% clinical success.

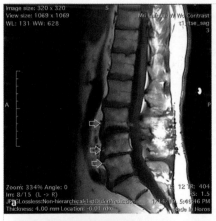
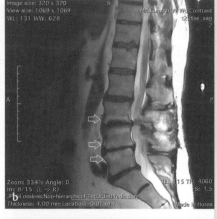
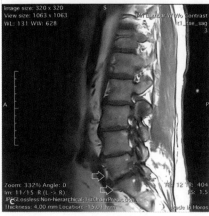
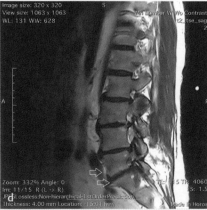

Fig. 30.1 Preprocedure magnetic resonance imaging (MRI). Utilizing T1-weighted (T1W) and T2-weighted (T2W) sequences, imaging of the lumbar spine is shown here. The bright signals expressed within the imaging (yellow arrows) are indicative of hyperintensity; with the combination of hyperintensity expression in both T1 W and T2 W, the patient was categorized to have Modic Type 2 end plate changes. **(a, b)** Bright signals were observed on the inferior end plate of L3 in L3–L4 and superior end plate of L4 in L4–L5 on both T1 W and T2 W sequences. **(c, d)** In the same patient, bright signals were again observed on the L5–S1 disk space adjacent end plates.

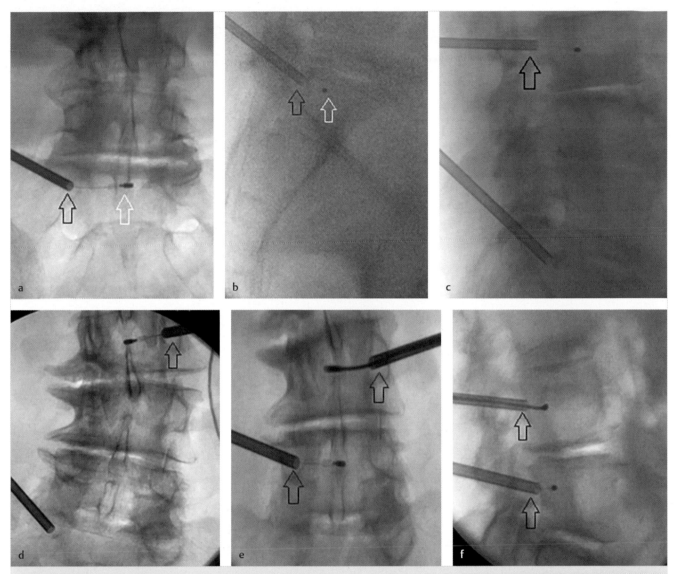

Fig. 30.2 Intraoperative fluoroscopic imaging. Prior to performing the radiofrequency ablation (RFA), trochars and probes were placed in multiple locations with the patient in prone position. **(a, b)** Placement of a trochar on S1 through a left transpedicular approach (black arrow) with the placement of a probe (white arrow) along the S1 center vertebral body. **(c, d)** Imaging was a continuation from **a** and **b** with the addition of another trochar on L3 through a right transpedicular approach (arrow). **(e, f)** Imaging now focused on L4–L5, with trochars (arrows) and probes placed with a right transpedicular approach on L4 and a left transpedicular approach on L5.

In recent years, there has been an advance in the knowledge of pain generators for chronic low back pain. In addition to traditional pain sources such as the myotendon, facet, annulus, and vertebral body, there is new evidence that innervation occurs within the end plates of each vertebral body through a network of basivertebral nerves.[2,3] The basivertebral nerve enters the vertebral body through the basivertebral foramen that also carries the basivertebral veins. The basivertebral nerve innervates the superior and inferior vertebral body end plates and transmits pain signals.[4] Nerve density increases in damaged and degenerated end plates.[5]

Vertebral body pathology, such as degenerative end plates and Modic changes, correlates with chronic low back pain.[6,7] Patients with low back pain who have Modic end plate changes are clinically worse that those patients with low back pain without Modic end plate changes.[8] Patients with low back pain

with Modic changes report a greater frequency and duration of low back pain episodes and seek medical care more often.[9] Patients with Modic 1 changes are associated with poor outcome with conservative treatment[10,11]; given these findings, Modic 1 and 2 changes are considered imaging surrogates to vertebrogenic end plate chronic pain.

To validate this hypothesis, the initial pivotal prospective, multicenter, randomized, double-blind, sham controlled SMART trial was undertaken.[12] There were 18 sites (15 US and 3 German); 225 patients (147 treatment arm and 78 sham) were enrolled. The results from this trial demonstrated the Oswestry Disability Index (ODI) decreased 20.5 points in the treatment arm compared to 15.2 in sham arm. At 3 months there were 75.6% of patients in treatment arm and 55.3% in the sham control arm who demonstrated meaningful improvements of ≥ 10 points based on the ODI scale.

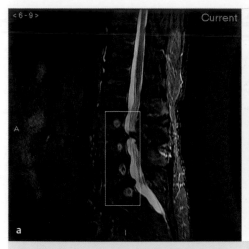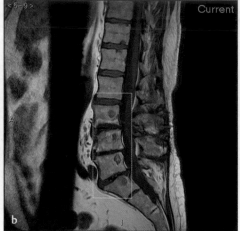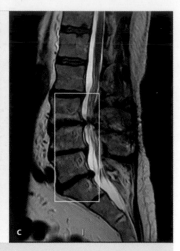

Fig. 30.3 (a–c) Postablation magnetic resonance imaging (MRI). Utilizing short tau inversion recovery (STIR), T1-weighted (T1W), and T2-weighted (T2W) MRI sequences, post–radiofrequency ablation (RFA) imaging was obtained. Within all treated vertebral bodies, there are oval-shaped signal changes (inside yellow boxes) apparent compared to the preoperative imaging (▶ Fig. 30.1) indicating the ablative zones.

In a second prospective, multicenter clinical trial (INTRACEPT),[13] a treatment arm was compared to a conservative treatment arm. An interim analysis in this trial showed statistically significant improvements at the primary end point of 3 months in both ODI and visual analog scale for basivertebral nerve ablation. The data were so overwhelming toward the treatment arm that the data management committee recommended to halt further enrollment and offered early cross-over for patients in the control group.

To conclude, chronic low back pain is ubiquitous. A potential subset of these patients who may be treated effectively has been under-recognized. MRI characteristics and description for Modic changes have become very important in identifying these subpopulations of patients who may benefit from treatment of basivertebral nerve ablation.

References

[1] Shmagel A, Foley R, Ibrahim H. Epidemiology of chronic low back pain in US adults: data from the 2009–2010 National Health and Nutrition Examination Survey. Arthritis Care Res (Hoboken). 2016; 68(11):1688–1694

[2] Antonacci MD, Mody DR, Heggeness MH. Innervation of the human vertebral body: a histologic study. J Spinal Disord. 1998; 11(6):526–531

[3] Fras C, Kravetz P, Mody DR, Heggeness MH. Substance P-containing nerves within the human vertebral body. An immunohistochemical study of the basivertebral nerve. Spine J. 2003; 3(1):63–67

[4] Bailey JF, Liebenberg E, Degmetich S, Lotz JC. Innervation patterns of PGP 9.5-positive nerve fibers within the human lumbar vertebra. J Anat. 2011; 218 (3):263–270

[5] Lotz JC, Fields AJ, Liebenberg EC. The role of the vertebral end plate in low back pain. Global Spine J. 2013; 3(3):153–164

[6] Carragee EJ. The surgical treatment of disc degeneration: is the race not to the swift? Spine J. 2005; 5(6):587–588

[7] Modic MT, Masaryk TJ, Ross JS, Carter JR. Imaging of degenerative disk disease. Radiology. 1988; 168(1):177–186

[8] Kjaer P, Korsholm L, Bendix T, Sorensen JS, Leboeuf-Yde C. Modic changes and their associations with clinical findings. Eur Spine J. 2006; 15(9):1312–1319

[9] Jensen TS, Karppinen J, Sorensen JS, Niinimäki J, Leboeuf-Yde C. Vertebral endplate signal changes (Modic change): a systematic literature review of prevalence and association with non-specific low back pain. Eur Spine J. 2008; 17(11):1407–1422

[10] Jensen OK, Nielsen CV, Sørensen JS, Stengaard-Pedersen K. Type 1 Modic changes was a significant risk factor for 1-year outcome in sick-listed low back pain patients: a nested cohort study using magnetic resonance imaging of the lumbar spine. Spine J. 2014; 14(11):2568–2581

[11] Jensen RK, Leboeuf-Yde C. Is the presence of modic changes associated with the outcomes of different treatments? A systematic critical review. BMC Musculoskelet Disord. 2011; 12:183

[12] Fischgrund JS, Rhyne A, Franke J, et al. Intraosseous basivertebral nerve ablation for the treatment of chronic low back pain: a prospective randomized double-blind sham-controlled multi-center study. Eur Spine J. 2018; 27(5):1146–1156

[13] Khalil JG, Smuck M, Koreckij T, et al. INTRACEPT Trial Investigators. A prospective, randomized, multicenter study of intraosseous basivertebral nerve ablation for the treatment of chronic low back pain. Spine J. 2019; 19 (10):1620–1632

31 CT-Guided Peripheral Nerve Blocks

Parham Pezeshk, Vibhor Wadhwa, and Avneesh Chhabra

31.1 Introduction

There is a large population of patients who present daily in outpatient clinics with the chief complaint of pain, or a functional disability due to pain. Image-guided perineural injections have high technical success rate and nearly 100% face validity. The frequency of image-guided injections is increasing relative to landmark-guided injections due to direct visualization of the target peripheral nerves and perineural fat planes. Cross-sectional anatomy, however, can be complicated, and many providers are not aware of the exact sites of nerve locations and their respective injections on imaging. It is essential that radiologists and interventionists familiarize themselves with the techniques of image-guided perineural injections in order to allow safe and accurate targeting to help their patients.

The main goal of perineural injections is not to provide permanent relief of pain but rather to improve quality of life for the patients by decreasing the level of the pain to the extent that they can regain routine daily function to a reasonable level, can undergo physical therapy exercises more comfortably and efficiently, and reduce the dosage of systemic pain medications and steroids to mitigate the possibility of long-term side-effects from these medications. Some patients might falsely expect to be pain-free for a long time; thus, it is important to have an honest discussion with the patient. It should be explained that the extent and duration of pain relief varies between individuals and depends on various factors including severity of the nerve inflammation, source of the pain, and the individual's physiologic response to the medication. For these reasons, while a perfectly performed perineural injection might significantly improve pain in one patient, it might not be as effective in another.

31.2 Causes of Peripheral Neuropathy and Their Evaluation

The list of etiologies of peripheral neuropathy is long and includes trauma, ischemia, inflammation, infection, side effects from medications, and involvement by infiltrative processes such as tumors, and systemic diseases including diabetes and sarcoidosis.[1] A detailed history and physical examination are needed to determine the pattern of involvement of the peripheral nerves. In more complicated cases, diagnostic tests such a nerve conduction velocity (NCV) and magnetic resonance neurography (MR neurography) might also be of help to further investigate the affected nerves as well as to evaluate the severity of the neuropathy.[2,3] These adjunctive tests should be correlated and interpreted in the light of clinical findings and history in order to narrow the differential diagnoses and to avoid pitfalls and confirmation bias. Apart from providing therapeutic relief, image-guided perineural injections can also be helpful as a diagnostic tool.

31.3 Types of Injections and Medications

Two main types of perineural injections are performed: diagnostic and therapeutic. Due to the complexity of innervation in some areas of the body, particularly the pelvis, it is sometimes challenging to identify the exact source of pain. This is especially true if there is referred pain or a predominant psychosomatic component. In these situations, the provider might consider performing a set of trial and error "diagnostic" injections to identify the nerve responsible for the patient's pain. Since the purpose of such procedures is diagnostic, a local anesthetic (typically a combination of lidocaine [1%] and bupivacaine [0.5%]) is used while steroids are avoided. If the patient's pain improves following a diagnostic test, future injections can be performed as "therapeutic" by adding steroid (4 mg dexamethasone/mL) to the local anesthetic for longer pain relief.

Hyaluronidase is a fibrinolytic agent that can be used in the setting of nerve entrapment with demonstrable postoperative fibrosis and scarring on imaging. The usual dosage is 100 to 150 units, and it can be combined with local anesthetics and steroids to additionally decrease the nerve inflammation. Botulinum toxin type A (Botox, Allergan, Parsippany, NJ) is another medication that is used to reduce muscle spasm or to shrink hypertrophied muscle, such as in the cases of piriformis syndrome or thoracic outlet syndrome.

There is controversy about using particulate versus nonparticulate steroids for perineural injections. Although particulate steroids might exhibit longer pain relief in some studies, some providers do not recommend their use in the cases of perineural injection due to possible occlusion of small vessels with resultant ischemia and fibrosis. At the authors' institution, nonparticulate steroids, such as dexamethasone, are used for perineural injections.

31.4 Types of Imaging

Depending on the depth of the nerve, ultrasound (US) or computed tomography (CT) scan can be used for image-guided injections of the peripheral nerves. The choice of imaging depends largely on operator's preference, availability of the respective imaging modality, and a risk–benefit assessment of radiation exposure depending upon the patient's age and frequency of the injections. Fluoroscopy is used by some providers for some perineural injections based on bony landmarks; however, due to its less accurate localization of the nerve compared to cross-sectional imaging, most perineural injections may be more accurately performed with US or CT. US can be used in cases of more superficial nerve injections, while CT scan is most helpful for visualization of the deeper pelvic and abdominal nerves.

31.5 Technique

The preprocedure steps for perineural injections are similar to any other interventional procedure. Reviewing available medical records and imaging studies to plan the appropriate approach for the injection is vital. The procedure with its risks and benefits should be explained to the patient, and consent should be obtained. As stated above, it is helpful to explain to the patient that the duration and degree of response to perineural injections may vary from patient to patient depending on the etiology of the pain and physiologic response to pain medications. Some patients might have an unrealistically high hope of complete and prolonged pain relief with injections; reasonable expectations must be explained at the beginning of the procedure that pain may decrease, stay the same, or occasionally even worsen following the procedure. The latter is especially possible for patients who are hypersensitive to steroids or who are on long-term narcotics. In some cases, such as perisciatic or posterior femoral cutaneous nerve injections, the patient should be cautioned about possible numbness, temporary leg weakness, and paresthesia of the leg, which may require extra safety measures by the patient and family during ambulation as well as potentially precluding driving for up to 48 hours.

A time-out should be performed before the procedure with the entire team present in the procedural area and at least two patient identifiers must be checked. For CT-guided procedures, a grid should be placed over the site of injection and the entry point marked on the skin. In cases of US-guided injections, the site of injection should be identified in two orthogonal planes and the entry point marked on the skin. After marking, the skin is prepped and draped in sterile fashion. As a general rule, injections are directed to the perineural fat plane and needle placement or injection within the nerve itself must be avoided. During CT-guided injections, a small amount of dilute contrast or air (in the cases of contrast allergy) is injected before the final injection of medication to demonstrate the expected spread of the medicated injectate. A postinjection image is finally obtained in order to document the distribution of the injectate. Pre- and postinjection pain levels are documented in the chart, and the patient is told to decrease activity for 24 hours with resumption of normal activities the day after. A pain diary is maintained, and the recorded data are brought by the patient during the follow-up visit to the provider. A repeat injection of the same nerve is avoided in our practice for 4 to 6 weeks, since some patients may experience delayed pain relief.

In the authors' practice, the same nerve is not injected more than twice if there is negative block (no pain relief is achieved). In case of definite positive blocks (more than 50% or at least a two-point pain reduction on visual analog scale of 1–10, sustained for at least 24 hours), repeat therapeutic injections can be performed up to a total of three to four times per year. A "possible positive block" is one that has an effect for less than 24 hours and/or demonstrates less than 50% pain reduction. For more sustained relief, radiofrequency ablation (RFA) or cryoablation can be further attempted in cases of definite or possible positive block. Pulsed RFA (42 °C for 120 seconds) is used for motor or mixed motor-sensory nerves, such as pudendal nerve, while continuous RFA (70–90 °C for 90 seconds) is used for purely sensory nerves, such as iliohypogastric, ilioinguinal, and lateral femoral cutaneous nerves.

31.6 Common Perineural Injections, Anatomy, and Technique

31.6.1 Sciatic Nerve

Originating from L4–S3 nerve roots of the lumbosacral plexus, the sciatic nerve courses out of the pelvis through the sciatic notch and passes under the piriformis muscle. For perineural injections of the sciatic nerve, the patient is positioned prone and the perineural fat of the nerve is targeted at the level of the ischial spine or ischial tuberosity (► Fig. 31.1). For piriformis syndrome (wallet-area pain or tenderness), the center of the piriformis muscle bulk is targeted and a combination of 50 to 100 units of Botox (depending upon the bulk of the muscle, especially with repeated injections) along with 6 mL of lidocaine 1% and 4 mL of bupivacaine 0.5% is injected intramuscularly. This injection is performed with the goal of shrinking the muscle mass (► Fig. 31.2). In the event of perineural scar from prior hamstring surgery or joint replacement, the injectate is supplemented with hyaluronidase.

31.6.2 Posterior Femoral Cutaneous Nerve (PFCN)

A pure sensory nerve, the posterior femoral cutaneous nerve (PFCN) originates from the S1–S3 nerve roots, exits the pelvis

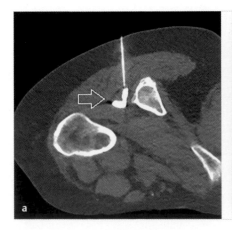
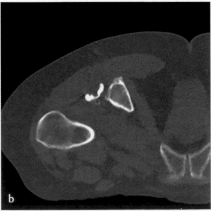

Fig. 31.1 Computed tomography (CT)-guided right sciatic nerve injection. (a) Axial CT image demonstrates the tip of the needle in the perisciatic fat at the level of the ischial tuberosity (arrow). Perisciatic nerve injection can be performed along the course of the nerve more proximally (as demonstrated here), or more distally in the proximal thigh where perineural fat can be safely targeted. (b) Axial image shows the injectate, surrounding the right sciatic nerve.

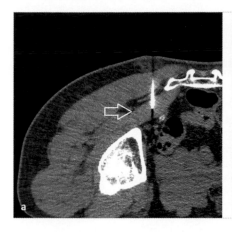
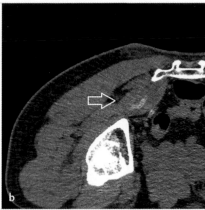

Fig. 31.2 Computed tomography (CT)-guided right piriformis intramuscular injection. (a) Axial CT image shows the middle of the piriformis muscle bulk (arrow) targeted for injection. (b) Axial CT image shows the final injection after administration of small amount of contrast and medication demonstrating the distribution of the injectate. Notice the increase in the size of the piriformis muscle (arrow) following injection.

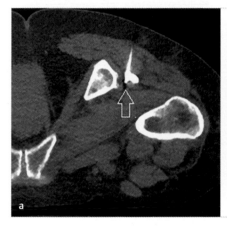
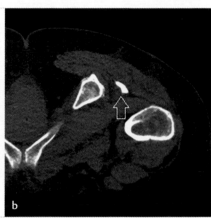

Fig. 31.3 Computed tomography (CT)-guided injection of the left posterior femoral cutaneous nerve (PFCN) at the level of ischial tuberosity. (a) Axial CT image demonstrates the tip of the needle (arrow) in the fat plane between the ischial tuberosity and the sciatic nerve where the PFCN resides. (b) Axial image shows contrast filling the perineural fat plane of the PFCN (arrow).

via the greater sciatic foramen, descends beneath the gluteus maximus muscle, and then lies superficial to the long head of the biceps femoris in the posterior aspect of the thigh. It eventually penetrates the fascia lata in the popliteal fossa. Patients with PFCN damage typically present with pain localized over the medial gluteal region, ischial tuberosity, or posteromedial perineum. The pain is typically worsened with sitting, but does not extend below the knee crease level. On cross-sectional imaging, the PFCN can be visualized between the sciatic nerve and ischial tuberosity; more distally, it lies at the inferolateral margin of the gluteus maximus muscle. For selective injection of the nerve, the patient lies prone and the fat plane between the sciatic nerve and ischial tuberosity, or alternatively the fat plane slightly more distally underneath the gluteus maximus, is targeted (▶ Fig. 31.3). One may apply slight angulation with the needle tip coursing medially toward the hamstring muscles to avoid distribution of the majority of the injectate along the sciatic nerve. The injection can also be combined with hamstring needling if there is predominant hamstring-related pain (ischial tuberosity pain or pain with hamstring stretch). Another option is hamstring needling with ischiogluteal bursa injection for the latter case.

31.6.3 Lateral Femoral Cutaneous Nerve (LFCN)

The lateral femoral cutaneous nerve (LFCN) is a pure sensory nerve formed from the L2 and L3 nerve roots. It originates

at the lateral margin of the psoas muscle and descends anterior to the iliacus and psoas muscles. The nerve courses underneath the inguinal ligament, and its two branches innervate the anterolateral aspect of the thigh. Patients with LFCN injury present with anterolateral thigh pain, tingling, or numbness (aka meralgia paresthetica). On cross-sectional imaging, the nerve can be visualized anterior to the iliopsoas muscle, coursing under the inguinal ligament approximately 1.0 to 1.5 cm medial to the anterior superior iliac spine (ASIS). For injection, the patient lies supine and the fat space 1.0 to 1.5 cm medial to the ASIS is targeted proximal to the inguinal ligament in the retroperitoneal fat plane (▶ Fig. 31.4). The injectate is dispersed along the course of the nerve by angling the needle along the direction of the nerve while injecting.

31.6.4 Pudendal Nerve and Inferior Rectal Nerve

A mixed motor and sensory nerve originating from S2–S4 nerve roots, the pudendal nerve courses inferolaterally along the anterior border of the piriformis muscle. It subsequently enters the space between the sacrotuberous and sacrospinous ligaments, before entering Alcock's canal under the obturator fascia. It gives the inferior rectal nerve branch in the ischiorectal space, multiple sensory perineal branches, as well as the dorsal nerve of the penis in man and clitoris in women. Patients with injury to this nerve present with perineal, clitoral, penile, or pelvic floor pain.

Pelvic floor muscle dysfunction is also commonly noted. Nantes criteria, MR neurography, or perineural injection can be used for diagnosis. For perineural injection of the pudendal nerve, the patient is positioned prone and the perineural fat is targeted at the level between the ischial tuberosity and ischial spine, under the sacrotuberous ligament where the nerve is located (▶ Fig. 31.5). The nerve is intermediate in density on CT as compared to bright or calcified vessels; sometimes the fascicles of the nerve can be visualized on CT. It is usually the posterior-most structure of the neurovascular bundle in the Alcock's canal. Ideally, the injectate would flow anteromedially along the course of the nerve into the Alcock's canal. For perineural injection of the inferior rectal nerve, the mid aspect of the ischiorectal fat is targeted, where the nerve passes medially toward the rectum.

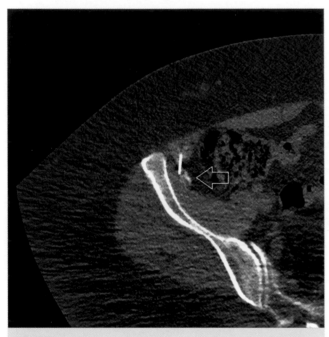

Fig. 31.4 Computed tomography (CT)-guided lateral femoral cutaneous nerve injection. Axial CT image demonstrates needle placement via an anterior approach, with the needle tip in the retroperitoneal fat medial to the anterior superior iliac spine and proximal to the inguinal ligament. A small amount of contrast confirms the distribution of the injectate (arrow).

31.6.5 Genitofemoral Nerve (GFN)

A mixed motor and sensory nerve, the genitofemoral nerve (GFN) originates from the ventral rami of the L1 and L2 nerve roots, and courses inferiorly along the anterior aspect of the psoas muscle. At the level of the L5 vertebra, the nerve divides into a genital branch, which courses through the inguinal canal to innervate the skin of the scrotum in men and labia majora in women, and a femoral branch that courses under the inguinal ligament to supply a small area in the anteromedial aspect of the upper thigh. Patients with GFN pain present with idiopathic pain, prior groin/pelvic trauma, or pain following groin/hernia surgery. The region of pain distribution is in the groin, scrotum, vulva, and anteromedial thigh. For injection, the patient lies supine and the perineural fat proximal to the deep inguinal ring is targeted for the genital branch (▶ Fig. 31.6). The femoral branch can be affected with scarring secondary to prior bleeding in the area from trauma or femoral vascular catheterization and, in such cases, injection with hyaluronidase in addition to local anesthetics and a steroid is recommended.

31.6.6 Iliohypogastric and Ilioinguinal Nerve

The iliohypogastric and ilioinguinal nerves originate from the L1 and L2 nerve roots, course together through the psoas muscle before coursing laterally. The nerves then penetrate the transversus abdominis muscle, course between the internal oblique and transversus abdominis muscles, and give rise to cutaneous branches to innervate the skin over the hypogastrium, inguinal ligament, groin, and upper thigh. These nerves can be injured during prior laparotomy, abdominal wall trauma, and inguinal hernia repair with scar entrapment. Patients with infiltration of these nerves present with hypogastric or groin pain. For injection, the patient lies in the supine position and the fat plane between the transverse abdominis and internal oblique muscles is targeted at the level of the ASIS where the iliohypogastric and ilioinguinal nerves course inferiorly (▶ Fig. 31.7). The iliohypogastric nerve can also be selectively injected more proximally where it courses along the anterior abdominal wall. The ilioinguinal nerve can be selectively injected in the left anterior groin along the inguinal ligament and between the internal oblique and transversus abdominis muscles.

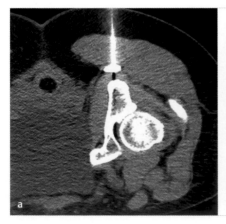
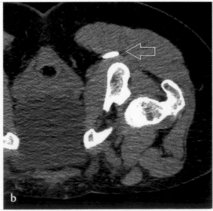

Fig. 31.5 Computed tomography (CT)-guided right pudendal nerve injection. (a) Axial CT image demonstrates the tip of the needle in the fat plane underneath the sacrotuberous ligament, midway between the ischial tuberosity and ischial spine. (b) Axial CT image post-procedure with the injectate (arrow) distributing medially and distally along the course of the pudendal nerve in the Alcock's canal.

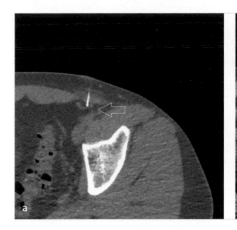

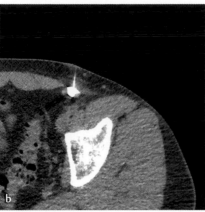

Fig. 31.6 Computed tomography (CT)-guided left genitofemoral nerve injection. (a) Axial CT image demonstrates needle insertion using an anterior approach with the needle tip (arrow) proximal to the deep inguinal ring. (b) The location of the needle tip in the inguinal canal is confirmed by the injection of contrast.

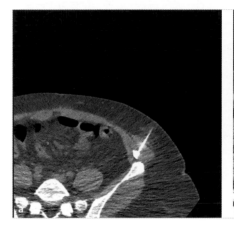

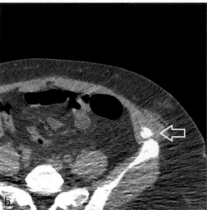

Fig. 31.7 Computed tomography (CT)-guided left ilioinguinal and iliohypogastric injection. (a) Axial image shows the tip of the needle in the fat plane between the transversus abdominis muscle (deep layer) and internal oblique muscle (middle layer), where the ilioinguinal and iliohypogastric nerves course together. The ilioinguinal nerve can also be injected more distally where it courses along the anterior abdominal wall. (b) Axial image demonstrates the distribution of contrast (arrow) following final injection.

31.6.7 Superior Gluteal Nerve

A mixed motor and sensory nerve from L4 to S1 nerve roots, the superior gluteal nerve exits the pelvis via the greater sciatic foramen, and in the gluteal region travels cephalad over the inferior border of the gluteus minimus muscle. The superior gluteal nerve courses laterally between the gluteus medius and minimus muscles.[4] Patients with superior gluteal nerve injury present with posterolateral gluteal pain. Additionally, a ganglion cyst may also be noted in this nerve following hip labrocapsular injuries. For injection, the patient is placed prone and the superior portion of the greater sciatic notch above the piriformis muscle is targeted. There must be careful avoidance of the fine neurovascular bundle in this region.

31.6.8 Femoral Nerve

The femoral nerve is a mixed sensory and motor nerve originating from the posterior divisions of the L2 to L4 nerve roots. It forms in the lateral aspect of the psoas muscle, courses caudally between the iliacus and psoas muscles, and enters the femoral triangle. The nerve may be affected by prior pelvic trauma, iatrogenic nerve block, perineural scarring from vascular catheterization and bleeding, and hip replacement surgery. For injection, the patient is positioned supine and the perineural fat is targeted in the femoral canal lateral to the femoral artery (▶ Fig. 31.8). Since the obturator nerve may be affected

concomitantly, the perineural fat of the obturator foramen can in addition be targeted for better pain relief.

31.6.9 Obturator Nerve

A mixed motor and sensory nerve, the obturator nerve arises from the anterior divisions of L2 to L4 nerve roots and courses inferiorly in the direct coronal plane of the pelvis, medial to the psoas major. It enters the obturator canal where it divides into its anterior and posterior divisions. The nerve can be affected by prior obturator ring fracture, obturator foramen fat hernia, obturator muscle hernia (baseball pitcher, hockey goalie syndrome), or in an idiopathic fashion. With the patient in the supine position, the perineural fat of the obturator foramen can be targeted for injection (▶ Fig. 31.9).

31.6.10 Cluneal Nerves

Superior, middle, and inferior cluneal nerves are pure sensory nerves that innervate the lumbar and gluteal regions and in some patients may contribute to low back pain.

The superior cluneal nerve originates from the lower thoracic and lumbar posterior nerve roots, penetrates the thoracolumbar fascia at the lateral margin of the quadratus lumborum muscle, and courses inferolaterally along the gluteus maximus muscle. For injection of the nerve, the patient is positioned

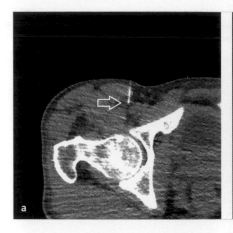

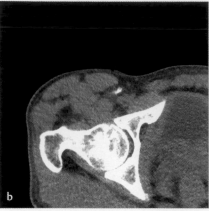

Fig. 31.8 Computed tomography (CT)-guided right femoral nerve injection. (**a**) Axial CT image shows the tip of the needle (arrow) adjacent to the right femoral nerve. (**b**) Final image after injection of contrast and medication.

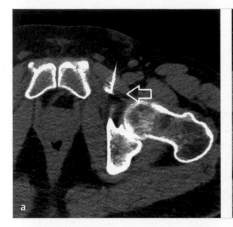

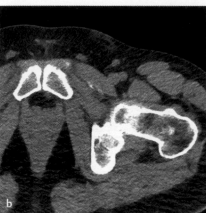

Fig. 31.9 Computed tomography (CT)-guided injection of the left obturator nerve. (**a**) Axial image demonstrates needle placement using an anterior approach, with the needle tip (arrow) in the fat plane of the distal obturator canal. (**b**) Injectate dispersed in the fat plane around the nerve.

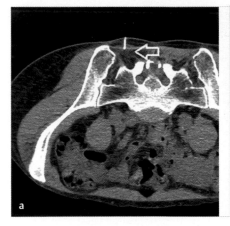

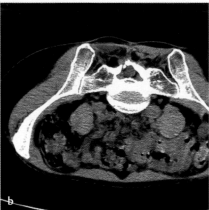

Fig. 31.10 Computed tomography (CT)-guided injection of the right middle cluneal nerve. (**a**) Axial CT image at S1–S2 level demonstrates needle placement (arrow) using a posterior approach, in the fascial planes between the retrosacral muscles. (**b**) Axial image following injection of medication and contrast shows obliteration of the respective fat plane.

prone and the lateral aspect of quadratus lumborum at the level of the superior iliac crest is targeted.

The middle cluneal nerve originates from the S1–S4 nerve roots, courses below the long posterior sacroiliac ligament between the posterior superior iliac spine (PSIS) and posterior inferior iliac spine (PIIS), and eventually courses over the iliac crest to the gluteal region.[5,6,7] For injection of the nerve, the patient lies prone and the fat plane deep to the sacroiliac ligament is targeted (▶ Fig. 31.10).

The inferior cluneal nerve is a terminal branch of the PFCN and innervates the inferior gluteal area.[4] The nerve courses inferiorly in the lateral aspect of the ischium at the level of the ischial tuberosity, and anterior to the gluteus maximus before perforating the fascia of the gluteus maximus at its lower margin. With more proximal injection of PFCN at the ischial tuberosity, the inferior cluneal nerve is also targeted (▶ Fig. 31.11).

The superior cluneal nerve can be injured during iliac graft harvests, the middle cluneal nerve by sacroiliac joint injuries or

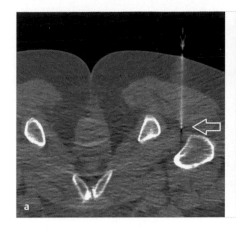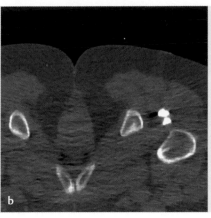

Fig. 31.11 Computed tomography (CT)-guided left inferior cluneal nerve injection. (**a**) Axial CT image demonstrates needle placement using a posterior approach, with the needle tip (arrow) deep to the gluteus maximus and in the lateral aspect of the fat plane between the obturator externus and gluteus maximus. (**b**) Final image demonstrates the distribution of injectate.

surgery, and the inferior cluneal nerve is implicated in lateral gluteal crease pain symptoms. For selective lateral gluteal crease pain symptoms, the fat plane underneath the inferior margin of the gluteus maximus is targeted.

31.6.11 Epidural or Selective Nerve Root Injections

Transforaminal epidural perineural injections can be performed under the guidance of fluoroscopy or CT. While fluoroscopy-guided injection using a C-arm is usually quicker and has less radiation exposure, CT scan provides cross-sectional anatomical views of the neural foramen for more accurate delivery of the injectate. The choice of guidance depends on the modality available and operator's preference. For fluoroscopy-guided transforaminal epidural injections, a C-arm is used to obtain a "Scotty dog view" of the vertebral body in an oblique view. In this projection, the superior aspect of the neural foramen underneath the neck of the Scotty dog is targeted. The needle is advanced intermittently under fluoroscopy guidance until the needle tip contacts the bone. A small amount of contrast is injected to confirm flow along the nerve root, and then medication is injected. For CT-guided injections, the patient is placed prone and the superior aspect of the neural foramen is targeted in a lateral to medial needle tip approach prior to the perineural fat being injected.

31.7 Potential Pitfalls

Despite care to target the fat adjacent to nerves, the needle tip might inadvertently enter the nerve itself. Possible major complications include nerve injury, hematoma formation, local anesthetic toxicity, and allergic reaction.[1] The majority of these complications are self-limiting. These injuries are usually transient and might result in temporary numbness, weakness, and paresthesias which typically resolve in a few months.[8,9] To avoid such nerve damage, a small-gauge needle (22-gauge or smaller) should be used, and the needle should be advanced slowly after measuring the distance of the needle tip to the target. The needle tip may not be in the expected location and the initial injection of contrast can help predict the distribution of the injectate. Adjustment of the course and depth of the needle can be made as needed.

References

[1] Wadhwa V, Scott KM, Rozen S, Starr AJ, Chhabra A. CT-guided perineural injections for chronic pelvic pain. Radiographics. 2016; 36(5):1408–1425

[2] Chhabra A, Chalian M, Soldatos T, et al. 3-T high-resolution MR neurography of sciatic neuropathy. AJR Am J Roentgenol. 2012; 198(4):W357-W364

[3] Chhabra A, Faridian-Aragh N, Chalian M, et al. High-resolution 3-T MR neurography of peroneal neuropathy. Skeletal Radiol. 2012; 41(3):257–271

[4] Isu T, Kim K, Morimoto D, Iwamoto N. Superior and middle cluneal nerve entrapment as a cause of low back pain. Neurospine. 2018; 15(1):25–32

[5] Tubbs RS, Levin MR, Loukas M, Potts EA, Cohen-Gadol AA. Anatomy and landmarks for the superior and middle cluneal nerves: application to posterior iliac crest harvest and entrapment syndromes. J Neurosurg Spine. 2010; 13(3):356–359

[6] Konno T, Aota Y, Saito T, et al. Anatomical study of middle cluneal nerve entrapment. J Pain Res. 2017; 10:1431–1435

[7] McGrath MC, Zhang M. Lateral branches of dorsal sacral nerve plexus and the long posterior sacroiliac ligament. Surg Radiol Anat. 2005; 27(4):327–330

[8] Löscher WN, Wanschitz J, Iglseder S, et al. Iatrogenic lesions of peripheral nerves. Acta Neurol Scand. 2015; 132(5):291–303

[9] Jeng CL, Torrillo TM, Rosenblatt MA. Complications of peripheral nerve blocks. Br J Anaesth. 2010; 105 Suppl 1:i97–i107

32 Peripheral Nerve Blocks (Ultrasound)

Nan Xiang and Vinita Singh

32.1 Case Presentation

A 65-year-old man presented with an 8-month history of right-sided groin pain. He had a history of coronary artery bypass, atrial fibrillation, and most recently underwent percutaneous coronary intervention 8 months previously. The patient reported that following his coronary procedure, he had bleeding at his right groin site that required manual compression by the interventionalist. He reports that he first began experiencing right groin and scrotal pain during the manual compression that persisted even after hemostasis was established and manual pressure had ceased. His right scrotal pain was initially most bothersome, but that has since resolved. His predominant pain is currently in the right lower abdomen in the L1 nerve distribution and in the inguinal region, and is significantly worse on the right compared to the left. He describes the pain as a constant dull ache, rated 10/10 at worst, that worsens with a distended bladder or tight belts. The pain improves when avoiding pressure to the area. He denies any sharp or shooting pain or paresthesia.

He denies experiencing the pain prior to the events described above. He denies any other trauma or possible infection, and has no history of sexually transmitted diseases. He previously had mild benefit from gabapentin 1800 mg daily that did not seem to last the entire day. He was not taking any opioid medications on a regular basis. On physical examination, the patient exhibited tenderness to palpation in the right inguinal region, the right lower quadrant of the abdomen, and in the medial thigh at the level of the scrotum. There was no skin discoloration, bruising, or edema. There were no sensory deficits with light touch and pinprick, though there may have been a mild degree of allodynia.

At this time, given the patient's description of symptoms, close correlation with his percutaneous coronary intervention complicated by manual compression at the right groin site, and physical examination findings, a right-sided ilioinguinal and/or iliohypogastric neuropathy was suspected. The ilioinguinal nerve provides innervation to the medial thigh and suprapubic region while the iliohypogastric nerve provides innervation to the inguinal canal, lateral thigh, and suprapubic region. The initial involvement of the right scrotum suggests possible involvement of the genitofemoral nerve, which can also be compressed at the inguinal canal.

An injection targeting the ilioinguinal and iliohypogastric nerves, at the location of the lateral transverse abdominus plane (TAP), with a combination of local anesthetic and steroid was performed. The lateral TAP is typically used perioperatively for surgeries involving lower abdominal incisions, providing T10–T12 dermatomal coverage. By starting at a more caudad location, closer to the anterior superior iliac spine, the ilioinguinal and iliohypogastric nerves could be addressed. These nerves are located in the plane above the transverse abdominus muscle and below the internal oblique muscle.

32.2 Technical Description

The block was performed in the right lower abdomen, after locating the umbilicus and palpation of the anterior superior iliac spine.[1] Chlorhexidine was used to cleanse the skin. A high-frequency linear ultrasound probe with a sterile probe cover was placed transversely to provide axial images of the abdominal wall. The probe was maneuvered laterally and posteriorly around the abdomen, until the three distinct layers that comprise the external oblique, internal oblique, and transverse abdominus muscles were visualized. The skin was anesthetized with 1 mL of 1% lidocaine. A 21-G 4″ Stimuplex needle was advanced from anteromedial to posterolateral direction, piercing through the external and internal oblique muscles until the layer just superficial to the transverse abdominus muscle was reached. Hydrodissection with sterile normal saline resulted in the appropriate "unzipping" of the internal oblique and transverse abdominus layers, creating a hypoechoic layer of fluid on the ultrasound (▶ Fig. 32.1a, b). Of note, if the hydrodissection occurs within the muscle fascia, the resulting fluid layer would appear more cloudy and heterogenous. At this point, after negative aspiration, an injectate comprised of 20 mL 0.25% bupivacaine and 10 mg of dexamethasone was administered at this location. The procedure was well tolerated, and the patient reported his abdominal and inguinal pain were significantly improved. The patient reported that his pain completely resolved for 2 days before returning back to baseline.

32.3 Discussion

32.3.1 Ultrasound Guidance

Ultrasonography (USG) is an inexpensive imaging modality without the risks related to radiation exposure. However, USG

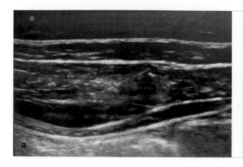
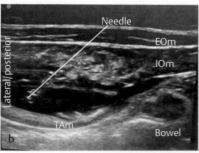

Fig. 32.1 (a, b) Transverse abdominus plane (TAP) block. EOm, external oblique muscle; IOm, internal oblique muscle; TAm, transversus abdominis muscle.

imaging skills are very operator-dependent, requiring appropriate levels of training and anatomical knowledge. The portable nature of USG allows the operator to perform USG-guided procedures in numerous settings, including perioperatively, at the bedside, and in an outpatient clinic. Additionally, blood vessels, soft tissue, pleura, peritoneum, and viscera are easily identified under USG, making it safer in situations where risk of puncture to these structures is present. Real-time visualization with USG allows for continuous visualization of the block needle for the entire duration of the procedure, especially while advancing through different tissue layers.[2]

32.3.2 What Is a Peripheral Nerve Block?

A peripheral nerve block entails injecting local anesthetic with or without steroid around or adjacent to a nerve. The local anesthetic blocks sodium channels, thus inhibiting the generation of an action potential. Sensory afferent fibers have longer action potential durations than motor neurons, and are therefore more sensitive to lower concentrations of local anesthetic. Blockade of the nerve conduction results in the stoppage of all signals carried by the nerve, including pain signals, for the duration of that medication's effect. Once the local anesthetic's effect has worn off, usually after five half-lives, the pain often returns. However, sometimes the nerve block can provide several weeks to months of pain relief, especially if steroids are added to the injectate. The mechanism of prolonged relief from a nerve block is unclear, but it may be a result of resetting the pain pathways during the temporary blockade. Steroids can provide additional relief by prolonging the block and reducing inflammation, especially when pain is secondary to entrapment or neuroma formation. However, the duration of relief is difficult to predict as it varies from person to person.

Risks of peripheral nerve blocks includes bleeding, infection, and damage to the nerve or nearby structures. The authors recommend following American Society of Regional Anesthesia and Pain Medicine (ASRA-PM) guidelines in patients receiving antithrombotic or thrombolytic therapy to reduce the risk of

bleeding.[3] Sterile precautions should be observed while performing the nerve block to reduce the risk of infection. Ultrasonography is able to reduce the risk of injury by allowing for better visualization of the soft tissue, musculoskeletal structures, fascial layers, pleura, and peritoneum. Furthermore, it allows for consistent visualization of the needle tip during advancement in the in-plane approach, which is also a key safety feature. Pain on injection and increasing pressure with injection might be signs of intraneural injection, which may lead to nerve damage and should be avoided. Use of the Doppler function of most ultrasounds allows for visualization of blood flow through vascular structures and helps minimize risk of bleeding or hematoma formation. Along with intermittent aspiration, it can also help avoid intravascular injection. If there is any concern that the needle is intraneural or intravascular, the needle tip should be withdrawn and redirected until a more reassuring location is established.

32.3.3 Clinical Scenarios

Given the temporary nature of these blocks, they are often utilized for acute pain, especially in the perioperative setting. However, they are also utilized for patients with chronic pain for diagnostic or therapeutic purposes (especially in cases of nerve entrapment). Examples include:

- Head and neck blocks: Occipital nerve, trigeminal nerve, glossopharyngeal nerve, superficial cervical plexus, stellate ganglion, etc.
- Upper extremity blocks: Brachial plexus, median nerve, radial nerve, suprascapular nerve, etc. ► Fig. 32.2 demonstrates a potential approach (interscalene) for brachial plexus block in the neck. A single shot or continuous brachial plexus block is often utilized for pain control for patients undergoing upper extremity surgery. ► Fig. 32.3 demonstrates the location of the median nerve just above the wrist. It can be blocked here easily for relief from median nerve entrapment related pain, such as carpal tunnel syndrome.
- Chest and thorax blocks: Intercostal nerve (► Fig. 32.4), paravertebral, Pec I and II, serratus anterior plane, erector spinae, etc. Ultrasound allows for ready visualization of the pleura, reducing the risk of pneumothorax. An intercostal nerve block can be utilized in the treatment of intractable chest wall pain of various etiologies, such as postherpetic neuralgia, postmastectomy pain syndrome, post-thoracotomy pain syndrome, etc.
- Abdomen, groin, and genitalia blocks: TAP, ilioinguinal nerve, genitofemoral nerve, pudendal nerve, etc.

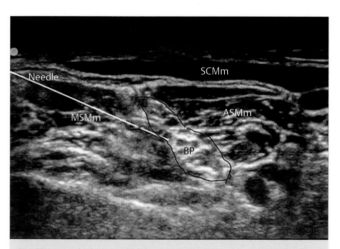

Fig. 32.2 Brachial plexus block with interscalene approach. ASMm, anterior scalene muscle; BP, brachial plexus; carotid artery; MSMm, middle scalene muscle; SCMm, sternocleidomastoid muscle.

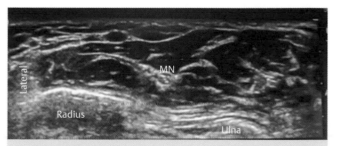

Fig. 32.3 Median nerve, just proximal to the wrist. MN, median nerve.

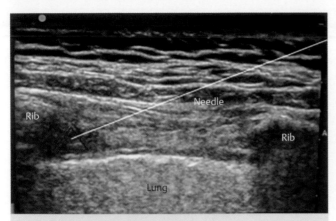

Fig. 32.4 Needle trajectory for intercostal nerve block. Intercostal groove containing intercostal neurovascular bundle is marked with a red triangle. Pleura can be easily visualized as white line above the lung.

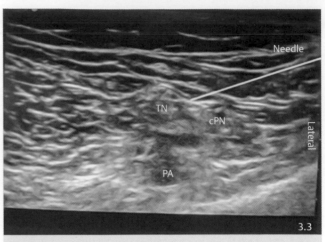

Fig. 32.5 Sciatic nerve block at the level of the popliteal fossa. The sciatic nerve can be visualized as dividing into tibial nerve (TN) and common peroneal nerve (cPN). PA, popliteal artery.

- Lower extremity blocks: lateral femoral cutaneous nerve, femoral/saphenous nerve, sciatic nerve (▶ Fig. 32.5), posterior tibial nerve, superficial peroneal nerve, obturator nerve, ankle, digital, etc.

32.3.4 Options in Cases of Short-Term Pain Relief with Temporary Nerve Block

Continuous peripheral nerve blockade using a perineural catheter can provide prolonged analgesia. This is often used when pain is expected to improve, such as for postoperative pain following joint surgery or cancer-related pain from a bony lesion that is about to undergo radiation therapy. If the relief from the nerve block is short lived, but significant, then other options can be considered for chronic pain such as nerve destruction or neuromodulation.

Neurolysis can be achieved via chemical or physical modalities. There is increased risk of neuritis with neurolysis of peripheral nerves as compared to neurolysis of a sympathetic plexus, such as celiac plexus or superior hypogastric plexus. Cryoablation is a physical modality of nerve destruction and has not been reported to result in neuritis. Radiofrequency ablation, in both conventional and pulsed settings, uses heat for destruction of nerve tissue. There are several chemical options for nerve destruction such as alcohol, phenol, and glycerol. Glycerol is preferred for head and neck while phenol is preferred for bigger somatic nerves (such as the femoral nerve), given its inherent local anesthetic properties.

There has been a recent upsurge in ultrasound-guided peripheral nerve stimulator (PNS) with the development of wearable external pulse generator (does not need to be implanted inside the body), allowing for a percutaneous approach for lead placement. This allows for implantation of the leads under ultrasound guidance while minimizing the size of skin incision. They are currently approved by the Federal Drug Administration (FDA) for chronic intractable pain of peripheral nerve origin. The ability to place the external pulse generator in the intended location should be taken into consideration when planning for PNS. Diagnostic nerve blocks help to identify the affected nerve as well as the location affected, though larger volumes of medication can result in higher rates of false positive responses. The biggest risk with the PNS is lead migration, followed by other device-related risks such as lead fracture and erosion.

32.4 Conclusion

Ultrasound-guided nerve block is a radiation-free, portable, and inexpensive method of pain control for many different pain pathologies.

References

[1] Narouze SN. Atlas of Ultrasound-Guided Procedures in Interventional Pain Management. 2nd ed. Springer; 2018

[2] Chan VWS. Ultrasound Imaging for Regional Anesthesia. 2nd ed. Toronto, ON: Toronto Printing Company; 2009

[3] Horlocker TT, Vandermeulen E, Kopp SL, Gogarten W, Leffert LR, Benzon HT. Regional anesthesia in the patient receiving antithrombotic or thrombolytic therapy: American Society of Regional Anesthesia and Pain Medicine Evidence-Based Guidelines (Fourth Edition). Reg Anesth Pain Med. 2018; 43 (3):263–309

33 Peripheral Nerve Blocks (MRI)

Danoob Dalili, Daniel E. Dalili, Amanda Isaac, and Jan Fritz

33.1 Case Presentations

A 56-year-old man who was an ex-professional cyclist presented to our institution with erectile dysfunction, perineal pain, and numbness worse on the left side. The pain scored 7 to 8 on an 11-point visual analog scale (VAS). Following normal magnetic resonance imaging (MRI) of the lumbar spine, a clinical diagnosis of pudendal neuralgia was suspected. A fluoroscopy-guided pudendal nerve block was performed (▶ Fig. 33.1).

A 38-year-old man presented with sharp burning pain with "pins and needles" in the left pelvic area and a sensation of a "golf ball" in the buttocks; the symptoms were worse on sitting and improved by standing and lying down. The pain scored 7 to 9 on an 11-point VAS. On clinical examination, his pain was recreated by palpating the nerve in the ischial region. A diagnosis of pudendal nerve entrapment was suspected; however, nerve conduction studies were inconclusive. MRI of the lumbosacral spine and pelvis was performed to exclude a neoplastic or infectious cause for his symptoms, after which a diagnostic and therapeutic pudendal nerve injection was performed (▶ Fig. 33.2).

A 28-year-old woman presented with left buttock pain, as well as shooting and burning sensations in the perineum. Symptoms were exacerbated by sitting for prolonged periods. On clinical examination, the pain was described as burning, reaching 6 to 8 on an 11-point VAS. Clinically, a diagnosis of pudendal neuralgia was suspected. Her past medical history included pelvic surgeries. Dedicated magnetic resonance neurography (MRN) of the lumbosacral plexus demonstrated pudendal perineural scarring at the entrance level of the Alcock's canal and pudendal nerve T2 signal hyperintensity, consistent with scar entrapment-related pudendal neuropathy (▶ Fig. 33.3).

33.2 Discussion

Interventional MRI has been integrated into routine clinical practice over the last two decades. This has been made possible by the increase in commercially available technical instruments, software solutions, and a widening range of clinical applications.[1,2,3,4,5,6] Interventional MRI can be performed on either low or high magnetic field (ranging from 0.2 T to 3 T) magnetic resonance (MR) scanners. Most centers perform interventional procedures with 1.5-T scanners, although 3-T scanners have been more recently utilized and may be considered advantageous. Clinical wide-bore scanners are broadly accepted as the preferred scanner type and have equipped many centers to perform MR-guided interventions with faster sequences and improved resolution, as well as generally larger bores when compared to traditional lower magnetic field and older generation scanners.[2,7,8,9]

Interventional MRN combines high-contrast and high-spatial resolution of MRN with the capabilities required to perform intricate high-resolution interventional techniques, particularly for nerves situated deep in the body. Established features on diagnostic MRN indicative of neuropathy include asymmetrical T2 hyperintensity, architectural distortion (loss of the normal fascicular structure), focal thickening, and perineural soft tissue scarring.[1,10,11,12,13,14,15] Detailed physical examination, nerve conduction studies, and diagnostic MRN together with targeted perineural blocks allow identification of the pain-mediating nerve in the context of a normal MRN examination.[5]

With MRN, the operator is able to clearly visualize and map the course of the nerve in its entirety from its origin in the spinal cord, identify possible variant courses, and visualize any associated focal abnormalities as the nerve branches peripherally. This is particularly relevant in the presence of anatomical variants,

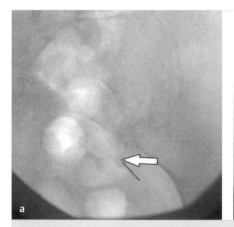
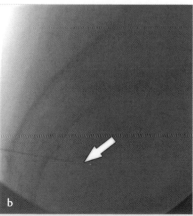
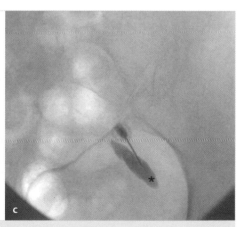

Fig. 33.1 Fluoroscopy-guided block of the left pudendal nerve. Posteroanterior (**a**) and lateral (**b**) fluoroscopic images with anatomic landmarks permit targeting the pudendal nerve in the Alcock's canal with a 22-gauge spinal needle (arrow). (**c**) Posteroanterior view demonstrating contrast mixed with 40 mg triamcinolone (*) distending the Alcock's canal and bathing the pudendal nerve. The patient's pain reduced to 3/10 at 2 weeks follow-up indicating a positive response and confirming the diagnosis of pudendal neuralgia.

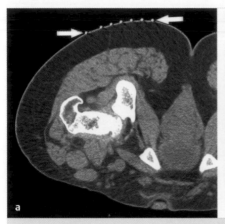
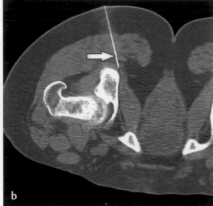
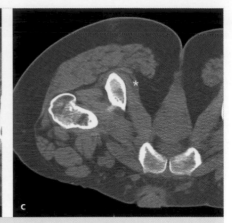

Fig. 33.2 Computed tomography-guided pudendal nerve injection. (**a**) Axial preprocedure planning image demonstrating placement of radio-opaque fiducial skin markers (arrows) at the level of the sacrotuberous ligament and entrance to the Alcock's canal. (**b**) Utilizing anatomical landmarks, a 22-G spinal needle (arrow) was inserted into the Alcock's canal just lateral to the sacrotuberous ligament. (**c**) A mixture of steroid and local anesthetic injectate distended the canal (*), bathing the pudendal nerve. A positive pain response was elicited at clinical follow-up and the patient proceeded to surgical decompression.

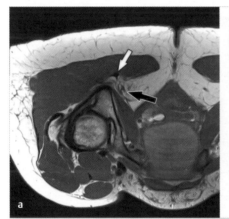
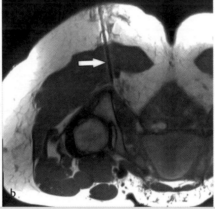
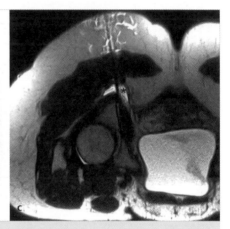

Fig. 33.3 Magnetic resonance neurography–guided pudendal nerve block utilizing a clinical wide-bore 3 Tesla magnetic resonance imaging (MRI) system. (**a**) Preprocedural, axial, PD-weighted, high-resolution magnetic resonance neurography with its exquisite soft tissue contrast permits clear identification and mapping of the pudendal nerve entering the Alcock's canal just lateral to the triangular sacrotuberous ligament (white arrow). The area of entrapment is clearly visualized as a result of perineural scarring (black arrow) at the proximal aspect of the canal. The trajectory is planned with fiducial markers (not shown), avoiding neighboring critical structures. (**b**) Axial, interventional, 12-second PD sequence demonstrates a 20-G magnetic resonance compatible needle (white arrow) cannulating the entrance to the Alcock's canal via a posterolateral approach, lateral to the sacrotuberous ligament and adjacent to the pudendal nerve. (**c**) Axial, interventional, 4-second, T2-weighted Half-Fourier Acquisition Single-shot Turbo spin Echo imaging (HASTE) sequence demonstrates the final distribution of the injectate (*), bathing the pudendal nerve with a mixture of 4 mL 1% ropivacaine, 40 mg triamcinolone acetonide, and 300 international units of hyaluronidase. Following the injection, there was perineal anesthesia and near-complete resolution of symptoms, indicating the pudendal nerve as the main pain generator.

postoperative distortion of anatomical beds, or in the presence of malignancy with locoregional infiltration.[16,17,18,19,20,21,22] MRN may also narrow the differential diagnosis, excluding neoplastic causes for the pain, localize any extrinsic neural compression, or post-traumatic/postoperative locoregional scarring around a nerve, visualize architectural distortion, and identify variant courses or focal neuromas. As demonstrated in the above examples, interventional MRI permits precise targeting of the nerve and understanding of the locoregional structures with better detail than other modalities such as computed tomography (CT), fluoroscopy, or ultrasound. This is particularly the case when

these modalities have failed in identifying any abnormality or when targeting deep pelvic or retroperitoneal nerves, or targets that require accurate drug delivery such as botulinum neurotoxin for piriformis syndrome.[5] Use of augmented reality and advanced interventional techniques, as well as application of fast imaging sequences, may further improve the accuracy and safety of interventional MRI.[1,4,11]

Unlike CT, with real-time MR fluoroscopy, the spread of the actual injectant can also be directly visualized without the need for additional contrast agents. As such, MRN-guided nerve blocks offer a high level of technical accuracy for the operator, while allowing objective evaluation of the adequacy of the blocks and pain outcomes.[3,7,8,11,13,23] Interventional MRI also allows precise imaging near metalwork with metal artifact reduction protocol modifications. These modifications improve imaging when compared to standard CT imaging techniques, particularly in the absence of dual energy CT technology which requires the purchase of dedicated hardware to allow metal suppression.[24,25] When compared to CT, MRI provides superior soft tissue contrast resolution while avoiding potentially harmful ionizing radiation, thus rendering it safe for repeated procedures as well as when treating pregnant women, women of childbearing age, or children.[3,7,25,26]

In addition to MR-guided spine interventions, peripheral (nonspinal) nerve blocks using MRI have been described for celiac nerve blocks,[27] sympathetic nerves,[9] posterior femoral cutaneous nerves,[7,28,29,30] pudendal nerves,[7,29] obturator and lateral femoral cutaneous nerve of the thigh,[7] ganglion impar,[31] genitofemoral nerve, iliohypogastric nerve, and ilioinguinal nerve.[32]

Patient-reported outcome measures are favorable with these techniques, as well as overall patient satisfaction.[3,4,7,14,32,33,34] Patient satisfaction with interventional MRI procedures is a key indicator of the impact of introducing such services and integrating them into mainstream treatment strategies. Majority of patients report immediate pain relief, comfortable and acceptable examination time, and favorable positioning. Intraprocedural MR-related complications include claustrophobia (albeit typically mild), intermittent nausea (minimal symptoms), minor headaches, disagreeable transient heat sensation, and mild intraprocedural pain, vertigo, and tinnitus.[32]

33.3 Conclusion

Interventional MRI has been validated to provide safe and effective treatment strategies for managing peripheral neuropathies, with improved patient satisfaction and superior precision technologies when compared to other imaging modalities. Interventional MRI blocks can help confirm the diagnosis of neuralgia and can alleviate patients' symptoms, either as a sole intervention or when combined with other interventions including cryoanalgesia or neurolysis.

References

[1] Fritz J, U-Thainual P, Ungi T, et al. Augmented reality visualization using image overlay technology for MR-guided interventions: cadaveric bone biopsy at 1.5 T. Invest Radiol. 2013; 48(6):464–470

[2] Garmer M, Grönemeyer D. Magnetic resonance-guided interventions of large and small joints. Top Magn Reson Imaging. 2011; 22(4):153–169

[3] Sequeiros RB, Sinikumpu JJ, Ojala R, Järvinen J, Fritz J. Pediatric musculoskeletal interventional MRI. Top Magn Reson Imaging. 2018; 27(1):39–44

[4] Fritz J, Thomas C, Clasen S, Claussen CD, Lewin JS, Pereira PL. Freehand real-time MRI-guided lumbar spinal injection procedures at 1.5 T: feasibility, accuracy, and safety. AJR Am J Roentgenol. 2009; 192(4):W161–7

[5] Dalili D, Ahlawat S, Rashidi A, Belzberg AJ, Fritz J. Cryoanalgesia of the anterior femoral cutaneous nerve (AFCN) for the treatment of neuropathy-mediated anterior thigh pain: anatomy and technical description. Skeletal Radiol. 2021; 50(6):1227–1236

[6] Murphy KJ, Nussbaum DA, Schnupp S, Long D. Tarlov cysts: an overlooked clinical problem. Semin Musculoskelet Radiol. 2011; 15(2):163–167

[7] Fritz J, Dellon AL, Williams EH, Belzberg AJ, Carrino JA. 3-Tesla high-field magnetic resonance neurography for guiding nerve blocks and its role in pain management. Magn Reson Imaging Clin N Am. 2015; 23(4):533–545

[8] Fritz J, Tzaribachev N, Thomas C, et al. Evaluation of MR imaging guided steroid injection of the sacroiliac joints for the treatment of children with refractory enthesitis-related arthritis. Eur Radiol. 2011; 21(5):1050–1057

[9] Sze DY, Mackey SC. MR guidance of sympathetic nerve blockade: measurement of vasomotor response initial experience in seven patients. Radiology. 2002; 223(2):574–580

[10] Papakonstantinou O, Isaac A, Dalili D, Noebauer-Huhmann IM. T2-weighted hypointense tumors and tumor-like lesions. Semin Musculoskelet Radiol. 2019; 23(1):58–75

[11] Sequeiros RB, Fritz J, Ojala R, Carrino JA. Percutaneous magnetic resonance imaging-guided bone tumor management and magnetic resonance imaging-guided bone therapy. Top Magn Reson Imaging. 2011; 22(4):171–177

[12] Fritz J, U-Thainual P, Ungi T, et al. MR-guided vertebroplasty with augmented reality image overlay navigation. Cardiovasc Intervent Radiol. 2014; 37(6):1589–1596

[13] Fritz J, U-Thainual P, Ungi T, et al. Augmented reality visualisation using an image overlay system for MR-guided interventions: technical performance of spine injection procedures in human cadavers at 1.5 Tesla. Eur Radiol. 2013; 23(1):235–245

[14] Fritz J, Sonnow L, Morris CD. Adjuvant MRI-guided percutaneous cryoablation treatment for aneurysmal bone cyst. Skeletal Radiol. 2019; 48(7):1149–1153

[15] Dalili D, Isaac A, Fayad LM, Ahlawat S. Routine knee MRI: how common are peripheral nerve abnormalities, and why does it matter? Skeletal Radiol. 2021; 50(2):321–332

[16] Lee TC, Guenette JP, Moses ZB, Chi JH. MRI-guided cryoablation of epidural malignancies in the spinal canal resulting in neural decompression and regrowth of bone. AJR Am J Roentgenol. 2019; 212(1):205–208

[17] Dalili D, Isaac A, Bazzocchi A, et al. Interventional techniques for bone and musculoskeletal soft tissue tumors: current practices and future directions - Part I. Ablation. Semin Musculoskelet Radiol. 2020; 24(6):692–709

[18] Cazzato RL, Garnon J, De Marini P, et al. French multidisciplinary approach for the treatment of MSK tumors. Semin Musculoskelet Radiol. 2020; 24(3):310–322

[19] Dalili D, Isaac A, Rashidi A, Åström G, Fritz J. Image-guided sports medicine and musculoskeletal tumor interventions: a patient-centered model. Semin Musculoskelet Radiol. 2020; 24(3):290–309

[20] Cazzato RL, Auloge P, De Marini P, et al. Spinal tumor ablation: indications, techniques, and clinical management. Tech Vasc Interv Radiol. 2020; 23(2):100677

[21] Garnon J, Meylheuc L, Auloge P, et al. Continuous injection of large volumes of cement through a single 10G vertebroplasty needle in cases of large osteolytic lesions. Cardiovasc Intervent Radiol. 2020; 43(4):658–661

[22] Carrino JA, Blanco R. Magnetic resonance-guided musculoskeletal interventional radiology. Semin Musculoskelet Radiol. 2006; 10(2):159–174

[23] Fritz J, Henes JC, Thomas C, et al. Diagnostic and interventional MRI of the sacroiliac joints using a 1.5-T open-bore magnet: a one-stop-shopping approach. AJR Am J Roentgenol. 2008; 191(6):1717–1724

[24] Khodarahmi I, Bonham LW, Weiss CR, Fritz J. Needle heating during interventional magnetic resonance imaging at 1.5- and 3.0-T field strengths. Invest Radiol. 2020; 55(6):396–404

[25] Khodarahmi I, Isaac A, Fishman EK, Dalili D, Fritz J. Metal about the hip and artifact reduction techniques: from basic concepts to advanced imaging. Semin Musculoskelet Radiol. 2019; 23(3):e68–e81

[26] Fritz J, Tzaribachev N, Thomas C, et al. Magnetic resonance imaging-guided osseous biopsy in children with chronic recurrent multifocal osteomyelitis. Cardiovasc Intervent Radiol. 2012; 35(1):146–153

[27] Hol PK, Kvarstein G, Viken O, Smedby O, Tønnessen TI. MRI-guided celiac plexus block. J Magn Reson Imaging. 2000; 12(4):562–564

[28] Fritz J, Bizzell C, Kathuria S, et al. High-resolution magnetic resonance-guided posterior femoral cutaneous nerve blocks. Skeletal Radiol. 2013; 42(4):579–586

[29] Fritz J, Chhabra A, Wang KC, Carrino JA. Magnetic resonance neurography-guided nerve blocks for the diagnosis and treatment of chronic pelvic pain syndrome. Neuroimaging Clin N Am. 2014; 24(1):211–234

[30] Joshi DH, Thawait GK, Del Grande F, Fritz J. MRI-guided cryoablation of the posterior femoral cutaneous nerve for the treatment of neuropathy-mediated sitting pain. Skeletal Radiol. 2017; 46(7):983–987

[31] Marker DR, U-Thainual P, Ungi T, et al. MR-guided perineural injection of the ganglion impar: technical considerations and feasibility. Skeletal Radiol. 2016; 45(5):591–597

[32] Fritz J, Dellon AL, Williams EH, Rosson GD, Belzberg AJ, Eckhauser FE. Diagnostic accuracy of selective 3-T MR neurography-guided retroperitoneal genitofemoral nerve blocks for the diagnosis of genitofemoral neuralgia. Radiology. 2017; 285(1):176–185:

[33] Fritz J, Dellon AL, Williams EH, Rosson GD, Belzberg AJ, Eckhauser FE. Diagnostic Accuracy of Selective 3-T MR Neurography-guided Retroperitoneal Genitofemoral Nerve Blocks for the Diagnosis of Genitofemoral Neuralgia. Radiology. 2017;285(1):176-185.

[34] Fritz J, Pereira PL. [MR-guided pain therapy: principles and clinical applications]. Röfo Fortschr Geb Röntgenstr Nuklearmed. 2007; 179(9):914–924

34 Nerve Ablations I (Genicular RF)

Felix M. Gonzalez, Samuel E. Broida, and Nima Kokabi

34.1 Introduction

Subchondral insufficiency fractures of the knee (SIFK) are painful, nontraumatic fractures that occur predominantly in the medial femoral condyle of postmenopausal osteoporotic women in their fifth and sixth decades of life. SIFK typically presents with acute knee pain localized to the area of the subchondral fracture.[1,2] These fractures can be recognized radiologically by the presence of a linear subchondral T1–T2 hypointense defect usually located on magnetic resonance imaging (MRI) underneath the articular cartilage with surrounding marrow and soft tissue edema.[3] Other articular pathology such as posterior root medial meniscus tears and resultant meniscal extrusion may also be noted on imaging.[4] A previously used term "spontaneous osteonecrosis of the knee (SONK)" is now considered a misnomer, given that histologically osteonecrosis is absent in this setting. Disease progression has been attributed to lesion size and continued weight-bearing following the initial fracture.[2,5] For this reason, immobilization, restricted weight-bearing, and physical therapy have been proposed as a way to manage the low-grade lesions that will most likely resolve.[6] Other conservative measures such as teriparatide supplementation and bisphosphonates have been employed in the treatment of SIFK, though the true benefit of these modalities has been a source of debate.[7,8,9,10,11] For patients who are unable to tolerate physical therapy and desire definitive treatment, arthroplasty has been shown to be an effective treatment option.[12,13,14] However, a conservative treatment regimen that provides adequate pain relief to allow for long-term rehabilitation and recovery has not previously been described.

Given the reported success of nerve ablations in the treatment of chronic pain,[15] the authors suggest that radiofrequency ablation (RFA) of the genicular nerve may be a viable minimally invasive treatment option in the management of patients with symptomatic SIFK. Here is reported a positive outcome in the case of SIFK in a woman who was managed conservatively with RFAs of the genicular nerves and a bisphosphonate regimen, leading to ultimate resolution of her symptoms and complete healing of her necrotic lesion.

34.2 Case Presentation

A 66-year-old woman presented for evaluation of bilateral knee pain, left worse than right, that had been happening for 10 years. The left knee pain developed without any trauma shortly after a hysterectomy, and it was described as low grade until it significantly worsened 1 year prior to presentation. The discomfort was located in the medial and anterior aspects of the left knee, and driving or standing up from the seated position worsened her pain. She sought orthopedic care and was treated with a cortisone injection. Although the injection provided symptomatic pain relief, she also developed palpitations, malaise, and insomnia and was therefore deemed unfit for further corticosteroid. She continued to complain of moderate pain in

the right knee and severe pain the left knee as well as decreasing walking tolerance.

A dual energy X-ray absorptiometry (DEXA) scan demonstrated osteoporosis (< or = −2.5), and an MRI of the left knee showed a degenerative tear involving the posterior horn, root attachment, and body of the medial meniscus, with patellofemoral articular cartilage degeneration and medial femoral condyle marrow edema (▶ Fig. 34.1. A total knee replacement was offered; however, the patient was interested in conservative treatment, so she was referred to interventional radiology (IR) for consideration of a genicular nerve block.

She was seen in the IR clinic 2 months later and continued to complain of worsening pain in both knees. At that point, she reported total modification of her lifestyle to avoid aggravating her knee pain. Her left knee remained her primary concern. She reported pain at rest that was 5/10 in severity and worsened to 9/10 with activity. She maintained full range of motion. On further review of her prior MRI, a small subchondral insufficiency fracture along the medial aspect of the left medial femoral condyle measuring 7 × 8 mm was visualized, accompanied by adjacent subchondral marrow edema and a complex meniscal tear (▶ Fig. 34.1). She was deemed to be an appropriate candidate for a left knee genicular nerve block procedure and pending relief with the nerve block of at least 50%, subsequent genicular nerve ablation utilizing cooled RFA technique. The patient agreed and underwent the nerve block 10 days later. She reported immediate improvement, stating her pain improved to 2–3/10 in severity for a few days afterwards. Details of the nerve block and ablation procedures are presented below.

Cooled RFAs of the genicular nerves were performed 2 weeks later. There were no immediate complications. The patient experienced pain relief within 2 weeks after the ablations. After the ablations, she was started on weekly high-dose vitamin D (20,000 IU) for 4 months in preparation for bisphosphate therapy. This was followed by two infusions of ibandronate, given 8 weeks apart. She was restricted to touch-down weight bearing for 3 months following the procedure, after which her activity was improved by physical therapy. There was marked, progressive improvement in her pain and functional status during her rehabilitation and treatment (▶ Table 34.1). At her 8-week follow-up, she reported no pain while at rest and slight discomfort (1–2/10) with limited activity. MRI of the left knee performed at 4.5 months postprocedure demonstrated a decreasing joint effusion and resolution of the subchondral marrow edema, with slight progression of the medial meniscus tear (▶ Fig. 34.2).

34.2.1 Diagnostic Genicular Nerve Block Procedure

The patient was placed supine on the fluoroscopy table with feet and ankles secured to the fluoroscopy table with sturdy tape in order to ensure leg immobility during the procedure. A skin wheal was first made utilizing 1 to 2 mL of 1% lidocaine for superficial local anesthesia in order to avoid involvement of the

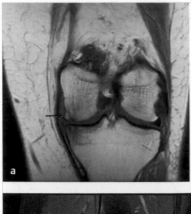
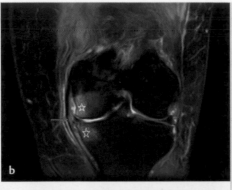
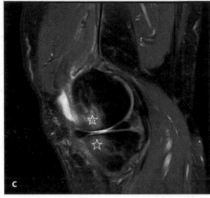
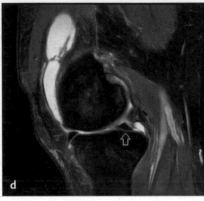

Fig. 34.1 Preablation magnetic resonance imaging (MRI) of the left knee: Coronal T1-weighted (**a**) images demonstrating the T1 hypointense subchondral insufficiency fracture line within the medial aspect of the medial femoral condyle measuring 7 mm (red arrow). (**b** and **c**) Coronal proton density fat saturation (PD FS) and sagittal PD FS images at the same level demonstrating the reciprocal bone marrow edema in the medial femoral condyle and medial tibial plateau (stars), as well as a tear of the medial meniscal body (orange arrow). Sagittal PD FS image (**d**) at the level of the posterior horn–root junction of the medial meniscus demonstrating blunting of the medial meniscus compatible with free edge radial tear (black arrow with white border).

Table 34.1 Functional outcome scores after radiofrequency ablation compared to baseline

	Baseline	2 weeks	1 month	3 months	6 months
KOOS	16.7	81	84	86	91
WOMAC	23	65	65	65	82
VAS	9–10	4	2	1	0

Abbreviations: KOOS, Knee Injury and Osteoarthritis Outcome Score; VAS, Visual Analog Scale; WOMAC, Western Ontario and McMaster Universities Osteoarthritis Index.

genicular nerves. Needle placement was confirmed in both the anteroposterior (AP) and lateral planes. Extra care was taken to ensure that the condyles of the femur were superimposed over one another on the lateral imaging (▶ Fig. 34.3). At each needle site, 1.0 mL of 2% lidocaine was injected without complications.

34.2.2 Genicular Nerve Radiofrequency Ablation Procedure

Similar steps were followed as during the diagnostic block procedure. Sedation and analgesia (midazolam 1–2 mg intravenous [IV] and/or fentanyl 25–100 µg IV) and supplemental nasal cannula oxygen were given. Skin and soft tissues were anesthetized with 1 to 2 mL of 1% lidocaine at each of the three anatomic sites for RFA probe placement. A 75-mm, 17-gauge introducer needle was placed in the three locations mentioned above. Once the introducer needle was placed, the 18-gauge, internally cooled, 4-mm, active-tip RFA electrode (Coolief, Halyard Health, Alpharetta, GA, USA) was placed into the introducer needle, and positioning was verified with AP and lateral fluoroscopic views. Testing at 2 Hertz at 1 mA was performed to test for motor

nerve activity. Then 1 mL of 2% lidocaine was injected through the introducer needles. Each target was sequentially treated for 2 minutes and 30 seconds at a set temperature of 60 °C, producing a tissue temperature of 77° to 80 °C surrounding the electrode. Electrode position is shown in ▶ Fig. 34.3.

34.3 Discussion

Given the relative infrequency with which subchondral insufficiency fractures of the knee are diagnosed, a consensus regarding classification and management does not currently exist. Outcomes vary widely even among patients who are managed with similar protocols, suggesting that treatment algorithms may benefit from further classification of these fractures based on prognosis. The authors previously proposed an SIFK grading system based on lesion size and associated pathology as viewed on MRI.[6] The size of SIFK lesions appears to be a valid indicator of outcome, with large size (mean sum of dimensions ≥ 26 mm; AP [anterior to posterior] mean values of 16.78 ± 7.88; and TR [transverse] dimensions of 13.14 ± 3.13) portending irreversibility with conservative management (sensitivity of 91%).

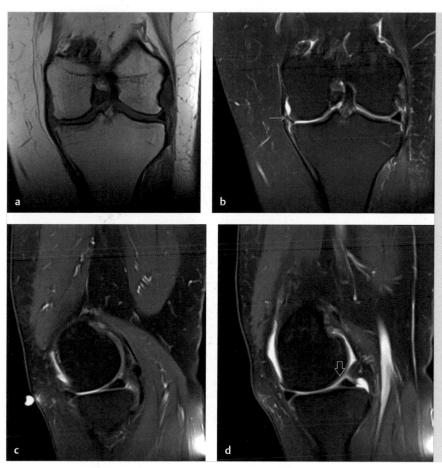

Fig. 34.2 Postablation magnetic resonance imaging (MRI) of the left knee: Coronal T1-weighted images (**a**) of the left knee post ablation demonstrating resolution of the previous subchondral insufficiency fracture within the medial femoral condyle. Coronal and sagittal proton density fat saturation (PD FS) images (**b** and **c**) at the same level also show complete resolution of the previously seen bone marrow edema, as well as progression of the medial meniscal tear (orange arrow). Sagittal PD FS image at the level of the medial meniscus posterior horn–root junction (**d**) also showing further blunting of the posterior horn when compared to ▶ Fig. 34.1 (arrow).

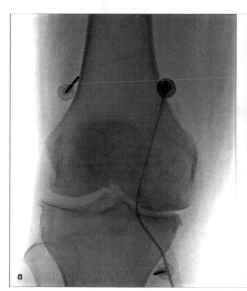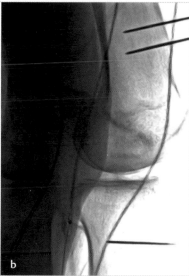

Fig. 34.3 Frontal and lateral views of the knee demonstrating proper needle placement.

Arthroplasty and joint-preserving procedures may be better reserved for these larger fractures.

Conservative management of patients with smaller lesions or those who opt against surgery is more challenging. Barriers to recovery include the severe pain typically associated with these fractures as well as a slow rate of healing, often requiring extensive periods of non-weight-bearing. Bisphosphonates have been proposed as an adjunct therapy to aid in healing and prevent subchondral collapse, though the use of bisphosphonates has been a source of debate, and further investigation must be done before an accurate conclusion regarding their efficacy can be drawn.[8,9] Pain management strategies to date have included oral and topical analgesics, immobilization, and physical therapy. However, these modalities may in some cases be insufficient to control symptoms for the long duration of rehabilitation. RFA of the genicular nerve has been previously demonstrated to be effective in other chronic pain disorders of the knee, although to the authors' knowledge it has never been used in symptomatic management of SIFK. In the case presented here, this was offered to a woman with a debilitating low-grade SIFK, who did not desire surgery.

The patient, a middle-aged, osteoporotic woman with a subchondral insufficiency fracture of the medial femoral condyle and medial meniscus tears with extrusion, is a classic presentation of SIFK. Her fracture dimensions totaled 15 mm, and therefore she was deemed a good candidate for nonoperative management. Cooled RFA of the genicular nerve provided sufficient pain relief to allow her to tolerate physical therapy after a prolonged non-weight-bearing protocol. Supplementation with vitamin D and ibandronate were used to improve bone density during rehabilitation. She had eventual resolution of her fracture within 4.5 months, and had subsequent return to baseline activity without limitation. The authors therefore submit this report to raise the possibility of cooled RFA as a conservative therapy to provide symptomatic relief for low-grade SIFK lesions. Larger studies with additional subjects would be an important next step in elucidating the role of nerve blocks in management of these fractures.

References

[1] Wilmot AS, Ruutiainen AT, Bakhru PT, Schweitzer ME, Shabshin N. Subchondral insufficiency fracture of the knee: a recognizable associated soft tissue edema pattern and a similar distribution among men and women. Eur J Radiol. 2016; 85(11):2096–2103

[2] Yamamoto T, Bullough PG. Spontaneous osteonecrosis of the knee: the result of subchondral insufficiency fracture. J Bone Joint Surg Am. 2000; 82(6):858–866

[3] Zywiel MG, McGrath MS, Seyler TM, Marker DR, Bonutti PM, Mont MA. Osteonecrosis of the knee: a review of three disorders. Orthop Clin North Am. 2009; 40(2):193–211

[4] Yamagami R, Taketomi S, Inui H, Tahara K, Tanaka S. The role of medial meniscus posterior root tear and proximal tibial morphology in the development of spontaneous osteonecrosis and osteoarthritis of the knee. Knee. 2017; 24(2):390–395

[5] Zanetti M, Romero J, Dambacher MA, Hodler J. Osteonecrosis diagnosed on MR images of the knee. Relationship to reduced bone mineral density determined by high resolution peripheral quantitative CT. Acta Radiol. 2003; 44(5):525–531

[6] Sayyid S, Younan Y, Sharma G, Singer A, Morrison W, Zoga A, Gonzalez FM. Subchondral insufficiency fracture of the knee: grading, risk factors, and outcome. Skeletal Radiology. 2019 Dec;48(12):1961–1974.

[7] Gourlay ML, Renner JB, Spang JT, Rubin JE. Subchondral insufficiency fracture of the knee: a non-traumatic injury with prolonged recovery time. BMJ Case Rep. 2015; 2015:bcr2015209399

[8] Kraenzlin ME, Graf C, Meier C, Kraenzlin C, Friedrich NF. Possible beneficial effect of bisphosphonates in osteonecrosis of the knee. Knee Surg Sports Traumatol Arthrosc. 2010; 18(12):1638–1644

[9] Meier C, Kraenzlin C, Friederich NF, et al. Effect of ibandronate on spontaneous osteonecrosis of the knee: a randomized, double-blind, placebo-controlled trial. Osteoporos Int. 2014; 25(1):359–366

[10] An VV, Broek MVD, Oussedik S. Subchondral insufficiency fracture in the lateral compartment of the knee in a 64-year-old Marathon runner. Knee Surg Relat Res. 2017; 29(4):325–328

[11] Zanetti M, Romero J, Dambacher MA, Hodler J. Osteonecrosis diagnosed on MR images of the knee: relationship to reduced bone mineral density determined by high resolution peripheral quantitative CT. Acta Radiologica. 2003 Sep;44(5):525–531.

[12] Mont MA, Rifai A, Baumgarten KM, Sheldon M, Hungerford DS. Total knee arthroplasty for osteonecrosis. J Bone Joint Surg Am. 2002; 84(4):599–603

[13] Radke S, Wollmerstedt N, Bischoff A, Eulert J. Knee arthroplasty for spontaneous osteonecrosis of the knee: unicompartimental vs bicompartimental knee arthroplasty. Knee Surg Sports Traumatol Arthrosc. 2005; 13(3):158–162

[14] Myers TG, Cui Q, Kuskowski M, Mihalko WM, Saleh KJ. Outcomes of total and unicompartmental knee arthroplasty for secondary and spontaneous osteonecrosis of the knee. J Bone Joint Surg Am. 2006; 88 Suppl 3:76–82

[15] Jamison DE, Cohen SP. Radiofrequency techniques to treat chronic knee pain: a comprehensive review of anatomy, effectiveness, treatment parameters, and patient selection. J Pain Res. 2018; 11:1879–1888

35 Nerve Ablations II—Intercostal Neuralgia

Kody Kleinrichert and James Morrison

35.1 Case Presentation

A 36-year-old woman with stage IV metastatic breast cancer was referred to palliative medicine for chest wall pain related to dermal invasion and ulceration. The initial diagnosis was invasive mammary carcinoma with metastatic disease to the liver and spine. She was treated with neoadjuvant chemotherapy, total mastectomy with lymph node dissection, and radiation therapy. At the time of mastectomy, positron emission tomography (PET) scan demonstrated no active residual disease in the breast or axilla; however, on histologic examination there was lymphovascular invasion with skin lesions. A skin rash developed along the right chest wall after completion of radiation therapy which was found to be residual/recurrent disease via punch biopsy. Repeat imaging (PET) around the time of presentation demonstrated radiopharmaceutical uptake in the right chest wall (▶ Fig. 35.1). Despite continued chemotherapy, the skin lesions enlarged and ulcerated with weeping bloody drainage (▶ Fig. 35.2).

At the time of presentation, physical examination demonstrated a right chest wall ulcer measuring 10.8 × 31 × 0.8 cm, with thick fibrinous slough covering the base. Her primary complaint was pain from this skin and chest wall lesion, described as both constant burning and stabbing pain (6/10) in the area. The pain was aggravated by activity, and was worse during daily dressing changes. At best her pain level was 2/10. Taking deep breaths raised the pain to 5/10, and dressing changes resulted in 10/10 pain. She was taking Morphine SR (30 mg twice daily) with Morphine IR (15 mg every 4 hours as needed and 45 minutes before dressing changes) for breakthrough pain. Ketamine spray was also applied to the wound with dressing changes. Despite this aggressive drug regimen, she continued to have ongoing uncontrolled pain along the right chest wall and axilla. Palliative care referred the patient to interventional radiology for adjunctive pain management.

A plan of care discussed with the patient included initial nerve block of the anticipated treatment area in order to confirm adequate pain relief and coverage. If the nerve block was successful, it was to be followed by cryoablation of the same nerves. Distribution of skin lesions and pain followed the 6th to 10th intercostal dermatomes. Intercostal nerve blocks were performed using a combination of ultrasound and fluoroscopic guidance at the target levels. These procedures were performed as an outpatient procedure under moderate sedation. Using ultrasound guidance, a 22-gauge spinal needle was directed toward the inferior margin of the rib at each target level (▶ Fig. 35.3a). After bone contact, the needle was repositioned inferiorly into the intercostal groove. Placement was confirmed with injection of a small amount of contrast material, looking for linear distribution along the nerve sheath (▶ Fig. 35.3b). Once appropriate placement was confirmed, 1 mL of 40 mg/mL Depo-Medrol mixed with 5 mL 0.5% bupivacaine was injected at each level. The patient had immediate relief of pain from these nerve blocks. The pain relief was sustained for approximately 4 weeks, after which it began to return to baseline. At that point, it was decided to proceed with cryoablation.

General anesthesia was administered during the cryoablation procedure. The patient was placed prone on the computed tomography (CT) table. An initial scan was performed with gridlines to identify the target levels. Local anesthesia was achieved with 0.1% lidocaine. Ultrasound was again used to provide guidance for needle placement. The cryoablation probe was advanced under ultrasound guidance to the intercostal to the intercostal groove, positioning was confirmed with CT, and

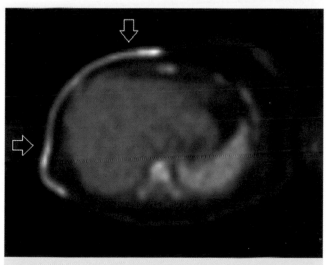

Fig. 35.1 Positron emission tomography–computed tomography (PET/CT) showing fluorodeoxyglucose (FDG)-avid disease in the right chest wall (arrows).

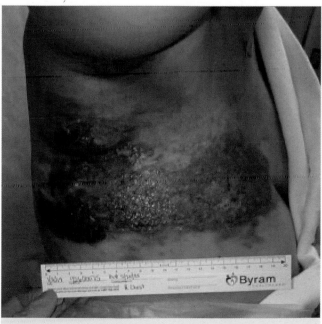

Fig. 35.2 Malignant skin ulceration.

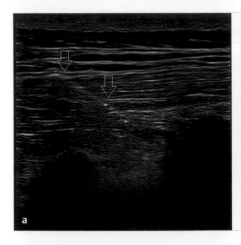

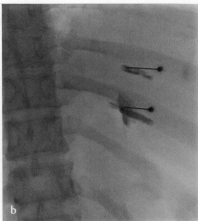

Fig. 35.3 (a) Ultrasound imaging is useful for needle placement (arrows) directed at the intercostal groove along the inferior rib. (b) Fluoroscopic image of the lower intercostal levels demonstrating linear spread of contrast along the nerve tract and a small amount of extravasation at the lower needle.

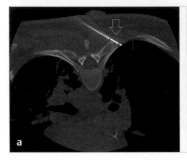

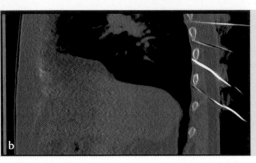

Fig. 35.4 (a) Axial computed tomography (CT) image showing probe placement (arrow) along the undersurface of the proximal rib. (b) Sagittal CT image demonstrating needle placement at four adjacent levels.

ablation was initiated. Ablation was performed in a serial fashion such that as freezing was initiated with the first needle, the second needle was being placed, etc. Each location underwent two 8 minutes freeze cycles, separated by a 5 minutes passive thaw. Short shaft needles were utilized given the short path through the tissue (▶ Fig. 35.4).

After recovery from anesthesia, the patient reported resolution of pain. She was discharged home the same day. After 4 months of treatment she reported new pain along the inferior margin of the previous treatment zone corresponding to expansion of her dermal disease. Nerve block with steroids and local anesthetic was again performed, this time at the 9th and 10th intercostal levels, which provided sufficient coverage and pain relief. Cryoablation followed 2 weeks after nerve block when the pain returned.

35.2 Companion Case

A 75-year-old man with small cell lung carcinoma was treated with radiation therapy and chemotherapy. The patient experienced a prolonged bout of shingles with postherpetic neuralgia lasting over one year. Radiation therapy is a risk factor for herpes zoster reactivation. An initial nerve block lasted for only approximately 12 hours before return of pain. Cryoablation at the same level was performed for prolonged pain relief with excellent results.

35.3 Discussion

Thoracic wall pain from intercostal neuralgia can be a significant source of morbidity related to both pain and functional

limitations with deep breathing or cough. These functional limitations can further lead to serious complications, including postoperative atelectasis, decreased sputum clearance, pneumonia, prolonged intubation, and respiratory failure. Given the morbidity associated with intercostal neuralgia, various modalities aimed at achieving adequate analgesia have been evaluated over the years.

Analgesic drugs, particularly opioids, can be used to provide some relief from intercostal neuralgia. Opioids, however, typically result in central nervous system and respiratory depression when administered in ample doses. This, coupled with their potential for dependence, makes them a poor candidate for long-term management of intercostal neuralgia.

Another option for pain control in this population is an intercostal nerve block. Intercostal blocks with local anesthetic, while effective, are typically short-acting and need to be frequently repeated by trained personnel. Longer-acting agents such as Efocaine and phenol have been studied for use in prolonged intercostal nerve blocks. Unfortunately, the use of these agents has resulted in severe complications, including paralysis and death due to spinal neurolysis and local tissue destruction following injection.[1,2]

Historically, surgical nerve transection has been performed in an attempt to provide analgesia for patients with intercostal neuralgia. Although surgical nerve transection alone provides denervation of the intercostal distribution, it has been long shown to result in painful neuroma formation. Despite this, some authors suggest that intercostal neurectomy with proximal nerve implantation into the latissimus dorsi may be a curative treatment for intercostal neuralgia. This prevents neuroma formation and may permanently decrease pain from intercostal

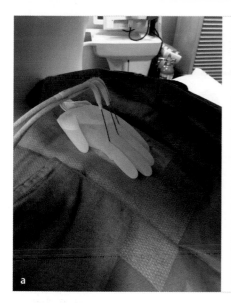
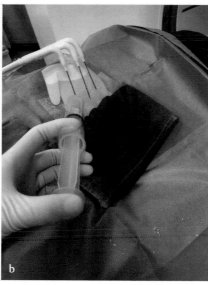

Fig. 35.5 (a) Sterile glove filled with warm saline and positioned around each of the cryoprobes. (b) Warm saline injected continuously over the probes and skin around the cryoprobes entry site.

neuralgia.[3] Nevertheless, this surgical approach is invasive, complex, and has demonstrated mixed results with some studies showing no improvement in pain postoperatively.[4]

Intercostal nerve cryoablation is a technique shown to provide effective short- and long-term pain control for intercostal neuralgia. It was first described in 1974 by Nelson et al, who demonstrated a reduction in analgesia use after thoracotomy when intraoperative intercostal nerve cryoablation was employed.[5] In 1976, Lloyd et al demonstrated its efficacy in the treatment of preexisting intractable pain.[6] Multiple studies during the 1970s and 1980s continued to describe the effectiveness of intercostal cryoablation, especially in the setting of postthoracotomy pain syndrome. Despite its efficacy, it was largely abandoned due to the high risk of complications, in part believed to be due to the use of landmark guidance only. However, in the 1990s, advances in imaging technology resulted in the reemergence of intercostal cryoablation.[7] The use of ultrasound or CT guidance resulted in a significant reduction in procedural complications due to the ability to verify needle placement, monitor for hemothorax or pneumothorax, and visualize ice-ball formation.[8] Continued studies have demonstrated the effective use of cryoablation for intercostal neuralgia of multiple etiologies.

Intercostal cryoablation can be performed as a minimally invasive procedure under local anesthesia or moderate sedation. Benefits include direct visualization of the ablation zone and minimal pain both during and after the procedure. It also carries a reduced risk of neuroma formation compared to surgical techniques, as it does not result in disruption of the acellular epineurium or perineurium. Unfortunately, for this same reason, nerve regeneration following cryoablation is possible, and if it occurs pain generally returns.[7] Nevertheless, intercostal cryoablation is not without risk. General risks include infection, postprocedural pain, bleeding from intercostal vessels, hemothorax, pneumothorax, skin hyper-/hypopigmentation, and frostbite if performed too superficially. Frostbite can be avoided by skin warming and continuous warm liquid irrigation (► Fig. 35.5). Although the risk is relatively low compared to other treatments, there are some reports of neuroma formation following cryoablation. Absolute contraindications to cryoablation include severe coagulopathy and superficial infection at the proposed site of ablation.[9]

Image-guided thermal radiofrequency ablation has been reported in recent studies to have utility in the treatment of intercostal neuralgia refractory to traditional treatments. By using heat generated from an alternating radiocurrent, this modality induces cell death via coagulation necrosis. This provides more definitive pain control than the traditional surgical approaches previously discussed. However, patients who undergo radiofrequency ablation are at higher risk for neuroma formation and increased postprocedural pain compared to cryoablation.[10]

References

[1] Angerer AL, Su HH, Head JR. Death following the use of efocaine; report of a case. J Am Med Assoc. 1953; 153(6):550–551

[2] Gollapalli L, Muppuri R. Paraplegia after intercostal neurolysis with phenol. J Pain Res. 2014; 7:665–668

[3] Williams EH, Williams CG, Rosson GD, Heitmiller RF, Dellon AL. Neurectomy for treatment of intercostal neuralgia. Ann Thorac Surg. 2008; 85(5):1766–1770

[4] Koryllos A, Althaus A, Poels M, et al. Impact of intercostal paravertebral neurectomy on post thoracotomy pain syndrome after thoracotomy in lung cancer patients: a randomized controlled trial. J Thorac Dis. 2016; 8 (9):2427–2433

[5] Nelson KM, Vincent RG, Bourke RS, et al. Intraoperative intercostal nerve freezing to prevent postthoracotomy pain. Ann Thorac Surg. 1974; 18(3): 280–285

[6] Lloyd JW, Barnard JDW, Glynn CJ. Cryoanalgesia. A new approach to pain relief. Lancet. 1976; 2(7992):932–934

[7] Bittman RW, Peters GL, Newsome JM, et al. Percutaneous image-guided cryoneurolysis. AJR Am J Roentgenol. 2018; 210(2):454–465

[8] Koethe Y, Mannes AJ, Wood BJ. Image-guided nerve cryoablation for post-thoracotomy pain syndrome. Cardiovasc Intervent Radiol. 2014; 37(3): 843–846

[9] Law L, Rayi A, Derian A. Cryoanalgesia. [Updated 2022 Aug 22]. In: StatPearls [Internet]. Treasure Island (FL): StatPearls Publishing; 2022 Jan. Available from: https://www.ncbi.nlm.nih.gov/books/NBK482123/. Accessed December 2022.

[10] Abd-Elsayed A, Lee S, Jackson M. Radiofrequency ablation for treating resistant intercostal neuralgia. Ochsner J. 2018; 18(1):91–93

36 Genicular Artery Embolization

Alexandra K. Banathy, Daniel P. Sheeran, and Luke R. Wilkins

36.1 Case Presentation

A 56-year-old man with past medical history of obesity, hypertension, and hyperlipidemia presented to his primary care physician with right knee pain. He rated the pain as 7 out of 10, and it has slowly worsened over many years. He complained of morning stiffness and pain while walking and using the stairs. He also had difficulty getting in and out of the car and was unable to continue his lifelong hobby of gardening. His WOMAC (Western Ontario and McMaster Universities Osteoarthritis Index) score was 26 out of 68. On physical examination, he had tenderness along the lateral right knee joint. Ligament testing was normal.

Weight-bearing knee radiograph demonstrated Kellgren-Lawrence Grade 2 osteoarthritis (▶ Fig. 36.1a). He had trialed nonsteroidal anti-inflammatory drugs (NSAIDs), physical therapy, and intra-articular corticosteroid injections over the previous year without relief. Radiographic findings and symptoms were not severe enough to warrant total knee arthroplasty, and the patient was not interested in a major surgery that would limit his activities. He was referred to interventional radiology to discuss a minimally invasive intervention for symptomatic relief of osteoarthritis, and was counseled regarding genicular artery embolization (GAE).

For the procedure, the left common femoral artery was accessed under ultrasound guidance. A 5-Fr sheath was placed and a catheter advanced to the right common femoral artery. Multistation arteriogram of the right lower extremity was performed. Hyperemia in the lateral compartment was identified as predominantly arising from the inferolateral genicular artery

(▶ Fig. 36.1b). A microcatheter was used to select the inferolateral genicular artery and embolization performed until stasis using 75uM Embozene microspheres (CeloNova BioSciences Inc., San Antonio, TX) (▶ Fig. 36.1c, d).

At 1-month follow-up appointment, the patient said that his pain had significantly improved. He rated it as 2 to 3 out of 10 and now only takes ibuprofen two to three times a month compared to five to six times a week prior to the procedure. He was able to return to his normal activities including gardening without pain. His WOMAC score was 6. On physical examination, there was splotchy purple-blue discoloration along the lateral knee, and motor and sensory examination was normal. The discoloration resolved at 2-month follow-up and the patient experienced continued clinical benefit

36.2 Discussion

Osteoarthritis is the most common form of arthritis and significantly affects the quality of life of ageing adults.[1] The cardinal symptoms are joint pain, stiffness, and physical limitations on activities of daily living. Symptoms can be clinically quantified with scoring scales such as the WOMAC and Knee Injury and Osteoarthritis Outcome Score (KOOS).[1,2,3] Radiographic evidence of knee osteoarthritis is commonly graded based on the Kellgren-Lawrence scale, which was first developed in 1957. The scale is based on the severity of osteophyte formation and joint space narrowing, the findings of which are summarized in ▶ Fig. 36.2.[4] According to recent epidemiologic studies, radiographic evidence of knee osteoarthritis is present in 37% of adults over the age of 60.[5] However, multiple studies have

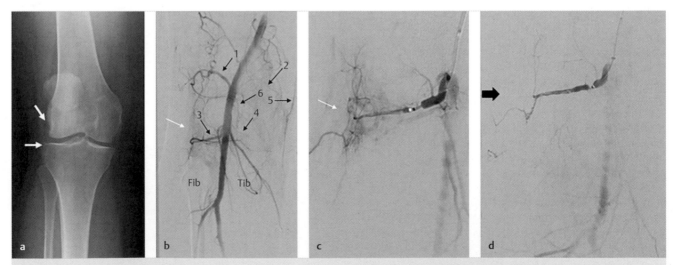

Fig. 36.1 Genicular artery embolization in a patient with mild osteoarthritis. (**a**) Standing anteroposterior (AP) radiograph of the right knee demonstrates Kellgren-Lawrence Grade 2 osteoarthritis with mild narrowing of the lateral compartment and osteophytes (thick white arrows). (**b**) Arteriogram of the popliteal artery demonstrates genicular artery anatomy (black arrows). 1, superolateral genicular artery; 2, superomedial genicular artery; 3, inferolateral genicular artery; 4, inferomedial genicular artery; 5, descending genicular artery; 6, middle genicular artery. There is hyperemia arising from the inferolateral genicular artery (white arrow). (**c**) Selective catheterization of the inferolateral genicular artery confirms neovessel proliferation (white arrow). (**d**) Postembolization arteriogram of the inferolateral genicular artery demonstrating devascularization (thick black arrow).

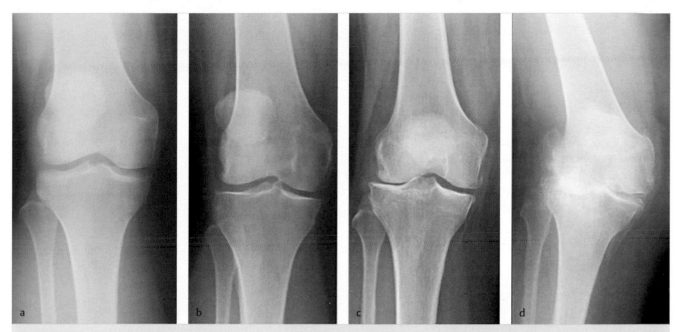

Fig. 36.2 Kellgren-Lawrence radiographic grading of osteoarthritis. (a) Grade 1: Doubtful narrowing of joint space and possible osteophytic lipping. (b) Grade 2: Definite osteophytes and possible narrowing of joint space. (c) Grade 3: Moderate multiple osteophytes, definite narrowing of joint space, some sclerosis, and possible deformity of bony ends. (d) Grade 4: Large osteophytes, marked narrowing of joint space, severe sclerosis, and definite deformity of bone ends.

demonstrated poor association between radiographic knee osteoarthritis and clinically symptomatic knee osteoarthritis.[6,7,8] This suggests that factors other than radiographic findings regarding the joint space contribute to pain and disability in osteoarthritis.

Osteoarthritis-related pain may be associated with abnormal new blood vessel formation (neovessels) and low-grade inflammation in the periarticular soft tissues including the synovium, infrapatellar fat pad, periosteum, and joint capsule.[9,10] The hypothesized pathophysiology is that vascular endothelial growth factor (VEGF) and inflammatory cytokines promote abnormal neovessel formation, which provides inflammatory cells access to the joint tissues where they can produce bone and cartilage destruction.[11] The osteochondral junction and the synovium have been implicated as the earliest sites of neovessel formation.[9,10,12] This is supported by histologic and magnetic resonance imaging (MRI) studies identifying the presence of low-grade synovitis in osteoarthritis patients.[13,14] In addition, angiogenesis is associated with perivascular sensory nerve fiber growth. Since cartilage does not contain sensory fibers, new nerve growth into the synovium may contribute to pain in osteoarthritis.[10,15,16]

GAE was developed based on the theory that permanent embolization of abnormal synovial neovessels might decrease inflammation and neuropathic pain in osteoarthritis.[17,18,19]

GAE has been safely used to treat spontaneous hemarthrosis after knee arthroplasty with clinical success, but GAE has just recently been used clinically for osteoarthritis.[20,21] The most common cause of hemarthrosis after knee arthroplasty is repetitive microtrauma to a hypertrophic vascular synovium, which is targeted for devascularization with GAE (▶ Fig. 36.3).[21]

Initial prospective studies for treatment of osteoarthritis with GAE were performed by Okuno et al in symptomatic patients with Kellgren-Lawrence Grade 1–3 osteoarthritis who failed conservative management. In a study of 72 patients, GAE improved clinical symptoms based on the WOMAC score in 80% of patients at 3 years post-procedure. They also found a statistically significant improvement in MRI-graded synovitis 2 years post-procedure, further implicating synovitis as a significant contributor to osteoarthritis.[17,18]

Knee arthroplasty is the definitive treatment for severe knee osteoarthritis that has failed conservative management and significantly affects the patient's quality of life.[22] However, there are few treatment options for patients with mild to moderate osteoarthritis resistant to conservative therapies or patients who are not surgical candidates. Evidence-based conservative treatments for osteoarthritis include topical and oral NSAIDs, intraarticular steroid injections, capsaicin cream, weight loss, and exercise. Although there is no evidence for opioid usage, 16% of patients are prescribed opioids for osteoarthritis-related pain.[23] GAE is a minimally invasive therapy that may provide symptomatic relief for this population of patients.

The procedure is typically performed through a common femoral artery access, followed by arteriography of the affected lower extremity. The primary blood supply to the knee joint is a network of arteries arising from the popliteal artery including the superolateral genicular, superomedial genicular, inferolateral genicular, inferomedial genicular, middle genicular, and descending genicular arteries, in addition to the anterior tibial recurrent artery (▶ Fig. 36.4). Genicular arteriogram is performed to identify branch arteries with associated hyperemia, which appears similar to a "blush" (▶ Fig. 36.1b). The normal arteriogram in ▶ Fig. 36.4 can be contrasted with the abnormal arteriogram performed on a patient with osteoarthritis in ▶ Fig. 36.1b, which demonstrates significantly more neovessels. The distribution of knee pain on preprocedure examination and

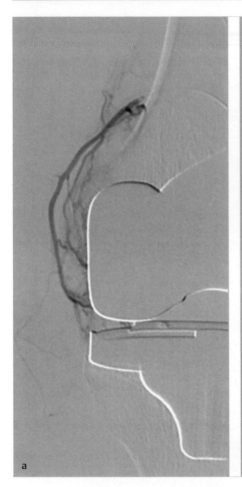

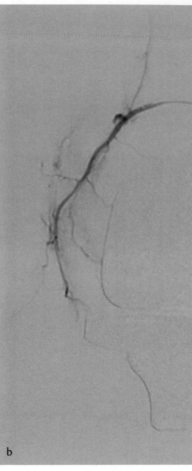

Fig. 36.3 Genicular artery embolization for post-arthroplasty recurrent spontaneous hemarthrosis. (**a**) Selective catheterization and arteriogram of the superomedial genicular artery demonstrates neovessel proliferation and hyperemia. Embolization of the hyperemic superomedial genicular artery was performed with Embozene microscopheres. (**b**) Postembolization arteriogram demonstrates improvement of the hyperemic "blush" and pruning of neovessels.

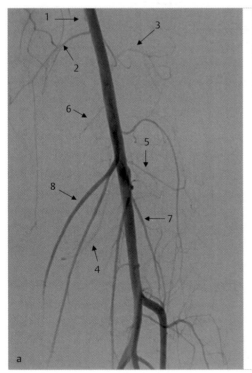

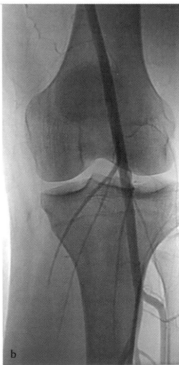

Fig. 36.4 Arteriogram of a normal patient demonstrating genicular artery anatomy. (**a**) Digital subtraction angiography of the popliteal artery (black arrows). 1, popliteal artery; 2, superomedial genicular artery; 3, superolateral genicular artery; 4, inferomedial genicular artery; 5, inferolateral genicular artery; 6, middle genicular artery; 7, anterior tibial recurrent artery; 8, cutaneous branch of the popliteal artery. (**b**) Unsubtracted angiogram for anatomic correlation.

angiographically demonstrated hyperemia directs the selection of the target vessel for embolization. Imipenem/cilastatin sodium particles or Embozene 75-μm particles are the most frequently used embolic agents. The embolic agent is given in increments until there is stasis in the abnormal neovessels.[17,18,19] Patients may feel pain or a tingling sensation in the region of embolization during the procedure, and many report an initial immediate decrease in pain followed by a sustained response weeks later. Okuno et al reported no major complications and no ischemic complications on follow-up MRI. Minor complications include puncture site hematoma and transient purple-blue cutaneous discoloration in the treated region, more commonly noted in patients treated with Embozene.[17,18] A second embolization can be considered for insufficient treatment response or pain recurrence.

At the time of this writing, there are no results of large randomized controlled trials evaluating GAE, although there is a double-blinded randomized controlled placebo trial in process.[19] Although initial studies are encouraging, more research is needed to establish the cellular effects of embolization on the knee joint soft tissues as well as the efficacy, safety, and role of GAE on a larger scale in order for the therapy to become an accepted minimally invasive therapy in knee osteoarthritis.

References

[1] Neogi T. The epidemiology and impact of pain in osteoarthritis. Osteoarthritis Cartilage. 2013; 21(9):1145–1153

[2] Roos EM, Toksvig-Larsen S. Knee injury and Osteoarthritis Outcome Score (KOOS)—validation and comparison to the WOMAC in total knee replacement. Health Qual Life Outcomes. 2003; 1:17

[3] Bellamy N, Kirwan J, Boers M, et al. Recommendations for a core set of outcome measures for future phase III clinical trials in knee, hip, and hand osteoarthritis. Consensus development at OMERACT III. J Rheumatol. 1997; 24(4):799–802

[4] Kellgren JH, Lawrence JS. Radiological assessment of osteo-arthrosis. Ann Rheum Dis. 1957; 16(4):494–502

[5] Lawrence RC, Felson DT, Helmick CG, et al. National Arthritis Data Workgroup. Estimates of the prevalence of arthritis and other rheumatic conditions in the United States. Part II. Arthritis Rheum. 2008; 58(1):26–35

[6] Hannan MT, Felson DT, Pincus T. Analysis of the discordance between radiographic changes and knee pain in osteoarthritis of the knee. J Rheumatol. 2000; 27(6):1513–1517

[7] Felson DT. The epidemiology of knee osteoarthritis: results from the Framingham Osteoarthritis Study. Semin Arthritis Rheum. 1990; 20(3) Suppl 1:42–50

[8] Pereira D, Severo M, Santos RA, et al. Knee and hip radiographic osteoarthritis features: differences on pain, function and quality of life. Clin Rheumatol. 2016; 35(6):1555–1564

[9] Ashraf S, Mapp PI, Walsh DA. Contributions of angiogenesis to inflammation, joint damage, and pain in a rat model of osteoarthritis. Arthritis Rheum. 2011; 63(9):2700–2710

[10] Mapp PI, Walsh DA. Mechanisms and targets of angiogenesis and nerve growth in osteoarthritis. Nat Rev Rheumatol. 2012; 8(7):390–398

[11] Pap T, Distler O. Linking angiogenesis to bone destruction in arthritis. Arthritis Rheum. 2005; 52(5):1346–1348

[12] Suri S, Gill SE, Massena de Camin S, Wilson D, McWilliams DF, Walsh DA. Neurovascular invasion at the osteochondral junction and in osteophytes in osteoarthritis. Ann Rheum Dis. 2007; 66(11):1423–1428

[13] Haywood L, McWilliams DF, Pearson CI, et al. Inflammation and angiogenesis in osteoarthritis. Arthritis Rheum. 2003; 48(8):2173–2177

[14] Roemer FW, Kassim Javaid M, Guermazi A, et al. Anatomical distribution of synovitis in knee osteoarthritis and its association with joint effusion assessed on non-enhanced and contrast-enhanced MRI. Osteoarthritis Cartilage. 2010; 18(10):1269–1274

[15] Ashraf S, Wibberley H, Mapp PI, Hill R, Wilson D, Walsh DA. Increased vascular penetration and nerve growth in the meniscus: a potential source of pain in osteoarthritis. Ann Rheum Dis. 2011; 70(3):523–529

[16] Walsh DA, Bonnet CS, Turner EL, Wilson D, Situ M, McWilliams DF. Angiogenesis in the synovium and at the osteochondral junction in osteoarthritis. Osteoarthritis Cartilage. 2007; 15(7):743–751

[17] Okuno Y, Korchi AM, Shinjo T, Kato S. Transcatheter arterial embolization as a treatment for medial knee pain in patients with mild to moderate osteoarthritis. Cardiovasc Intervent Radiol. 2015; 38(2):336–343

[18] Okuno Y, Korchi AM, Shinjo T, Kato S, Kaneko T. Midterm clinical outcomes and MR imaging changes after transcatheter arterial embolization as a treatment for mild to moderate radiographic knee osteoarthritis resistant to conservative treatment. J Vasc Interv Radiol. 2017; 28(7):995–1002

[19] Landers S, Hely A, Harrison B, et al. Protocol for a single-centre, parallel-arm, randomised controlled superiority trial evaluating the effects of transcatheter arterial embolisation of abnormal knee neovasculature on pain, function and quality of life in people with knee osteoarthritis. BMJ Open. 2017; 7(5):e014266

[20] van Baardewijk LJ, Hoogeveen YL, van der Geest ICM, Schultze Kool LJ. Embolization of the geniculate arteries is an effective treatment of recurrent hemarthrosis following total knee arthroplasty that can be safely repeated. J Arthroplasty. 2018; 33(4):1177–1180.e1

[21] Luyckx EGR, Mondelaers AMP, van der Zijden T, Voormolen MHJ, Van den Bergh FRA, d'Archambeau OC. Geniculate artery embolization in patients with recurrent hemarthrosis after knee arthroplasty: a retrospective study. J Arthroplasty. 2020; 35(2):550–556

[22] Dieppe P, Basler HD, Chard J, et al. Knee replacement surgery for osteoarthritis: effectiveness, practice variations, indications and possible determinants of utilization. Rheumatology (Oxford). 1999; 38(1):73–83

[23] DeMik DE, Bedard NA, Dowdle SB, Burnett RA, McHugh MA, Callaghan JJ. Are we still prescribing opioids for osteoarthritis? J Arthroplasty. 2017; 32(12):3578–3582.e1

37 Osteoid Osteoma I

Venkata Macha, A. Michael Devane, and Andrew J. Gunn

37.1 Case Presentation

A 3-year-old girl initially presented to the pediatric orthopedics clinic with a chief complaint of limping and left thigh pain. The patient and her parents reported several months of mild-to-moderate left thigh pain associated with alterations in gait. The patient primarily experienced the pain at night. There was no history of trauma or constitutional symptoms. The remainder of the patient's medical, family, and social histories were otherwise normal. Physical examination revealed normal vital signs, a healthy-appearing female child, and a limp gait. Laboratory values included normal C-reactive protein (CRP; < 0.5 mg/dL) and sedimentation rate (6 mm/h). Radiographs of the left leg were obtained (▶ Fig. 37.1a, b), which did not reveal an abnormality. Subsequently, an unenhanced magnetic resonance imaging (MRI) study of the left hip and thigh demonstrated an osteoid osteoma along the proximal portion of the anterior femur (▶ Fig. 37.1c, d). The patient was referred to interventional radiology for consultation for percutaneous ablation. No significant changes in the patient's history were noted at the time of the consultation, and after obtaining informed consent the

patient was scheduled for radiofrequency ablation (RFA) of her osteoid osteoma.

General anesthesia was used in this young child, and a weight-based dose of cefazolin was administered. Preprocedural computed tomography (CT) study demonstrated the osteoid osteoma and appropriate percutaneous access was planned (▶ Fig. 37.2a). After local anesthesia, a bone biopsy device (Bonopty®; AprioMed; Uppsala, Sweden) was advanced into the lesion under CT fluoroscopic guidance. Once in position, operators obtained a biopsy sample for surgical pathology. An 11-G needle was inserted through the trocar needle to create space for the RFA probe. After removal of the 11-G needle, the RFA probe (Cool-tip™; Medtronic; Minneapolis, MN) was inserted through the trocar; then ablation was performed using a 7-mm tip which was exposed for 6 minutes and 30 seconds (▶ Fig. 37.2b, c). Of note, Cool-tip™ is a bipolar RFA probe; hence, grounding pads are unnecessary. A postprocedure scan demonstrated no immediate complication (▶ Fig. 37.2d), and a sterile dressing was applied. Surgical pathology confirmed the lesion to be an osteoid osteoma.

After the procedure, the patient was admitted for overnight observation, as is routine at the authors' institution for pediatric

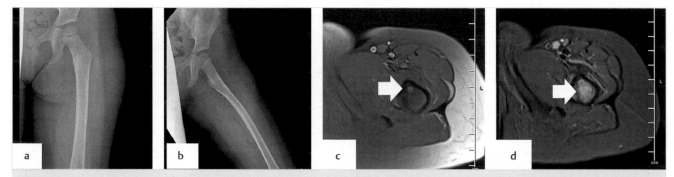

Fig. 37.1 Osteoid osteoma in a 3-year-old girl. Anteroposterior (AP) (**a**) and frog leg (**b**) radiographs of the left femur do not show a definite abnormality. (**c**) Axial, T1-weighted magnetic resonance imaging (MRI) of the upper left thigh demonstrates a small, focal, T1 hyperintense focus in the anterior femur (arrow). (**d**) Axial short tau inversion recovery (STIR) MRI of the upper left thigh demonstrates T2 hyperintensity in the adjacent bone (arrow), consistent with edema.

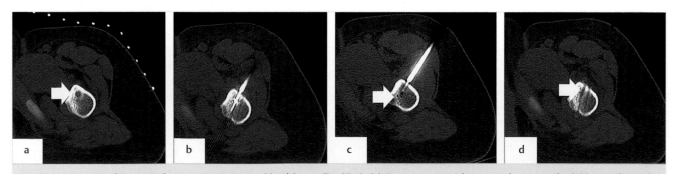

Fig. 37.2 Treatment of an osteoid osteoma in a 3-year-old girl (see ▶ Fig. 37.1). (**a**) Pretreatment axial computed tomography (CT) scan shows the osteoid osteoma in the anterior upper left thigh (arrow). A localizing grid is on top of the patient's skin. (**b**) Axial CT obtained during the procedure shows the ablation needle within the lesion. (**c**) Axial CT shows small gas bubbles in the bone (white arrow) during ablation. (**d**) Axial CT obtained immediately after the procedure shows the course of the ablation needle in the bone (arrow). An area of prior needle placement is seen immediately lateral to the treatment tract. The needle was repositioned from this area before treatment.

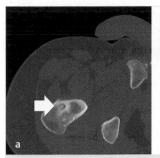 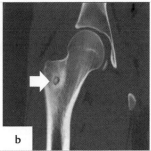 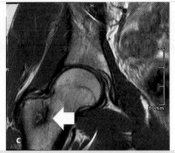 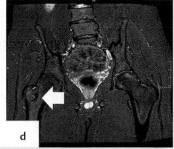

Fig. 37.3 Osteoid osteoma in a 17-year-old male. (**a**) Axial computed tomography (CT) of the right thigh demonstrates a radiolucent nidus with a dense central focus surrounded by reactive cortical bone (arrow). (**b**) Coronal reformat CT of the upper right thigh shows the characteristic finding of an osteoid osteoma (arrow). (**c**) Coronal, T1-weighted magnetic resonance imaging (MRI) of the right hip demonstrates hypointensity associated with the reactive cortical bone and central focus of the nidus (arrow). The remainder of the nidus is T1 isointense. (**d**) Coronal short tau inversion recovery (STIR) image of the pelvis demonstrates T2 hyperintensity surrounding the osteoid osteoma (arrow).

patients. Her stay was uneventful, and she was discharged the following morning with minimal soreness at the ablation site. At 1-month follow-up, the patient's parents were happy to report that the patient's limp disappeared almost immediately following the procedure, and she no longer had pain or a limp. She returned to full activity within a few days after the procedure and experienced no postprocedure complications. The patient has now been without complaint for more than a year.

37.2 Discussion

Osteoid osteomas represent approximately 12% of all benign skeletal neoplasms.[1] Although they can present later in life, osteoid osteomas usually present at a young age, with approximately half of cases being discovered in patients between the ages of 10 to 20.[2] Males are nearly four times as likely as females to be diagnosed with an osteoid osteoma[3]; Caucasian patients also have a higher incidence when compared to the general population.[4] As in this case, patients classically present with a dull, chronic pain in the location of the osteoid osteoma that worsens at night but is relieved by aspirin. It is most commonly located in the long bones of the lower extremity (i.e., tibia, femur, and fibula) (approximately 50%), typically within the bony cortex in the region of the diaphysis or meta-diaphysis.[2] Outside of the lower extremities, osteoid osteomas are most often found in the foot, hand, or spine.[2] In the spine, they are a well-recognized cause of painful scoliosis in the adolescent population.[5] The ischium, patella, mandible, ribs, and skull are atypical locations.[2]

Osteoid osteomas contain distinct regions, which contribute to their radiographic appearance.

The outer reactive zone consists of thickened, woven, and lamellar bone, while the inner region contains a nidus composed of osteoid trabeculae with osteoblasts.[2] Radiographically, this is characterized by a lucent cortical nidus with sclerosis and thickening of the adjacent bony cortex (▶ Fig. 37.2b and ▶ Fig. 37.3a, b). CT demonstrates the nidus in more detail as a rounded or ovoid lucency containing a dense central focus, consisting of mineralized osteoid. MRI is less sensitive than CT in detecting the nidus, but better demonstrates associated marrow changes (▶ Fig. 37.1d and ▶ Fig. 37.3c, d).[6] The nidus has

heterogeneous, high T2 signal intensity with low to intermediate T1 signal on MRI.[7] Osteoid osteoma can also cause joint effusion, and marrow and soft tissue edema all depicted as increased T2 signal.[6] Tc99 bone scintigraphy can localize osteoid osteoma with near 100% sensitivity.[8] The appearance on bone scintigraphy has been described as the "double density" sign with focal uptake of radiotracer within the nidus and halo of activity in the surrounding bone.[9]

Osteoid osteomas express high levels of prostaglandins, particularly PGE2 and PGI2.[10] In fact, prostaglandins in the nidus are 100 to 1000 times greater than normal bone.[11,12] Due to this, patients often experience high blood pressure, tachycardia, and pain during the ablation itself. These symptoms are common and usually resolve as soon as the operator turns off the ablation probe. Regardless, this is useful information to share with the patient, procedure nurse, and/or anesthetist. Outside of the ablation procedure, prostaglandins can lead to increased vascular pressures that stimulate adjacent nerves, resulting in the perception of pain by the patient.[13,14]

37.3 Companion Case

A 17-year-old man presented to interventional radiology with a symptomatic osteoid osteoma in the inter-trochanteric region of the right femur (▶ Fig. 37.3). He had a history of chronic right thigh pain, worse at night, which had failed conservative therapy with nonsteroidal anti-inflammatory drugs (NSAIDs). After a thorough history, physical examination, and review of the patient's laboratory work and imaging, the patient and his parents consented for percutaneous ablation using general anesthesia on an outpatient basis.

On the day of the procedure, the patient was placed in the supine position, and a preprocedure CT scan revealed the osteoid osteoma in the anterior aspect of the proximal right femur (▶ Fig. 37.4). A weight-based dose of cefazolin was given. After identifying a safe percutaneous route, local anesthesia was administered. Utilizing CT fluoroscopy guidance, a 13-gauge Osteo-Site® needle (Cook Medical; Bloomington, IN) was inserted into the nidus of the osteoid osteoma. The inner stylus was removed. Next, a 17-gauge, 15-cm microwave antenna (Neuwave™; Madison, WI) was inserted through the coaxial

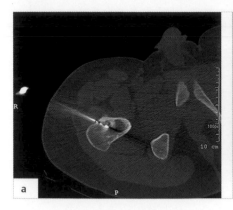
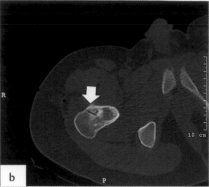

Fig. 37.4 Treatment of an osteoid osteoma in a 17-year-old male (see ▶ Fig. 37.3). (**a**) Axial computed tomography (CT) obtained during the procedure shows the ablation probe in the lesion. (**b**) Axial CT obtained immediately after the procedure shows the course of the ablation needle in the bone (arrow).

bone needle. The coaxial needle was retracted outside of the bone over the antenna to prevent thermal injury to the skin and soft tissues. Microwave ablation was performed at 30 Watts with a 2.45-GHz generator for 30 seconds alternating with a 30-second period of cooling. The total ablation time was 3 minutes. After removing all the needles, a sterile dressing was applied. The patient was discharged 2 hours after the procedure. On follow-up, the patient had near-immediate relief of symptoms and remains clinically well.

37.4 Discussion

The first-line therapy for osteoid osteomas consists of conservative medical therapy with NSAIDs.[10] In fact, some authors report that up to 75% of patients will respond to conservative therapy alone.[1,13] Medical therapy is therefore a viable option for many patients, especially in those who may be high-risk surgical candidates or who have lesions in difficult-to-ablate areas. For patients who do not respond to medical therapy, surgical resection was previously considered the standard of care.[15,16] However, surgical resection can be limited in its ability to identify the nidus, leading to recurrence of symptoms.[2,17,18,19,20] Additionally, the postsurgical recovery period is longer than that of ablation with a potentially higher rate of procedure-related complications. Recently, CT-guided mini-incision surgery has been proposed as a less invasive, more targeted surgical approach for osteoid osteomas.[21] In this procedure, CT imaging is used to help the surgeon localize the nidus, which lowers the amount of bone removed during the procedure and decreases the risks associated with excessive bone removal.

Image-guided percutaneous ablation of osteoid osteomas uses radiographs, CT, or MRI to help direct the interventional radiologist in placing an ablation probe directly into the lesion. Since its inception in the 1990s, percutaneous ablation has consistently demonstrated high levels of both efficacy and safety in osteoid osteoma ablation.[22,23,24,25,26,27] The use of imaging guidance to locate the nidus removes the uncertainty associated with surgical excision. Moreover, since the probes are placed percutaneously, the procedure is overall much less invasive than surgery. This results in lower rates of complications and shorter postprocedural hospital stays when compared to traditional surgical approaches. Adults typically tolerate the procedure using conscious sedation, thereby eliminating the risks associated with general anesthesia.

There are several ablation modalities available for clinical use. The most commonly employed technique for osteoid osteomas is RFA, which destroys adjacent tissue by using an alternating current that generates heat from the oscillation of nearby water molecules. Microwave ablation is a newer ablation technology that generates heat in a similar fashion to RFA, but can generate higher temperatures more rapidly.[28] There is less literature supporting its use in osteoid osteomas compared to RFA but the authors' institutional experiences with microwave ablation have shown promise. Cryoablation is an ablation modality that relies on the expansion of pressurized gas to generate lethal freezing temperatures in adjacent tissues. There are small case series showing its efficacy in osteoid osteomas.[29] Overall, image-guided ablation has replaced surgery as the primary therapeutic option for osteoid osteomas with near-immediate results when successful.

References

[1] Dahlin D, Unni K. Bone Tumors: General Aspects and Data on 8,542 Cases. 4th ed. Springfield, IL: Thomas; 1987:88–101. Available from: https://inis.iaea.org/search/search.aspx?orig_q=RN:19041134. Accessed January 21, 2020

[2] Kransdorf MJ, Stull MA, Gilkey FW, Moser RP, Jr. Osteoid osteoma. Radiographics. 1991; 11(4):671–696

[3] Athwal P, Stock H. Osteoid osteoma: a pictorial review. Conn Med. 2014; 78 (4):233–235

[4] Kendrick JI, Evarts CM. Osteoid-osteoma: a critical analysis of 40 tumors. Clin Orthop Relat Res. 1967; 54:51–59

[5] Pettine KA, Klassen RA. Osteoid-osteoma and osteoblastoma of the spine. J Bone Joint Surg Am. 1986; 68(3):354–361

[6] Chai JW, Hong SH, Choi JY, et al. Radiologic diagnosis of osteoid osteoma: from simple to challenging findings. Radiographics. 2010; 30(3):737–749

[7] Iyer RS, Chapman T, Chew FS. Pediatric bone imaging: diagnostic imaging of osteoid osteoma. AJR Am J Roentgenol. 2012; 198(5):1039–1052

[8] Sharma P, Mukherjee A, Karunanithi S, et al. 99mTc-methylene diphosphonate SPECT/CT as the one-stop imaging modality for the diagnosis of osteoid osteoma. Nucl Med Commun. 2014; 35(8):876–883

[9] Helms CA. Osteoid osteoma. The double density sign. Clin Orthop Relat Res. 1987(222):167–173

[10] Mungo DV, Zhang X, O'Keefe RJ, Rosier RN, Puzas JE, Schwarz EM. COX-1 and COX-2 expression in osteoid osteomas. J Orthop Res. 2002; 20(1):159–162

[11] Ciabattoni G, Tamburrelli F, Greco F. Increased prostacyclin biosynthesis in patients with osteoid osteoma. Eicosanoids. 1991; 4(3):165–167

[12] Makley JT, Dunn MJ. Prostaglandin synthesis by osteoid osteoma. Lancet. 1982; 2(8288):42

[13] Healey JH, Ghelman B. Osteoid osteoma and osteoblastoma. Current concepts and recent advances. Clin Orthop Relat Res. 1986(204):76–85

[14] Schulman L, Dorfman HD. Nerve fibers in osteoid osteoma. J Bone Joint Surg Am. 1970; 52(7):1351–1356

[15] Rosenthal DI, Hornicek FJ, Wolfe MW, Jennings LC, Gebhardt MC, Mankin HJ. Percutaneous radiofrequency coagulation of osteoid osteoma compared with operative treatment. J Bone Joint Surg Am. 1998; 80(6):815–821

[16] Papathanassiou ZG, Megas P, Petsas T, Papachristou DJ, Nilas J, Siablis D. Osteoid osteoma: diagnosis and treatment. Orthopedics. 2008; 31(11):1118

[17] Sim FH, Dahlin CD, Beabout JW. Osteoid-osteoma: diagnostic problems. J Bone Joint Surg Am. 1975; 57(2):154–159

[18] Swee RG, McLeod RA, Beabout JW. Osteoid osteoma. Detection, diagnosis, and localization. Radiology. 1979; 130(1):117–123

[19] Freiberger RH, Loitman BS, Helpern M, Thompson TC. Osteoid osteoma; a report on 80 cases. Am J Roentgenol Radium Ther Nucl Med. 1959; 82(2):194–205

[20] Norman A. Persistence or recurrence of pain: a sign of surgical failure is osteoid-osteoma. Clin Orthop Relat Res. 1978; 130(130):263–266

[21] Yang WT, Chen WM, Wang NH, Chen TH. Surgical treatment for osteoid osteoma—experience in both conventional open excision and CT-guided mini-incision surgery. J Chin Med Assoc. 2007; 70(12):545–550

[22] Tillotson CL, Rosenberg AE, Rosenthal DI. Controlled thermal injury of bone. Report of a percutaneous technique using radiofrequency electrode and generator. Invest Radiol. 1989; 24(11):888–892

[23] Rosenthal DI, Alexander A, Rosenberg AE, Springfield D. Ablation of osteoid osteomas with a percutaneously placed electrode: a new procedure. Radiology. 1992; 183(1):29–33

[24] Rosenthal DI, Hornicek FJ, Torriani M, Gebhardt MC, Mankin HJ. Osteoid osteoma: percutaneous treatment with radiofrequency energy. Radiology. 2003; 229(1):171–175

[25] Vanderschueren GM, Taminiau AHM, Obermann WR, Bloem JL. Osteoid osteoma: clinical results with thermocoagulation. Radiology. 2002; 224(1):82–86

[26] de Berg JC, Pattynama PMT, Obermann WR, Bode PJ, Vielvoye GJ, Taminiau AHM. Percutaneous computed-tomography-guided thermocoagulation for osteoid osteomas. Lancet. 1995; 346(8971):350–351

[27] Lindner NJ, Ozaki T, Roedl R, Gosheger G, Winkelmann W, Wörtler K. Percutaneous radiofrequency ablation in osteoid osteoma. J Bone Joint Surg Br. 2001; 83(3):391–396

[28] Skinner MG, Iizuka MN, Kolios MC, Sherar MD. A theoretical comparison of energy sources—microwave, ultrasound and laser—for interstitial thermal therapy. Phys Med Biol. 1998; 43(12):3535–3547

[29] Coupal TM, Mallinson PI, Munk PL, Liu D, Clarkson P, Ouellette H. CT-guided percutaneous cryoablation for osteoid osteoma: initial experience in adults. AJR Am J Roentgenol. 2014; 202(5):1136–1139

38 Osteoid Osteoma II: Pediatric Hip Pain

Will S. Lindquister and Anne Gill

38.1 Case Presentation

A 15-year-old boy presented to his pediatrician for chronic right hip pain that had been present for 6 months. The pediatrician believed the hip pain was related to overuse injury or sprain/strain in the anterior hip. Pelvic radiographs were ordered to evaluate for slipped capital femoral epiphysis but pelvic radiographs were negative. Recommendations were given for rest and physical therapy; neither therapy nor rest improved his pain. The patient was referred to an orthopedic surgeon who ordered a magnetic resonance imaging (MRI). The MRI findings were consistent with an osteoid osteoma (OO) at the right femoral neck (▶ Fig. 38.1).

The patient was referred to interventional radiology (IR) for biopsy and treatment of the OO. At the time of the IR clinic visit, the patient had experienced severe right hip pain for 1 year. On physical examination, the patient was unable to walk without a significant limp. He was extremely hesitant to bear full weight on the lower extremity and often used a single crutch. The hip pain was always worse at night, and he rated the pain as 8 out of 10. Often, the pain would wake him from sleep, and he would not be able to get relief until the morning. He tried nonsteroidal anti-inflammatory drugs (NSAIDs) for pain relief which worked early on in his course, but eventually the pain became too great and the NSAIDs were no longer helpful. The patient was scheduled for a percutaneous biopsy of the lesion, cryoablation, and postprocedure nerve block.

The procedure was performed under general anesthesia. Once the patient was anesthetized, he was positioned supine to allow access to the anterior lesion. Cone-beam computed tomography (CT) scan was performed of the right hip for planning (▶ Fig. 38.2).

The cone-beam CT images were reviewed and a percutaneous approach for targeting the lesion was chosen. Using a combination of cone-beam CT and fluoroscopy, the introducer needle was advanced to the cortex. A drill was used to cross the cortex with the introducer needle (OnControl Powered Bone Access System, Arrow-Teleflex, North Carolina). A 1- to 2-cm biopsy instrument was centered on the OO nidus, and a core biopsy specimen obtained. The biopsy not only confirmed the histologic diagnosis, but provided the tract through which the ablation probe was placed. The ablation probe was advanced through the introducer needle, and the position of the ablation probe was verified with a second cone-beam CT (▶ Fig. 38.3).

The OO was treated with two 10-minute freeze cycles; each freeze cycle was followed by a 5-minute active thaw. The probe was removed from the patient after the last thaw, and manual compression was used to obtain hemostasis. A nerve block was performed to anesthetize the anterior thigh compartment. In the postanesthesia recovery area, the patient had no pain in the right lower extremity, and he reported complete numbness. He was discharged home after 3 hours observation. He was only allowed to walk short distances for the first 3 weeks following the ablation, then was allowed to walk longer distances for

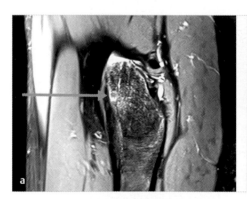
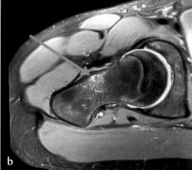

Fig. 38.1 (a) Sagittal view of the right femoral neck with an ovoid lesion (solid arrow) measuring 5.7 mm with low T2 signal in the center of the lesion and increased T2 signal around the lesion suggesting edema. (b) Axial view of the right femoral neck with redemonstration of the ovoid lesion and thickened cortex over the lesion (solid arrow).

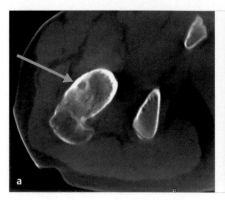
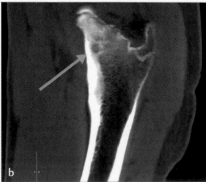

Fig. 38.2 (a) Axial cone-beam computed tomography (CT) image of the right femoral neck prior to needle localization. The osteoid osteoma is just beneath the thickened cortex (solid arrow) and the central portion of the lesion is lucent (darker) on CT. (b) Sagittal cone-beam CT reconstruction of the right proximal femur demonstrates the full cranial caudal extent of the lesion (solid arrow) as well as surrounding edema posterior to the lesion.

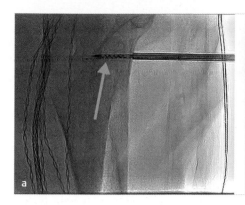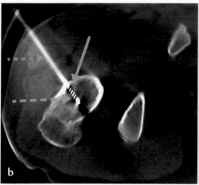

Fig. 38.3 (a) Fluoroscopic image of the ablation probe (solid arrow) crossing the osteoid osteoma while the introducer needle (dashed arrow) remains embedded in the cortex. (b) Axial cone-beam computed tomography (CT) with the introducer needle (dotted arrow) coursing through the muscle to the bony cortex. The osteoid osteoma (solid arrow) is completely covered by the ablation probe (dashed arrow).

weeks 4 to 6. Finally, he returned to full physical activity after week 6, at which point he reported no pain. At the 6-week post-procedure clinic visit, he reported the pain was completely resolved, and he was trying to go back to playing soccer. He was also working with a physical therapist to strengthen the right lower extremity so his limping will completely resolve.

38.2 Discussion

OO is a benign bone tumor, representing approximately 5% of all bone tumors.[1,2,3] With a male predilection, they usually present in the second decade of life.[1] OOs typically occur in the long bones, particularly in the lower extremities, but less frequently can occur in the axial skeleton. Although most OOs are extra-articular, some are intra-articular, most commonly involving the hip joint. The most frequent presenting symptom is dull nocturnal pain gradually increasing in intensity, which improves with NSAIDs.[1]

Imaging workup usually includes a radiograph, which demonstrates a central radiolucent intracortical nidus typically smaller than 2 cm surrounded by cortical thickening and periosteal reaction.[4,5] CT is typically diagnostic, demonstrating a well-defined low-attenuation nidus surrounding a smaller high-density focus representing mineralized osteoid.[1,4] Although MRI may be helpful in demonstrating the tumor's relationship to intra-articular structures and may better delineate associated marrow and soft tissue edema, synovitis, or joint effusions, it sometimes fails to show a small nidus and consequently can be misleading.[4,6,7] Therefore, CT is the imaging modality of choice for the diagnosis of OO.

The necessity of a biopsy prior to treatment is controversial. Some authors advocate this as an unnecessary step because of the high specificity of cross-sectional imaging in the diagnosis of OO and negative or inconclusive biopsy results in many cases.[1,2] Nevertheless, some lesions such as chronic nonbacterial osteomyelitis and osteoblastoma can mimic OOs on imaging.[8] Therefore, biopsy may have a role less in diagnosing of OO, but more in ruling out other pathology. This is particularly important as treatment (either surgery or ablation) changes the imaging appearance of the lesion and may confound subsequent evaluation. The lesions are therefore typically biopsied during the ablation procedure, following the introduction of the needle and immediately preceding the ablation.

First-line treatment for OO is medical management with NSAIDs. Studies have demonstrated that the natural history of

OO is spontaneous regression, with symptoms typically resolving between 6 to 15 years of age.[1,9,10] However, because of the severity of symptoms, this is frequently not a viable option for patients and may lead to long-term gait or other motor disturbances.

Historically, the definitive treatment for OO was en bloc resection, with removal of the entire nidus. Although recurrence rates following resection are reportedly low, the procedure can be morbid with a significant risk of subsequent fracture, sometimes requiring internal fixation or bone grafting.[1,11] Additionally, the patient's activity is restricted for a significant amount of time which can be particularly challenging in pediatric populations. Surgical excision of intra-articular lesions can be especially morbid, often requiring prophylactic internal fixation of the bone.[12]

For patients with chronic pain refractory to medical management, percutaneous ablation is the treatment of choice due to its high success rate, minimally invasive approach, and favorable side effect profile.[1] This procedure involves percutaneous placement of an ablation probe under CT guidance in the center of, or adjacent to, the tumor and using either rapid heating or freezing–thawing to treat the lesion.

Radiofrequency ablation (RFA) was the first ablation technology used for the treatment of OOs, originally described in the early 1990s.[11,13,14] RFA uses radiofrequency waves to induce coagulation necrosis of the tumor surrounding the probe. Many retrospective and prospective trials have been performed since the initial reports, with a systematic review reporting successful symptom resolution in 95% of patients treated with RFA.[15] Major complications are exceedingly rare, and minor complications are seen in 2% of patients, most commonly consisting of skin and muscle burns, soft tissue infections, broken bone drill, and superficial thrombophlebitis.[15]

Intra-articular lesions occur in approximately 13% of patients and present particular therapeutic challenges.[12,16] Although there are theoretical complications associated with the ablation of intra-articular lesions such as joint damage and injury to cartilage, studies have shown high success rates in treatment of intra-articular lesions with RFA.[12,17] Spinal OOs occur in approximately 10% of patients with OO.[2,3] Ablation of spinal OOs presents additional risk for nerve injury, especially in cases located close to nerve roots or the thecal sac. Studies have demonstrated similar high success and low complication rates with RFA of spinal OOs with only one reported episode of transient, self-resolving lower limb paresthesia.[18,19,20]

More recently, new ablation technologies have been used to treat OOs. Microwave ablation, first described for OO treatment in 2014, uses microwaves to rapidly heat tumors.[21,22] Microwave ablation enables larger ablation zones and is less affected by the type of tissue or tissue impedance than RFA.[23] Cryoablation, first described for the treatment of OOs in 2010, uses argon gas to freeze the tumor with a temperature below −40°C with cycles of rapid freezing and thawing, causing tissue necrosis.[24]

During cryoablation, a coaxial needle is directed into the OO nidus under imaging guidance using a cortical drill. This can be performed with either axial thin section CT, or on newer fluoroscopy units, cone-beam CT with navigational overlay. The process to target the lesion and obtain a biopsy is the same as described above in the case example. The number of probes as well as the number and length of freeze–thaw cycles depends on lesion size and location. This procedure can be performed either with sedation and analgesia, or, particularly in younger pediatric populations, with general anesthesia.

Several small retrospective studies have demonstrated high success and low complication rates with cryoablation of OOs. These studies report greater than 90% success with no major complications, results similar to RFA.[24,25,26,27,28,29,30] These findings are particularly salient, given the additional theoretical benefits of cryoablation over other ablation technologies, including decreased pain during and after the procedure that may limit the need for postprocedure pain medication. Additionally, the proceduralist can monitor the ablation zone by CT during the procedure. Recent studies have also suggested that cryoablation can promote an immune response to tumor cells outside the ablation zone, known as an abscopal effect, by causing the tissue necrosis without causing destruction of the intracellular contents.[31] Finally, there is evidence that nerves regenerate at a predictable rate when inadvertently (or intentionally) exposed to cryoablation, potentially rendering cryoablation a safer option for tumors in close proximity to nerves and the spinal cord.[32]

Long-term follow-up after ablation is important in this patient population. Although the clinical success rate of this procedure is greater than 90%, most failures are due to recurrent disease. Although most recurrences occur in the first few months following the initial ablation, some occur years later.[8,13,26,27] In many cases, a second ablation is successful in treating recurrent disease.[26] This highlights the importance of long-term clinical follow-up in this patient population.

References

[1] Noordin S, Allana S, Hilal K, et al. Osteoid osteoma: contemporary management. Orthop Rev (Pavia). 2018; 10(3):7496

[2] Ghanem I. The management of osteoid osteoma: updates and controversies. Curr Opin Pediatr. 2006; 18(1):36–41

[3] Rimondi E, Mavrogenis AF, Rossi G, et al. Radiofrequency ablation for non-spinal osteoid osteomas in 557 patients. Eur Radiol. 2012; 22(1):181–188

[4] Chai JW, Hong SH, Choi JY, et al. Radiologic diagnosis of osteoid osteoma: from simple to challenging findings. Radiographics. 2010; 30(3):737–749

[5] Papathanassiou ZG, Megas P, Petsas T, Papachristou DJ, Nilas J, Siablis D. Osteoid osteoma: diagnosis and treatment. Orthopedics. 2008; 31(11):1118–1127

[6] Davies M, Cassar-Pullicino VN, Davies AM, McCall IW, Tyrrell PN. The diagnostic accuracy of MR imaging in osteoid osteoma. Skeletal Radiol. 2002; 31(10):559–569

[7] Assoun J, Richardi G, Railhac JJ, et al. Osteoid osteoma: MR imaging versus CT. Radiology. 1994; 191(1):217–223

[8] Becce F, Theumann N, Rochette A, et al. Osteoid osteoma and osteoid osteoma-mimicking lesions: biopsy findings, distinctive MDCT features and treatment by radiofrequency ablation. Eur Radiol. 2010; 20(10):2439–2446

[9] Golding JS. The natural history of osteoid osteoma; with a report of twenty cases. J Bone Joint Surg Br. 1954; 36-B(2):218–229

[10] Moberg E. The natural course of osteoid osteoma. J Bone Joint Surg Am. 1951; 33 A(1):166–170

[11] Lindner NJ, Scarborough M, Ciccarelli JM, Enneking WF. [CT-controlled thermocoagulation of osteoid osteoma in comparison with traditional methods] [in German]. Z Orthop Ihre Grenzgeb. 1997; 135(6):522–527

[12] Papagelopoulos PJ, Mavrogenis AF, Kyriakopoulos CK, et al. Radiofrequency ablation of intra-articular osteoid osteoma of the hip. J Int Med Res. 2006; 34 (5):537–544

[13] Rosenthal DI, Hornicek FJ, Wolfe MW, Jennings LC, Gebhardt MC, Mankin HJ. Percutaneous radiofrequency coagulation of osteoid osteoma compared with operative treatment. J Bone Joint Surg Am. 1998; 80(6):815–821

[14] Simon MA. Percutaneous radiofrequency coagulation of osteoid osteoma compared with operative treatment. J Bone Joint Surg Am. 1999; 81(3): 437–438

[15] Lanza E, Thouvenin Y, Viala P, et al. Osteoid osteoma treated by percutaneous thermal ablation: when do we fail? A systematic review and guidelines for future reporting. Cardiovasc Intervent Radiol. 2014; 37(6): 1530–1539

[16] Allen SD, Saifuddin A. Imaging of intra-articular osteoid osteoma. Clin Radiol. 2003; 58(11):845–852

[17] Albisinni U, Bazzocchi A, Bettelli G, et al. Treatment of osteoid osteoma of the elbow by radiofrequency thermal ablation. J Shoulder Elbow Surg. 2014; 23 (1):e1–e7

[18] Albisinni U, Facchini G, Spinnato P, Gasbarrini A, Bazzocchi A. Spinal osteoid osteoma: efficacy and safety of radiofrequency ablation. Skeletal Radiol. 2017; 46(8):1087–1094

[19] Martel J, Bueno A, Nieto-Morales ML, Ortiz EJ. Osteoid osteoma of the spine: CT-guided monopolar radiofrequency ablation. Eur J Radiol. 2009; 71(3): 564–569

[20] Morassi LG, Kokkinis K, Evangelopoulos DS, et al. Percutaneous radiofrequency ablation of spinal osteoid osteoma under CT guidance. Br J Radiol. 2014; 87(1038):20140003

[21] Kostrzewa M, Diezler P, Michaely H, et al. Microwave ablation of osteoid osteomas using dynamic MR imaging for early treatment assessment: preliminary experience. J Vasc Interv Radiol. 2014; 25(1):106–111

[22] Basile A, Failla G, Reforgiato A, et al. The use of microwaves ablation in the treatment of epiphyseal osteoid osteomas. Cardiovasc Intervent Radiol. 2014; 37(3):737–742

[23] Hinshaw JL, Lubner MG, Ziemlewicz TJ, Lee FT , Jr, Brace CL. Percutaneous tumor ablation tools: microwave, radiofrequency, or cryoablation—what should you use and why? Radiographics. 2014; 34(5):1344–1362

[24] Liu DM, Kee ST, Loh CT, et al. Cryoablation of osteoid osteoma: two case reports. J Vasc Interv Radiol. 2010; 21(4):586–589

[25] Coupal TM, Mallinson PI, Munk PL, Liu D, Clarkson P, Ouellette H. CT-guided percutaneous cryoablation for osteoid osteoma: initial experience in adults. AJR Am J Roentgenol. 2014; 202(5):1136–1139

[26] Santiago E, Pauly V, Brun G, Guenoun D, Champsaur P, Le Corroller T. Percutaneous cryoablation for the treatment of osteoid osteoma in the adult population. Eur Radiol. 2018; 28(6):2336–2344

[27] Shah J, Gill A, Laporte J, et al. Long-term results and durability of cryoablation of osteoid osteoma in the pediatric and adolescent population. Pediatr Radiol. 2019; 49 Suppl 1:S75

[28] Miyazaki M, Saito K, Yanagawa T, Chikuda H, Tsushima Y. Phase I clinical trial of percutaneous cryoablation for osteoid osteoma. Jpn J Radiol. 2018; 36(11): 669–675

[29] Wu B, Xiao YY, Zhang X, Zhao L, Carrino JA. CT-guided percutaneous cryoablation of osteoid osteoma in children: an initial study. Skeletal Radiol. 2011; 40(10):1303–1310

[30] Whitmore MJ, Hawkins CM, Prologo JD, et al. Cryoablation of osteoid osteoma in the pediatric and adolescent population. J Vasc Interv Radiol. 2016; 27(2):232–237, quiz 238

[31] Aarts BM, Klompenhouwer EG, Rice SL, et al. Cryoablation and immunotherapy: an overview of evidence on its synergy. Insights Imaging. 2019; 10(1):53

[32] Prologo JD, Johnson C, Hawkins CM, Singer A, Manyapu SR, Chang-Yeon K, Mitchell J. Natural History of Mixed and Motor Nerve Cryoablation in Humans—A Cohort Analysis. J Vasc Interv Radiol. 2020 Jun;31(6):912–916.

39 Joint Injections

Dimitrios Filippiadis and Alexis Kelekis

39.1 Case Presentation

An 81-year-old woman was referred to the interventional radiology (IR) department due to left knee pain and mobility impairment. The patient was taking oral analgesics and nonsteroidal anti-inflammatory drugs (NSAIDs), but still reported a pain score of 9/10 numeric visual scale (NVS) units. Clinical examination demonstrated significant mobility impairment of the left knee. Furthermore, local pain and tenderness were noted upon palpation of the medial knee compartment. Standard knee anteroposterior and lateral radiographs illustrated signs of degenerative osteoarthritis including multiple osteophytes, joint space narrowing, a moderate degree of sclerosis, and deformity of the bone ends (grade III on Kellgren–Lawrence classification). The patient had refused knee arthroplasty operation on multiple occasions. A combined intra-articular approach with pulsed radiofrequency (RF) neuromodulation and viscosupplementation was decided upon.

During the procedure, the knee was placed in 45 degrees flexion. Under sterile conditions and with fluoroscopic guidance, the entrance skin point was determined (approximately 1 cm below and 1 cm lateral to the lateral border of the patella), and local anesthesia was applied. A 20 gauge/10 cm RF trocar was percutaneously inserted at a 45 degrees angulation from the anterolateral region of the knee joint (▶ Fig. 39.1).

For appropriate placement, in both anteroposterior and lateral fluoroscopy projections, the final position of the RF trocar should be in the midline between tibial and femoral bones and not beyond the intercondylar eminence of the tibia (▶ Fig. 39.2).

Coaxially, an RF electrode with a 10-mm "active tip" was introduced and a 10 minutes neurolysis session was performed with pulsed mode application of the RF energy. Subsequently, viscosupplementation was performed through the same trocar by intra-articular injection of 60 mg/6 mL of sodium hyaluronate. The patient was observed in the hospital for 30 to 45 minutes, and was discharged with instructions to rest for 1 day. After this 1-day recovery period, she was allowed to engage in normal activities, with resumption of sport activities delayed for at least 10 days.

Clinical examination 1 week post-procedure revealed a pain score of 1/10 NVS units (significant pain reduction of 8 NVS units) and significant mobility improvement. The clinical improvement lasted for 11 months, after which symptoms reappeared although significantly fewer than those of the baseline. At 12 months post procedure, the patient was retreated with a second combined approach.

39.2 Discussion

The most common cause of chronic knee pain in middle-aged and elderly patients is degenerative osteoarthritis, with the most common symptoms including pain and mobility impairment.[1] Therapeutic options for degenerative osteoarthritis of the knee includes: conservative means such as physical therapy and oral pharmacologic therapy, intra-articular injections,

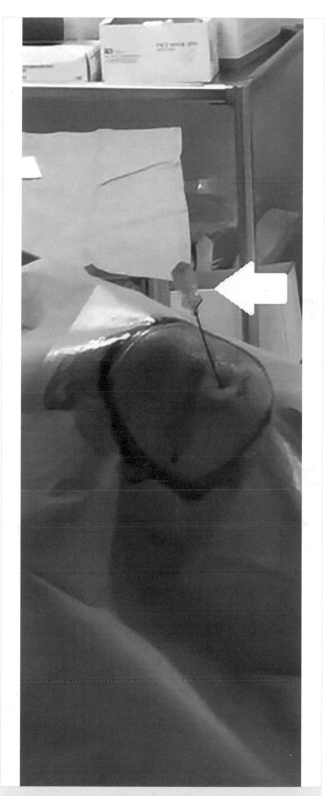

Fig. 39.1 The radiofrequency (RF) trocar (arrow) is percutaneously inserted from the anterolateral region of the knee joint at a 45 degrees angulation.

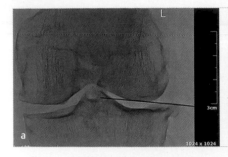
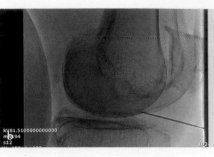

Fig. 39.2 Anteroposterior (**a**) and lateral (**b**) fluoroscopy projections verifying the final position of the radiofrequency (RF) trocar in the midline between tibial and femoral bones, not beyond the intercondylar eminence of the tibia.

nerve ablation or modulation, transcatheter arterial embolization, minimally invasive arthroscopic treatment, and partial or total knee arthroplasty. Interventional radiology techniques include intra-articular injections, neurotomy, and neuromodulation techniques as well as transcatheter intra-arterial therapies. Most recently, intra-arterially delivered cell-based therapies are applied in order to provide regenerative repair of bone and cartilage.[2]

Hyaluronic acid derivatives, especially those of high molecular weight, are recommended for intra-articular applications in symptomatic knee osteoarthritis patients with mild to moderate clinically and radiologically confirmed disease.[3,4] This type of viscosupplementation is governed by a 2 to 3 weeks delayed onset of action, with the effects lasting an average of 6 months, while retreatment can be considered in the event of recurrence of symptoms.[3,4]

In order to provide quicker and longer pain relief, by using the same intra-articular approach, operators can initially perform percutaneous neuromodulation followed by viscosupplementation.[5] By using a pulsed application of RF energy, the long silent phases (480 milliseconds) between the short bursts of energy deposition (10–20 milliseconds) maintain tissue temperature below the irreversible tissue damage threshold.[5,6] Intra-articular application of pulsed RF is related to excitatory C-fiber response suppression as well as blockade of the synaptic transmission, resulting in immediate pain relief.[5,6]

Factors such as obesity, advanced disease stage, and major malignment negatively affect the outcome of both techniques.[4,5,6] Due to the excellent safety profile and favorable risk/benefit ratio, intra-articular neuromodulation and viscosupplementation are considered an attractive approach for elderly or frail patients who refuse or cannot withstand surgical approaches.[7,8] Even in the setting of repeat injections, the overall rate of adverse events remains very low. A history or radiographic evidence of calcium pyrophosphate dihydrate arthropathy is considered a relative contraindication for viscosupplementation.[9]

Alternative agents for intra-articular injection include corticosteroids, platelet-rich plasma, mesenchymal stem cells, onabotulinumtoxin A, and ozone gas.[2] The alternative to intra-articular neuromodulation is standard genicular nerve neurolysis, during which continuous RF energy or cryoablation increase or decrease the temperature, respectively, to irreversible tissue damage thresholds.[2]

References

[1] Garstang SV, Stitik TP. Osteoarthritis: epidemiology, risk factors, and pathophysiology. Am J Phys Med Rehabil. 2006; 85(11) Suppl:S2–S11, quiz S12–S14

[2] Filippiadis D, Charalampopoulos G, Mazioti A, et al. Interventional radiology techniques for pain reduction and mobility improvement in patients with knee osteoarthritis. Diagn Interv Imaging. 2019; 100(7–8):391–400

[3] Bhadra AK, Altman R, Dasa V, et al. Appropriate use criteria for hyaluronic acid in the treatment of knee osteoarthritis in the United States. Cartilage. 2017; 8(3):234–254

[4] Raman R, Henrotin Y, Chevalier X, et al. Decision algorithms for the retreatment with viscosupplementation in patients suffering from knee osteoarthritis: recommendations from the EUROpean VIScosupplementation COnsensus Group (EUROVISCO). Cartilage. 2018; 9(3):263–275

[5] Filippiadis D, Velonakis G, Mazioti A, et al. Intra-articular application of pulsed radiofrequency combined with viscosupplementation for improvement of knee osteoarthritis symptoms: a single centre prospective study. Int J Hyperthermia. 2018; 34(8):1265–1269

[6] Masala S, Fiori R, Raguso M, Morini M, Calabria E, Simonetti G. Pulse-dose radiofrequency for knee osteoartrithis. Cardiovasc Intervent Radiol. 2014; 37(2):482–487

[7] Abdulla A, Adams N, Bone M, et al. British Geriatric Society. Guidance on the management of pain in older people. Age Ageing. 2013; 42 Suppl 1:i1–i57

[8] Bannuru RR, Brodie CR, Sullivan MC, McAlindon TE. Safety of repeated injections of sodium hyaluronate (SUPARTZ) for knee osteoarthritis: a systematic review and meta-analysis. Cartilage. 2016; 7(4):322–332

[9] Peterson C, Hodler J. Adverse events from diagnostic and therapeutic joint injections: a literature review. Skeletal Radiol. 2011; 40(1):5–12

40 Image-Guided (Fluoroscopic and Ultrasound) Joint, Tendon, and Bursal Injections

Vibhor Wadhwa, Uma Thakur, Parham Pezeshk, and Avneesh Chhabra

40.1 Introduction

The ability to perform technically successful image-guided joint and tendon injections is a valuable skill for the interventional physicians and musculoskeletal radiologists. Joint injections can be performed for diagnostic and/or therapeutic purposes, such as pain relief or computed tomography (CT) or magnetic resonance imaging (MRI) arthrograms. Tendon injections performed for tendinopathy include injection of corticosteroids and/or local anesthetic, or therapeutic substances such as platelet-rich plasma (PRP) and autologous blood following needle fenestration and/or tenotomy. This chapter provides an overview of such techniques for joint and tendon injections with relevant case examples.

40.2 General Technical Considerations for Joint Injections/ Aspirations

Joint injections or aspirations can be performed using fluoroscopic or ultrasound guidance. These interventions are performed under sterile conditions and following informed consent. After a time-out is performed with the patient in supine or prone position, the intended site is marked. Fluoroscopic guidance relies on appropriate patient and C-arm positioning, generally aligning the X-ray beam with the needle trajectory, and the needle entering the skin in a perpendicular fashion. This creates the so-called "bull's eye" appearance, with the needle tip and hub being superimposed on each other on the fluoroscopic image. Such an approach avoids parallax and distortion artifacts and helps adjust the needle hub in directing the needle tip to its target. Depth perception is generally achieved using a bony background, which is initially used as the target. Once the appropriate depth is reached, the needle can be redirected slightly to enter the joint cavity. A small amount of nonionic iodinated contrast, gadolinium, or alternatively air in the event of a documented severe allergy to iodinated contrast, can be injected to ensure that it flows away from the needle tip and opacifies the joint cavity or its recesses. If the contrast remains static and globular at the needle tip or fills an unintended space (such as iliopsoas bursa during a hip injection), the tip needs to be redirected to enter the joint. Care is needed during a pre-MRI arthrogram so that air is not inadvertently introduced into the joint as it will lead to blooming artifacts and can mimic an intra-articular loose body.

Alternatively, the injection or aspiration can be performed under ultrasound guidance. Ultrasound guidance has several advantages over fluoroscopic guidance. Most notably, during ultrasound-guided procedures the needle can be visualized in real-time instead of intermittently, and the needle trajectory can be easily manipulated to enter the joint recess or tendon avoiding vital structures such as vessels and nerves (due to the high soft tissue contrast). Ultrasound guidance also avoids exposure of the patient and operators to ionizing radiation. The parallel needle positioning is preferred (in-plane technique) to better visualize the entire needle throughout the procedure. Improved needle visualization can be achieved by using a shallower needle trajectory (less than 60-degree angle), beam steering, "jiggling" the needle, and hydro-dissection using a local anesthetic. The intra-articular position of the needle tip is confirmed by direct visualization and injection of the local anesthetic, which moves away from the needle tip into the joint recess without resistance. In addition, sonopalpation (pressing on the skin with the ultrasound probe) can be used to interrogate the site of tenderness over the tendon, bursa, or joint during diagnostic or therapeutic injections. In general, in most practices fluoroscopy-guided injections and arthrograms are favored over ultrasound guidance due to cost, lack of widespread musculoskeletal ultrasound operator skill, and more time needed for ultrasound probe preparation.[1]

40.3 Arthrography

Arthrography refers to imaging of a joint using contrast media. Isolated fluoroscopic arthrography is rarely performed after the advent of more advanced cross-sectional (CT/MRI) modalities. Arthrography is currently performed as an intra-articular injection of contrast followed by cross-sectional imaging. This provides adequate distension of the joint and assessment of internal joint structures, which could otherwise be obscured by cross-sectional imaging alone. CT arthrography is performed with iodinated contrast, while MR arthrography is performed by injecting diluted gadolinium into the joint (typically 1:100 or 1:200 dilution with saline). Following needle placement into the joint, the authors recommend rotating the needle to free the capsule, followed by injection of 1 to 2 cc 1% lidocaine. Free flow of the injectate confirms an intra-articular location of the needle and in addition provides comfort to the patient. The local anesthetic injection is followed by confirmation and documentation of intra-articular location with iodinated contrast agent. Care should be taken to exclude air from the tubing and needle to avoid susceptibility artifacts on MRI.

40.4 Therapeutic Joint Injections

Corticosteroid joint injections are commonly performed in a musculoskeletal or interventional pain practice. Steroids theoretically reduce synovial inflammation and provide short- or medium-term pain relief. Repeat steroid injections can be performed as clinically indicated. The authors limit the number of steroid injections to three to four per year to avoid adverse effects from systemic absorption of the injected steroid. Triamcinolone acetonide (Kenalog, 40 mg/mL or 80 mg/2 mL; Bristol-Myers Squibb Company, Princeton, NJ) is an insoluble steroid, which is commonly used for intra-articular injections. The steroid is typically combined with local anesthetic (1% lidocaine and/or 0.25–0.5% bupivacaine), which increases the injectate volume, provides better distribution of the steroid, and provides postprocedural comfort to the patient. The only point of caution is to mix particulate steroids with preservative-free anesthetics or normal saline to prevent precipitation of the particulate. In addition to steroids, intra-articular injection of hyaluronic acid (hyaluronan) can be used to provide pain relief from osteoarthritis refractory to steroids.

40.5 Specific Joint Considerations

40.5.1 Shoulder

The glenohumeral joint can be injected from anterior, rotator interval, and posterior approaches. The anterior anterosuperior rotator interval (▶ Fig. 40.1) or inferior glenohumeral (▶ Fig. 40.2) approaches are most commonly used under fluoroscopic guidance. Approximately 12 to 14 cc of injectate is administered into the joint for optimal distention. The patient is laid supine on the table with the arm in external rotation to expose the joint. The patient's hand is supinated (palm facing the ceiling) and a weight may be placed on the palm to maintain the external rotation position. A fluoroscopic image is obtained, and the needle site is marked. For the rotator interval approach, the needle is inserted to the cortex of the medial humeral head at and above the level of coracoid process; for the inferior glenohumeral approach it is directed toward the medial anteroinferior humeral head. Once the

needle contacts the bone, it is retracted slightly and directed medially to enter the joint. The rotator interval approach avoids the subscapularis tendon and thereby reduces patient discomfort. If the patient is not able to externally rotate the shoulder, the needle trajectory may be blocked by the coracoid process and contrast may fail to enter the joint or may selectively enter the biceps tendon sheath. The rotator interval approach may help to avoid this pitfall. Extension of contrast into the subacromial or subdeltoid bursa from the shoulder joint injection confirms a full-thickness tear. A pitfall to this diagnosis includes prior surgery, where a small amount of fluid extension into the bursa is normal. Ultrasound can also be used to perform the anterior glenohumeral joint access, whereby the transducer is placed in transverse plane at the level of coracoid process and parallel to the subscapularis tendon. The humeral head is identified, and the needle is inserted under direct visualization from the medial approach toward the medial edge of humeral head.

The posterior approach to the glenohumeral joint may be preferred in patients with anterior instability and to avoid obscuring anterior labral pathology. Fluoroscopic guidance can be used in a similar fashion for anterior approach; however, this approach is more commonly used with ultrasound. The transducer is aligned in an oblique-axial direction along the long axis of infraspinatus muscle. The needle is advanced from medial to lateral approach to avoid the suprascapular nerve and vessels, which run medially along the scapular spine. As the needle penetrates the infraspinatus, the patient may experience some pain and discomfort.

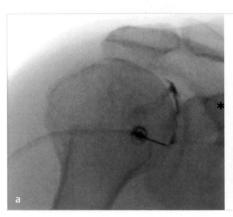
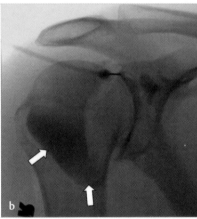

Fig. 40.1 Rotator interval approach for shoulder joint injection. (a) The needle (arrow) is inserted at the edge of humeral head, at and above the level of coracoid process (star). (b) Contrast opacification of the shoulder joint outlining the capsule (arrows) confirms intra-articular position of the needle tip.

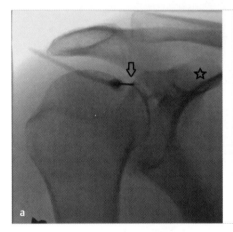
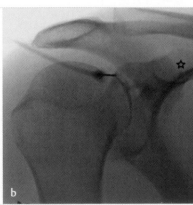

Fig. 40.2 Anterior inferior approach for glenohumeral injection. (a) The needle is inserted at the edge of humeral head, inferior one-third. (b) Rotator interval approach at the level of the coracoid (star) again demonstrated for comparison.

40.5.2 Knee

The commonly used approaches to access the knee joint are lateral patellofemoral, medial patellofemoral, and anterior approaches (▶ Fig. 40.3). The patient is placed supine on the procedure table with the knee in partial flexion and supported by a bolster. In the lateral patellofemoral approach, the patella is pushed and tilted manually medially, and the needle is passed under the patella between the patella and femoral condyle. Intra-articular position can be confirmed with loss of resistance to injection of local anesthetic, followed by injection of small volume of contrast. The medial patellofemoral approach is similar, where the sub-patellar joint space is accessed from the medial side of the knee. Care should be taken to avoid the Hoffa's fat pad, which may occur if the needle is inserted too inferiorly (caudal) in relation to the patella. The suprapatellar approach can be performed using ultrasound, where the probe is parallel to the long axis of the quadriceps tendon and the distal femur is identified. The needle is passed into the suprapatellar recess by a lateral-to-medial or medial-to-lateral approach. The lateral approach is generally preferred due to the presence of saphenous nerve branches in the medial subcutaneous tissues. Approximately 30 to 45 cc of injectate is administered into the joint for optimal distention. Contrast extension can be seen in the meniscus confirming meniscus tear or re-tear following a previous surgical repair.

The anterior approach (▶ Fig. 40.3) is advocated by some radiologists as an alternative in obese patients, and in patients with severe patellofemoral osteoarthritis and joint space narrowing. In this approach, the patellar tendon is palpated and the skin medial or lateral to it is identified to access the knee joint. The needle is inserted parallel to the procedure table, directed toward the contralateral femoral condyle. Care should be taken to avoid the respective knee menisci.

40.5.3 Wrist

Injections of the wrist joint can be performed as single compartment (radiocarpal), double compartment (radiocarpal and midcarpal), or triple compartment (radiocarpal, midcarpal, and distal radioulnar joint [DRUJ]). The radiocarpal joint is most commonly accessed for wrist arthrography to assess the integrity of the triangular fibrocartilage complex (TFCC) and intrinsic ligaments. Complete tears of the TFCC leads to communication between radiocarpal joint and DRUJ. If there is no communication seen on fluoroscopic arthrograms, the DRUJ can be directly injected for complete evaluation of partial tears of the TFCC. For optimal distention, 3 to 4 cc of injectate is administered into the joint. Contrast extension from the radiocarpal joint to the midcarpal joint indicates scapholunate or lunotriquetral ligament tear. Midcarpal joint injections show normal communication to the carpometacarpal joint.

For wrist arthrography, the patient sits on a chair next to the fluoroscopy table with the wrist on the table in the prone position. If the patient is apprehensive, he/she can be laid prone on the table, with the arm abducted and the hand pronated (palm facing the table). The wrist is held in slight flexion by placing a bolster under the wrist joint. A dorsal approach (▶ Fig. 40.4) is typically used to access the wrist, as many vital structures pass along the palmar aspect of the wrist. Slight flexion and ulnar deviation are useful to open the radiocarpal aspect of the joint. The needle is passed between the proximal cortex of the scaphoid and distal radius, lateral to the tubercle, at about 10- to 13-degree angle from the distal to the proximal wrist. Since the joint is small, caution should be taken not to over-distend and extravasate contrast into adjacent joint compartments, thereby mimicking full-thickness tears. The DRUJ is accessed using the radial aspect of the distal ulna proximal to the physeal scar as the target. The midcarpal compartment is targeted at the confluence of the triquetrum, lunate, capitate, and hamate bones.

Both fluoroscopic and ultrasound guidance can be used to inject the wrist joint compartments. With ultrasound guidance, injury to the sensory radial nerve branches, which may inadvertently course along the needle trajectory, can be avoided.

40.5.4 Elbow

The elbow joint can be accessed using either lateral or posterior approaches. For the lateral approach, the anterior half of the radiocapitellar joint is targeted fluoroscopically (▶ Fig. 40.5a). The patient sits on a chair beside the fluoroscopy table with the elbow in prone position on the table. If the patient is apprehensive, he/she can be placed prone with the arm over the head, with the elbow flexed 90 degrees. Partial supination of the hand with thumb facing up is used to maximally open the joint. The radiocapitellar joint is positioned parallel to the X-ray beam to avoid overlap of the radial head and capitellum; this joint is used as the fluoroscopic target. Approximately 5 to 6 cc of injectate is administered into the joint for optimal distention (▶ Fig. 40.5b). The posterior approach involves traversing the needle through the triceps superolateral to the olecranon, with the needle directed toward the olecranon fossa. The posterior

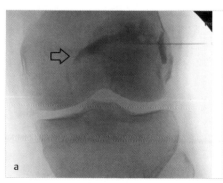
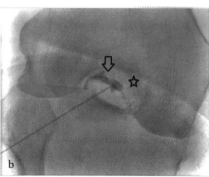

Fig. 40.3 Knee arthrogram, lateral and anterior approaches. The needle is inserted toward the lateral femoral condyle (**a**) in the lateral approach and toward the medial femoral condyle (star in **b**) in the anterior approach. Contrast (arrows) is injected in both the approaches to confirm intra-articular position.

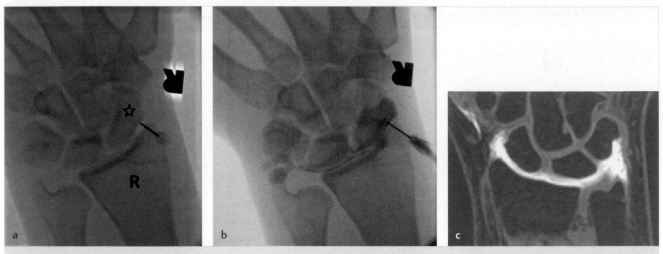

Fig. 40.4 Dorsal approach for wrist injection. The needle is passed between the proximal scaphoid (star) and distal radius (R) (**a**) and contrast injected to confirm the intra-articular position (**b**). T1, fat-saturated (FS), coronal plane magnetic resonance (MR) arthrogram showing capsular distension (**c**).

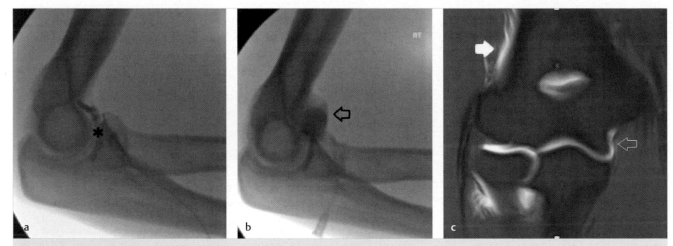

Fig. 40.5 Elbow arthrogram. A 29-year-old man with concern for ulnar collateral ligament (UCL) tear. The needle is passed at the radiocapitellar articulation with initial filling (*, **a**) followed by capsular distension (arrow, **b**) with magnetic resonance imaging (MRI) correlate, T1 coronal FS (**c**) demonstrating intact UCL (open arrow). Mild extravasation of contrast along lateral distal humerus is also noted (solid arrow).

approach decreases the likelihood of contrast extravasation along the lateral aspect of elbow, which may mimic full-thickness tears of the lateral collateral ligament on subsequent CT/MRI. Contrast extension across the ulnar collateral ligament confirms tear or re-tear. Ultrasound can be used to inject the elbow using lateral or posterior approaches. Ultrasound is especially useful for joint aspiration as it can evaluate the recesses (especially the olecranon recess) for fluid and allows appropriate targeting of the needle.

40.5.5 Hip

The hip joint is most commonly accessed using an anterior approach (▶ Fig. 40.6). The patient is placed supine on the procedure table and the lower extremity is internally rotated approximately 10 to 15 degrees. The femoral artery is palpated and marked with a skin marker and should be medial to the

skin entry site. The lateral aspect of the femoral head and neck junction is the optimal fluoroscopic target site. The bull's-eye approach is used to target the needle along the lateral edge of the bone and advance it into the joint after contacting the bone. In obese patients or patients with a hip prosthesis, an oblique inferior-to-superior or lateral-to-medial approach can be helpful. Patchy contrast collections or extension in a linear fashion in the iliopsoas tendon indicates the need to reposition of the needle; outlining of the zona orbicularis (dark band without surrounding bright contrast) confirms an intra-articular position (▶ Fig. 40.6b). Extension of contrast in the labrum confirms tear or re-tear. Ultrasound can be used to access the hip joint with the anterior approach, especially in children. The transducer is placed parallel to the long axis of femoral neck (▶ Fig. 40.7). The needle is advanced in distal-to-proximal direction, targeting the femoral head and neck junction.

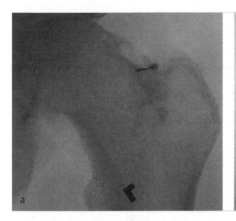
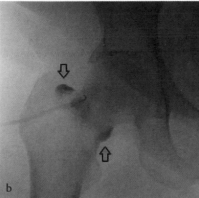

Fig. 40.6 Anterior approach for hip joint injection. The needle is inserted at the edge of femoral neck. Needle position may need to be altered due to osteophytosis as in this case (**a**). Contrast (arrows) flows freely along the zona orbicularis (**b**) in a different patient.

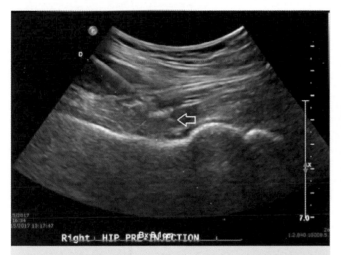

Fig. 40.7 Ultrasound-guided injection of hip. The needle (arrow) is inserted at the proximal femoral neck.

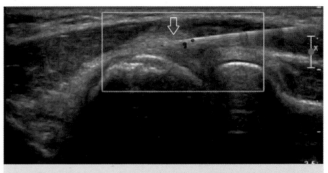

Fig. 40.8 Ultrasound-guided needling of lateral epicondylitis with needle (arrow) directed to the common extensor tendon.

40.5.6 Ankle

The ankle joint is commonly accessed from an anterior approach targeting the talar dome between the extensor hallucis longus and the extensor digitorum longus tendons. Care should be taken to avoid the dorsalis pedis artery. An alternative to the anterior approach to the ankle is to target the medial or lateral clear space. The mortise view is achieved by angulating the X-ray beam in 15 to 20 degrees of internal rotation, delineating the medial and lateral clear spaces. Ultrasound guidance can be used to target the ankle joint by obtaining a long-axis view of the tibialis anterior tendon and moving the transducer slightly medially to localize the anterior recess. The needle is passed under direct visualization to target the talar dome. Extension of fluid in the medial or lateral ankle (e.g., outlining the peroneal tendon sheath) confirms collateral ligament injuries.

40.6 General Considerations for Tendon Needling and Injections

Tendinopathy refers to pathologies involving the tendons, primarily due to incomplete or altered healing responses and decreased mechanical integrity. Image-guided tendon therapies include peritendinous steroid injections, percutaneous needle fenestration and tenotomy, prolotherapy, sclerotherapy, hydrodissection, sodium hyaluronate, and barbotage for calcific tendinopathy. In addition, PRP, autologous blood, bone marrow–derived stem cells, and biopharmaceutical agents are being increasingly used and investigated in this setting. Tendon injections are typically performed under ultrasound guidance.[2]

40.6.1 Steroid Injections

Corticosteroid injections are widely used for tendinopathies with similar mechanism of action as in joints (i.e., by decreasing the inflammatory cascade). Although short-term pain relief has been demonstrated in several studies, long-term effects of steroids are not known. Rat studies have shown an increased incidence of Achilles tendon tears with steroid injections. Therefore, direct Achilles tendon injection with steroids is avoided.

40.6.2 Percutaneous Tenotomy

"Dry needling" or percutaneous needle fenestration (tenotomy) refers to fenestration of the affected tendon, targeting the abnormal low-echogenic areas and neovascularity (▶ Fig. 40.8). The procedure encourages localized hemorrhage and subsequent healing response with fibroblast proliferation and collagen formation. Dry needling is performed under ultrasound guidance, typically with single skin insertion and redirection of the needle as needed. Typically, 10 to 20 needle passes are made.

40.6.3 Autologous Blood Injection

Autologous blood stimulates collagen regeneration and an ordered angiogenic response through cellular and humoral mediators within a diseased tendon. Blood (3–5 cc) is withdrawn from an appropriate vein, diluted with 1 to 2 cc of lidocaine, and injected into the site of tendon needling.

40.6.4 Platelet-Rich Plasma (PRP) Injection

PRP is prepared by centrifugation of whole blood to remove red blood cells and concentrate platelets to a degree of 1,000,000/μL. PRP augments tendon healing by introducing an increased number of cytokines locally. PRP injections increase cell count, stimulate cell differentiation, and restore tissue architecture. It is generally believed that PRP injections provide beneficial effect of alleviating pain in the intermediate to long term compared to other interventions. Although this therapy lacks the deleterious effects that may hypothetically occur due to repeat steroid injections, there is controversy in the literature as to the use of leukocyte-poor or leukocyte-rich PRP, and whether either of them offers more pain relief than steroid injections.

40.6.5 Barbotage

Calcific tendinitis occurs secondary to calcium hydroxyapatite crystals within or around the tendons, causing inflammation, bursitis, chronic pain, and loss of function. Percutaneous barbotage refers to ultrasound-guided needling of calcium deposit, and injection and aspiration of fluid to remove the calcific deposit (▶ Fig. 40.9). Removal of calcification from the tendon results in improvement in symptoms with high long-term success rate. The technique, typically used in the shoulder, involves repeated injection and aspiration of fluid (hot or normal temperature normal saline mixed with a local anesthetic), followed by injection of steroid or local anesthetic into the subacromial-subdeltoid (SASD) bursa. The soft calcium deposits can be easily

aspirated while the hardened and more mature calcium is often not amenable to aspiration. A 20- to 22-G needle is used for needling and 10 to 20 passes are typically made into the calcific areas. The patients may experience a flare of pain over the following 24 to 48 hours which may be relieved with acetaminophen. Rarely, chemical reactions may occur leading to prolonged pain. Most patients feel better with improved range of motion and pain relief for prolonged periods whether the calcium is aspirated or the tendon just fenestrated with needling. Over time, the local tissue reaction resorbs the majority of the calcium deposits.

40.7 Bursal Injections and Aspirations

Bursae are fluid-filled synovial spaces around joints and tendons which can become inflamed with repetitive trauma, termed bursitis. Congenital bursae are present at birth (e.g., iliopsoas bursa), while adventitial bursae form at friction sites (e.g., over osteochondroma or bunion). Image-guided bursal injections or aspirations are commonly performed in interventional and musculoskeletal practices to provide pain relief to these patients, or for the diagnosis of crystal arthropathy or suspected infections. The most commonly involved bursae are SASD bursa, iliopsoas bursa (▶ Fig. 40.10), greater trochanter bursa (▶ Fig. 40.11), and bicipitoradial bursa. In acute bursitis, there is presence of a hypoechoic effusion on ultrasound which distends the hyperechoic bursal walls. In chronic inflammation, the bursal walls become thickened, hypoechoic, and there may or may not be an effusion (▶ Fig. 40.12). Image-guided therapeutic bursal injections using corticosteroids (with or without local anesthetics) can be performed to reduce local inflammation and pain (▶ Fig. 40.12).

40.7.1 Subacromial-Subdeltoid Bursa

The SASD bursa covers the rotator cuff around the shoulder, which prevents friction between tendons and facilitates the movement of the supraspinatus during abduction. The bursa is located between the supraspinatus tendon and acromion, and is normally not in communication with the joint space when the rotator cuff is intact.[3] SASD bursitis may be secondary to rotator cuff degeneration (most common), rheumatoid arthritis,

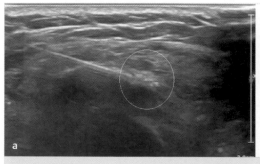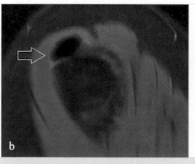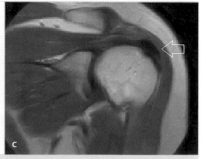

Fig. 40.9 Barbotage for calcific tendinitis. (**a**) Ultrasound guidance demonstrating needle penetrating echogenic focus of calcification (circle). (**b, c**) Magnetic resonance imaging (MRI) correlate demonstrating supraspinatus calcification (arrow) in sagittal (**b**) and coronal (**c**) planes.

gout, or other rheumatological conditions. SASD injections are performed under ultrasound guidance with the patient seated or in the supine position (► Fig. 40.13). The bursa is visualized best in longitudinal view with the probe positioned over the acromion process, and the needle is inserted in a lateral-to-medial and inferior-to-superior approach. Care should be taken not to contact the bone or tendons, which may result in an extra-bursal injection.[4] Fluoroscopic guidance can be used to target the SASD bursa in the subacromial space from an anterior approach.

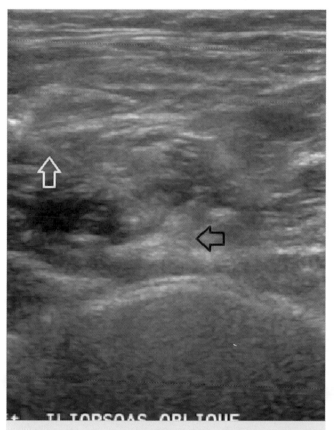

Fig. 40.10 Iliopsoas ultrasound-guided injection in a 63-year-old woman with anterior impingement. Black arrow shows tendon; white arrow shows the needle.

40.7.2 Iliopsoas/Iliopectineal Bursa

The iliopsoas/iliopectineal bursa is located between the anterior capsule of the hip and the iliopsoas muscle, and between the inguinal ligament superiorly and the lesser trochanter inferiorly. The femoral artery and vein are in close relation to the bursa and must be avoided during interventions. Iliopsoas bursitis may present as a painful groin mass and/or anterior hip pain that worsens with activity. Patients may also complain of a reproducible "snapping" sensation around the hip.[5] Aspiration or injections of iliopsoas may be performed using fluoroscopic, CT, or ultrasound guidance (► Fig. 40.10). Using fluoroscopic guidance, the acetabulum is targeted over the center of the femoral head and a test injection is performed to confirm contrast opacification of the bursa.[6] Under ultrasound guidance, the iliopsoas tendon is identified anterior to the femoral head and iliopectineal eminence of the acetabulum using oblique axial imaging along the inguinal ligament. The needle is passed with lateral approach deep to the tendon, where the bursa is located (► Fig. 40.10).

40.7.3 Bicipitoradial Bursa

The bicipitoradial bursa surrounds the distal tendon of the biceps brachii and is located between the tendon and the radial tuberosity. As with other bursae in the body, its function is to reduce friction between the tendon and bone, and it can get inflamed with overuse or rheumatological conditions. Clinical presentation is generally a reduced range of motion, pain, and a cystic palpable mass at the antecubital fossa; this mass may further lead to compressive neuropathy.[7] Injections are generally performed using ultrasound guidance, with the probe placed transversely over the antecubital fossa. The biceps tendon is identified, and the inflamed bursa can be identified originating deep to the biceps tendon at the level of radial tuberosity. The needle can be inserted from either a medial or lateral approach, with care taken not to transverse any superficial veins or nerves in this region.

40.8 Conclusion

To summarize, image-guided joint, tendon, and bursal injections are safe and have a high technical success rate. These can be used for both diagnostic and therapeutic purposes and are effective for patient management purposes.

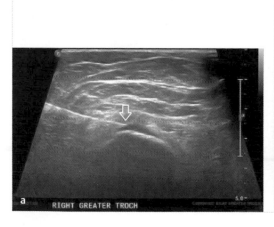

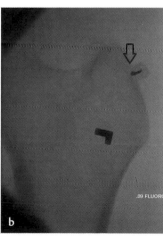

Fig. 40.11 Greater trochanteric bursal injection via sonographic (**a**) and fluoroscopic (**b**) guidance. The needle (arrows) is passed at the edge of the greater trochanter (expected location of greater trochanter bursa) and directed laterally when the bone is reached.

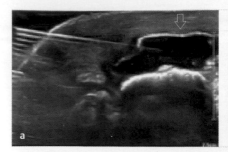
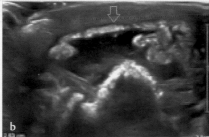

Fig. 40.12 Ultrasound-guided aspiration of olecranon bursitis in a 72-year-old man with chronic bursitis showing thickened echogenic bursal walls (arrows, **a** and **b**).

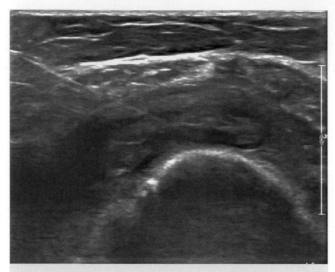

Fig. 40.13 Subacromial-subdeltoid bursal injection via sonographic guidance distending the bursa with injectate.

References

[1] Rastogi AK, Davis KW, Ross A, Rosas HG. Fundamentals of joint injection. AJR Am J Roentgenol. 2016; 207(3):484–494

[2] Burke CJ, Adler RS. Ultrasound-guided percutaneous tendon treatments. AJR Am J Roentgenol. 2016; 207(3):495–506

[3] Bureau NJ, Dussault RG, Keats TE. Imaging of bursae around the shoulder joint. Skeletal Radiol. 1996; 25(6):513–517

[4] Messina C, Banfi G, Orlandi D, et al. Ultrasound-guided interventional procedures around the shoulder. Br J Radiol. 2016; 89(1057):20150372

[5] Adler RS, Buly R, Ambrose R, Sculco T. Diagnostic and therapeutic use of sonography-guided iliopsoas peritendinous injections. AJR Am J Roentgenol. 2005; 185(4):940–943

[6] Maher P, Cardozo E, Singh JR. Technique for fluorscopically guided injection for iliopsoas bursitis. Am J Phys Med Rehabil. 2014; 93(12):1105–1106

[7] Sofka CM, Adler RS. Sonography of cubital bursitis. AJR Am J Roentgenol. 2004; 183(1):51–53

41 Appendicular Fracture Stabilizations (Cement and/or Screw Fixation)

Dimitrios Filippiadis and Alexis Kelekis

41.1 Case Presentation

A 59-year-old woman with oligometastatic breast cancer was referred to the interventional radiology (IR) department for local therapy of a metastatic lesion. The abnormality was in the right acetabulum with extension to the iliac bone, and was associated with a pathologic fracture. The patient was receiving analgesics, opioids, and reported a pain score of 9/10 numeric visual scale (NVS) units. Neurological examination demonstrated neither sensory nor motor deficit affecting the right lower extremity. Approximately 4 months prior the patient had undergone radiotherapy sessions (external beam radiation therapy [EBRT]) with no significant pain reduction. Furthermore, 3 weeks previously she reported a significant pain exacerbation. Positron emission tomography–computed tomography (PET-CT)

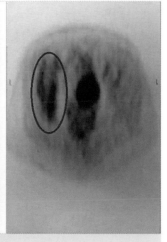

Fig. 41.1 Positron emission tomography–computed tomography (PET-CT) revealed an avid, mixed osteolytic-osteoblastic lesion in the right acetabulum (circles) along with the presence of a pathologic fracture (arrows).

revealed a PET-avid, mixed osteolytic-osteoblastic lesion in the right acetabulum along with the presence of a pathologic fracture (▶ Fig. 41.1).

Percutaneous augmented osteoplasty (cement injection combined with cannulated screw insertion), along with microwave ablation, was decided as the best therapeutic option. Under fluoroscopic guidance and sterile conditions, and after prophylactic intravenous (IV) antibiotics, two bone trocars were inserted inside the lesion. The two trocars were placed perpendicular to one another by means of a direct lateral approach and through the anterior superior iliac spine directed toward the acetabular lesion. A microwave antenna was inserted coaxially through each trocar, and an ablation session (40 Watts × 5 minutes) was performed at both sites. During ablation the trocars were retracted outside the expected ablation zone to prevent heat conduction. After ablation, the trocars were reinserted into the ablation zones and cement was injected, followed immediately by cannulated screw placement with sequential exchanges over Kirshner wires (▶ Fig. 41.2 and ▶ Fig. 41.3). The entire procedure was performed uneventfully.

41.2 Discussion

Although standard polymethylmethacrylate (PMMA) cement constitutes a stable material for the spine where mainly axial forces are applied upon the vertebrae, in the peripheral skeleton (and especially in the long bones) the presence of rotational and torsional forces complicates structural support. This results in the necessity for a more stable re-enforcement during interventions.[1] Furthermore, the presence of lytic lesions and cortical defects are considered risk factors for secondary fractures when only the cement is injected without hardware insertion.[2] Combining cement and cannulated screws in these locations provides enhanced structural support; cement injection also prevents screw migration and contributes to local tumor control due to various factors (e.g., direct toxicity, increased temperature produced during the exothermic reaction, anoxic

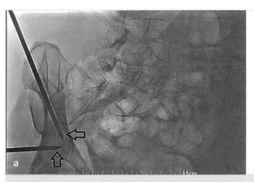
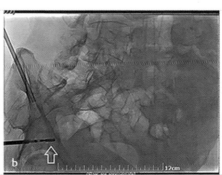
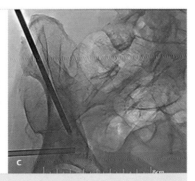

Fig. 41.2 (a) Anteroposterior fluoroscopy view showing the two bone trocars inside the acetabular lesion (black arrows). (b) A microwave antenna was inserted, and ablation was performed through each trocar (white arrow shows one of the antennae). During ablation both the trocars were retracted from the expected heated zone. (c) Advancement of cannulas and cement injection followed the ablation.

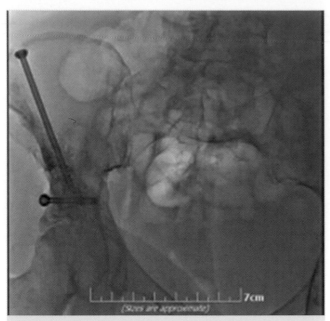

Fig. 41.3 Anteroposterior fluoroscopy view showing the two cannulated, partially threaded screws in position and the lesion filled with the injected cement.

environment).[3,4] Ablation, apart from local tumor control, may prevent tract seeding while transarterial embolization may be added to the combination therapy as well to both create an ischemic effect and decrease bleeding during subsequent therapies.[4]

The decision on which treatment to pursue is based upon lesion characteristics, classification scores (e.g., Mirels' score for long bones or Hurrington's classification for acetabular lesions), performance status, and life expectancy of the patient.[4,5] Indications include prevention of impending pathologic fracture, pain reduction in symptomatic patients, and local tumor control. In the cases of ablation or radiotherapy, stabilization should follow in order to avoid a secondary fracture due to post-therapeutic osteonecrosis and bone weakening.[3,4,5] The choice of materials (partially or fully threaded screws, or ablation technique) is based upon lesion characteristics and location, type of bone (e.g., flat, long) as well as operator's preference. Flat bones such as acetabular roof, femoral condyles, tibial end plates, and talus can be treated effectively with percutaneous osteoplasty. In the case presented here, the decision to treat with augmented osteoplasty combining cement to cannulated screws was based upon the presence of a pathologic fracture, postradiation necrosis, and the extent of the lesion.

In the literature there are numerous case series reporting augmented osteoplasty with cannulated screws and cement. They report significant efficacy concerning stabilization, pain

reduction, mobility improvement, and local tumor control with a good safety profile.[6,7] Variations to the standard cement–screw combination include a mesh of metallic micro-needles or wires (rebar concept) as well as stents, needles, and polyether ether ketone (PEEK) polymer implants.[8,9,10] Variations of the cement injection technique have also been reported, including inflation of kyphoplasty balloons or a simultaneous injection through two needles as performed here in order to produce a more compact and solid block of cement, while concurrently reducing radiation exposure at the same time.[11,12]

Complications are rare and include needle access complications (e.g., direct traumatic injury to artery, nerve, or muscular tendon), tumor seeding, periosteal cement extrusion or leakage causing symptoms due to direct compression on adjacent nerves or muscle, and cardiopulmonary events, including cement emboli, fat embolism, transient hypotension, or bradycardia.[13]

References

[1] Cazzato RL, Palussière J, Buy X, et al. Percutaneous long bone cementoplasty for palliation of malignant lesions of the limbs: a systematic review. Cardiovasc Intervent Radiol. 2015; 38(6):1563–1572

[2] Deschamps F, Farouil G, Hakime A, et al. Cementoplasty of metastases of the proximal femur: is it a safe palliative option? J Vasc Interv Radiol. 2012; 23 (10):1311–1316

[3] Deschamps F, de Baere T, Hakime A, et al. Percutaneous osteosynthesis in the pelvis in cancer patients. Eur Radiol. 2016; 26(6):1631–1639

[4] Kelekis A, Cornelis FH, Tutton S, Filippiadis D. Metastatic osseous pain control: bone ablation and cementoplasty. Semin Intervent Radiol. 2017; 34 (4):328–336

[5] Yevich S, Tselikas L, Kelekis A, Filippiadis D, de Baere T, Deschamps F. Percutaneous management of metastatic osseous disease. Linchuang Zhongliuxue Zazhi. 2019; 8(6):62

[6] Cazzato RL, Koch G, Buy X, et al. Percutaneous image-guided screw fixation of bone lesions in cancer patients: double-centre analysis of outcomes including local evolution of the treated focus. Cardiovasc Intervent Radiol. 2016; 39 (10):1455–1463

[7] Deschamps F, Farouil G, Hakime A, Teriitehau C, Barah A, de Baere T. Percutaneous stabilization of impending pathological fracture of the proximal femur. Cardiovasc Intervent Radiol. 2012; 35(6):1428–1432

[8] Kelekis A, Filippiadis D, Anselmetti G, et al. Percutaneous augmented peripheral osteoplasty in long bones of oncologic patients for pain reduction and prevention of impeding pathologic fracture: the rebar concept. Cardiovasc Intervent Radiol. 2016; 39(1):90–96

[9] Szpalski M, Gunzburg R, Aebi M, et al. A new approach to prevent contralateral hip fracture: evaluation of the effectiveness of a fracture preventing implant. Clin Biomech (Bristol, Avon). 2015; 30(7):713–719

[10] Nakata K, Kawai N, Sato M, et al. Bone marrow nails created by percutaneous osteoplasty for long bone fracture: comparisons among acrylic cement alone, acrylic-cement-filled bare metallic stent, and acrylic-cement-filled covered metallic stent. Cardiovasc Intervent Radiol. 2011; 34(3):609–614

[11] Kurup AN, Morris JM, Schmit GD, et al. Balloon-assisted osteoplasty of periacetabular tumors following percutaneous cryoablation. J Vasc Interv Radiol. 2015; 26(4):588–594

[12] Moser TP, Onate M, Achour K, Freire V. Cementoplasty of pelvic bone metastases: systematic assessment of lesion filling and other factors that could affect the clinical outcomes. Skeletal Radiol. 2019; 48(9):1345–1355

[13] Yevich S, Tselikas L, Gravel G, de Baère T, Deschamps F. Percutaneous cement injection for the palliative treatment of osseous metastases: a technical review. Semin Intervent Radiol. 2018; 35(4):268–280

42 Pudendal Interventions

Jordan Castle

42.1 Case Presentation

A 79-year-old woman with advanced metastatic vulvar cancer was referred to interventional radiology (IR) by the palliative care service. Her primary complaint was constant excruciating labial pain due to an ulcerating tumor. She was admitted strictly for pain management and required frequent high dose intravenous (IV) opioids. She was considering home hospice care if her pain could not be controlled.

On physical examination, the patient reported 10/10 vaginal pain that was nearly constant and burning, worse on the left, but did involve the right side. She had no motor deficits or urinary or fecal incontinence, but was bedridden due to exacerbation of the pain with minor movements and ambulation. Visual inspection confirmed an ulcerating left labial malignant tumor. Computed tomography (CT) imaging confirmed metastatic disease in the chest, abdomen, and pelvis.

The patient had limited options for pain relief given that she was a nonsurgical candidate, essentially bedridden, and dependent on IV narcotics. In IR, a diagnostic pudendal nerve block was initially performed. Using CT guidance, 22-gauge Chiba needles were advanced to the pudendal canals via a transgluteal approach (▶ Fig. 42.1). After the stylet was removed and a test aspiration yielded no blood, 0.5 mL of dilute contrast was injected to confirm spread within the pudendal canal and confirm there was no arterial or venous opacification (▶ Fig. 42.2). Following the diagnostic test, approximately 10 mL of 0.5% ropivacaine was injected through each needle.

Since the patient achieved significant relief from the block without any significant side effects, pudendal nerve cryoablation was performed 2 days later. Using CT guidance, via a transgluteal approach, one cryoablation probe was placed on each side parallel to the pudendal canal (▶ Fig. 42.3). Two freeze–thaw (8 minutes freeze, 4 minutes passive thaw) cycles were performed with intermittent CT scanning to visualize the iceball and confirm adequate coverage of the treatment zone.

Immediately after the procedure the patient reported significant pain relief with associated vaginal numbness. Her narcotic needs were drastically reduced over the next 3 days, and she was discharged on oral pain medication. At 1-month follow-up, her pain was rated as dull, intermittent, and 2/10 intensity with persistent vaginal numbness, all of which continued until she entered hospice 3 months later due to progressive metastatic disease.

42.2 Discussion

The pudendal nerve is a mixed sensory and motor nerve composed of fibers from the ventral rami of the S2–S4 nerve roots. It exits the greater sciatic foramen, courses around the ischial spine within the sacrospinous ligaments, enters the perineum through the lesser sciatic foramen, and courses along the pudendal (Alcock) canal between the medial aspect of the obturator internus and ischiorectal fat.[1,2,3] The pudendal nerve is the main sensory supply to the perianal region, perineum, and external genitalia, as well as the motor fibers to the pelvic floor muscles, and the external anal and urethral sphincters.[4] The pudendal nerve ultimately divides into three terminal branches:

- *The inferior rectal nerve*, which provides cutaneous innervation of the external anal sphincter and perianal region.
- *The perineal nerve*, which splits into superficial and deep branches.
  - The *superficial branch* innervates the posterior two-thirds of the genitalia, as the posterior scrotal nerve in men and the posterior labial nerve in women (the anterior scrotal/labial nerve arises from the ilioinguinal nerve).
  - The *deep branch*, also known as the muscular branch, innervates the muscles of the perineum (superficial transverse

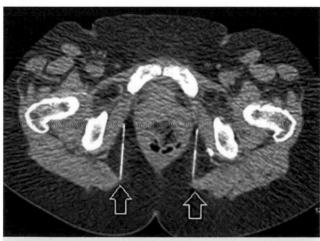

Fig. 42.1 Axial computed tomography (CT). Two 22-gauge Chiba needles (arrows) targeting the pudendal nerve at the medial border of the obturator internus.

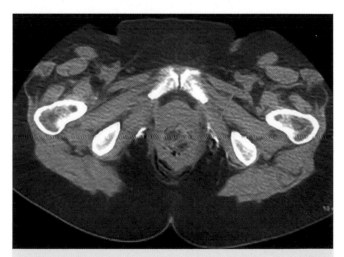

Fig. 42.2 Axial computed tomography (CT) after contrast injection into the pudendal canal demonstrating neurovascular bundle (arrow) along the medial wall of the obturator internus muscle.

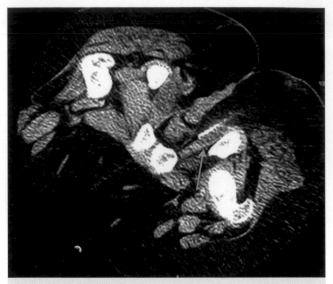

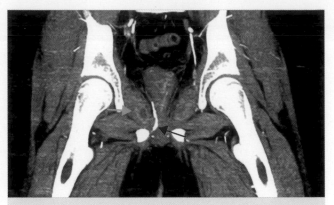

Fig. 42.5 Coronal computed tomography (CT) obtained 10 days after pudendal nerve cryoablation demonstrates a rare complication of a right pudendal arteriovenous fistula (orange arrow). Postablation changes are seen in the obturator internus muscle (green arrow).

Fig. 42.3 Axial computed tomography (CT) during cryoablation demonstrating ice-ball formation (green arrow) to target the pudendal nerve in the pudendal canal.

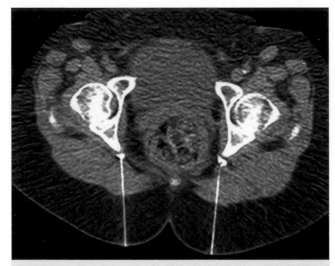

Fig. 42.4 Axial computed tomography (CT) after contrast injection targeting the pudendal nerve as it wraps around the ischial spine between the sacrospinous and sacrotuberous ligaments.

perineal muscle, bulbospongiosus, ischiocavernosus, and the external urethral sphincter).

- *The dorsal nerve of the penis/clitoris*, which supplies sensory innervation.

Pudendal neuralgia (PN) is a clinical syndrome defined as pain in the distribution of the pudendal nerve (e.g., vaginal, labial, perianal, and perineal regions). PN can be caused by a variety of etiologies, including trauma, pregnancy/childbirth, surgery, malignancy, and nerve entrapment among others. The Nantes criteria were originally developed to specifically diagnose pudendal nerve entrapment as a cause of PN. Diagnosis requires that all five characteristics are present: (1) pain in the territory of the pudendal nerve, (2) pain worsened by sitting, (3) not woken up at night by pain, (4) no objective sensory loss, and (5) a positive response to a pudendal nerve block.[5] However, there is no evidence that supports the presence of the clinical syndrome of PN with a diagnosis of nerve entrapment.[6] Pudendal nerve block is a valuable tool to diagnose the condition and manage the symptoms initially, preceding more invasive or permanent interventions such as neurolysis or surgical nerve decompression.

The pudendal nerve is typically targeted percutaneously along its path in the pudendal canal. An alternative potential target location is at the ischial spine, where the nerve is located between the sacrospinous and sacrotuberous ligaments (▶ Fig. 42.4). There are reports suggesting that performing the nerve block at both locations in a single session increases its effectiveness.[7] Steroids may also be injected with the anesthetic, but they are not required; they are most useful if there is suspicion of an inflammatory or entrapment etiology. The desired outcome is a pronounced sensory blockade for palliation from numbness along the nerve distribution. Several methods to achieve long-term pain relief have been employed and include neurolysis by chemodenervation, pulsed radiofrequency ablation, and cryoablation, as well as neuromodulation of the pudendal nerve and sacral nerve roots.[4,8,9]

If a patient's pain is predominantly lateralized, a unilateral nerve block may reduce the likelihood of unwanted side effects.[10,11] Complications are rare, but typically occur due to the close proximity of the pudendal nerve to the pudendal artery and vein, and include intravascular injection of anesthetic, bleeding, and vessel injury (▶ Fig. 42.5).

References

[1] Standring S. Gray's Anatomy: The Anatomical Basis of Clinical Practice. 39th ed. Elsevier; 2004

[2] Wolff BG, Fleshman JW, Beck DE, Pemberton JH, Wexner SD, eds. The ASCRS Textbook of Colon and Rectal Surgery. New York: Springer; 2007

[3] Robert R, Prat-Pradal D, Labat JJ, et al. Anatomic basis of chronic perineal pain: role of the pudendal nerve. Surg Radiol Anat. 1998; 20(2):93–98

[4] Hunter CW, Stovall B, Chen G, Carlson J, Levy R. Anatomy, pathophysiology and interventional therapies for chronic pelvic pain: a review. Pain Physician. 2018; 21(2):147–167

[5] Labat JJ, Riant T, Robert R, Amarenco G, Lefaucheur JP, Rigaud J. Diagnostic criteria for pudendal neuralgia by pudendal nerve entrapment (Nantes criteria). Neurourol Urodyn. 2008; 27(4):306–310

[6] Stav K, Dwyer PL, Roberts L. Pudendal neuralgia. Fact or fiction? Obstet Gynecol Surv. 2009; 64(3):190–199

[7] Kastler A, Puget J, Tiberghien F, Pellat J-M, Krainik A, Kastler B. Dual site pudendal nerve infiltration: more than just a diagnostic test? Pain Physician. 2018; 21(1):83–90

[8] Prologo JD, Lin RC, Williams R, Corn D. Percutaneous CT-guided cryoablation for the treatment of refractory pudendal neuralgia. Skeletal Radiol. 2015; 44 (5):709–714

[9] Richard HM, Marvel RP. CT-guided pulsed radiofrequency treatment for pudendal neuralgia. J Vasc Interv Radiol. 2014; 3):S109

[10] Vancaillie T, Eggermont J, Armstrong G, Jarvis S, Liu J, Beg N. Response to pudendal nerve block in women with pudendal neuralgia. Pain Med. 2012; 13(4):596–603

[11] Kurup AN, Morris JM, Schmit GD, et al. Neuroanatomic considerations in percutaneous tumor ablation. Radiographics. 2013; 33(4):1195–1215

43 Pelvic Congestion Syndrome

Roger Williams and Thomas Murphy

43.1 Case Presentation

A 37-year-old woman gravida 2, para 4 presented with a 12-year history of noncyclical pelvic pain. The patient was a Division 1 college athlete until 4 years ago, and recently was an active CrossFit athlete 5 days per week. Her exercise diminished to 1 day per week during her "attacks." Over the last 2 years her pain seemed to be more on the left than right. There was no history of trauma. She experienced only minimal relief with Advil. She had been hospitalized twice in the prior 18 months. During her second hospitalization, the obstetrician–gynecologist (OB/Gyn) physician ordered a pelvic ultrasound with Doppler evaluation, which made the diagnosis of pelvic congestion syndrome (PCS) (later confirmed by computed tomography [CT]) (▶ Fig. 43.1a, b).

43.2 Treatment

The patient presented to interventional radiology for treatment of her pelvic varicosities. Initial selective left gonadal venography demonstrated an incompetent vein and pelvic varicosities, which crossed the midline into the right pelvis (▶ Fig. 43.2). Coil embolization of the left gonadal/ovarian vein was performed using standard technique with a series of multiple detachable fibered coils ranging in size from 8 to 20 mm (▶ Fig. 43.3).

Retrograde embolization of the right gonadal vein was then performed, embolizing back to the more proximal pelvis using multiple detachable fibered coils ranging in size from 8 to 14 mm (▶ Fig. 43.4).

At 1-month, 3-month, 6-month, and 1-year follow-up evaluation, the patient reported near-complete resolution of her symptoms. She did report two episodes of pelvic pain: one during the 3-month follow-up, and the second at 1-year follow-up. Upon further questioning, both episodes correlated with menstruation.

43.3 Discussion

Currently, chronic pelvic pain in women has been defined as noncyclical pelvic pain lasting for more than 6 months.[1] Pelvic pain may be caused by a multitude of conditions, thus making a specific diagnosis difficult. The incidence of chronic pelvic pain in women aged between 18 and 50 years of age has been estimated to be approximately 15%.[1] In the USA, it is estimated that 35% of diagnostic laparoscopies and 15% of all hysterectomies have been performed because of chronic pelvic pain.[1]

In the majority of cases, symptoms are associated with the pelvic visceras: intestinal, urologic, gynecologic, and vascular etiologies. Higher resolution imaging techniques, as well as increased utilization of such imaging, has made diagnosis more accurate and less invasive than years past. This is especially so with vascular causes, affording referring clinicians the ability to correlate observed symptoms with imaging, thereby rapidly excluding other viscera from the differential.

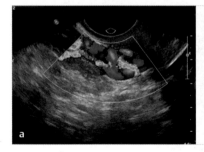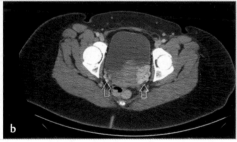

Fig. 43.1 Cross-sectional preprocedure imaging. (a) Ultrasound of the pelvis demonstrating extremely dilated pelvic venous structures likely representing ovarian veins. (b) Contrast-enhanced computed tomography (CT) scan of the pelvis demonstrating markedly dilated enhancing veins—left greater than right (arrows).

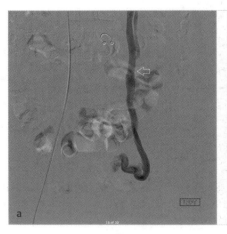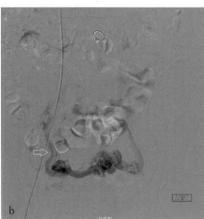

Fig. 43.2 Left gonadal venogram demonstrating an incompetent left ovarian vein (a, arrow) with communication to the right ovarian venous system (b, arrow).

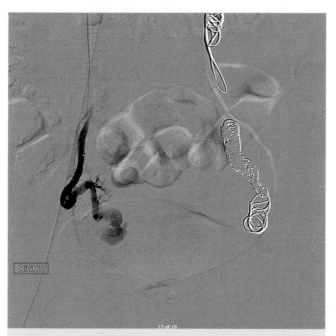

Fig. 43.3 Coil embolization of the left ovarian venous system with more proximal embolization to amputate tributary arcuate drainages.

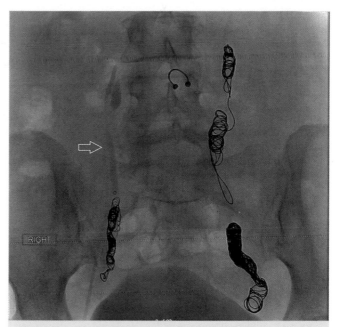

Fig. 43.4 Post distal embolization of the right gonadal vein with stasis of contrast (arrow) secondary to complete distal occlusion.

Pelvic varicose veins were first identified by Richet, in 1857. Subsequently, the term "pelvic venous congestion syndrome" was coined by Taylor in 1949.[2] In 1950, Topolanski-Sierra coined the term "chronic pelvic congestion" and demonstrated the relationship between chronic abdominal pain and pelvic varicose veins, as well as stressed the necessity of treatment.[3]

PCS results from incompetence of the gonadal veins, resulting in distention of pelvic veins; subsequent pain lasts longer than 6 months.[4,5,6] Although nonspecific, the suggested etiologies for PCS include physiologic, mechanical, vascular, and hormonal factors. PCS occurs most frequently in premenopausal multiparous women, and least commonly in postmenopausal women.[7] After menopause, the pain frequently subsides. During pregnancy, hormonal changes can cause massive dilation of up to 60 times the normal diameter of pelvic veins.[4] This significant distention of the pelvic venous system may persist for up to 6 months postpartum, as well as worsen with subsequent gestations.[4] As with varicosities of the lower extremities, venous hypertension causes reflux through the valves and leads to subsequent venous incompetence over time.

Pelvic varicosities are usually identified with pelvic ultrasound, CT, or magnetic resonance imaging (MRI). Because of the dependence on intrapelvic pressures for visualization of these venous structures, patients in the supine position may not generate enough hydrostatic pressure to cause venous distention, and the varices therefore may not be visualized on static imaging. If clinical suspicion persists, a dynamic (Valsalva) conventional diagnostic venogram can demonstrate the lack of valves or valvular insufficiency. In normal anatomic studies, the absence of valves in the left ovarian vein is noted in 13 to 15% of women; such an absence of valves is noted in only 6% in the right ovarian vein.[8] This is juxtaposed to valvular incompetence and reflux in 43% of symptomatic patients, with 31% occurring in the left and 41% in the right gonadal vein.[9]

A secondary cause of PCS is nutcracker syndrome, which is caused by the compression of the left renal vein by the superior mesenteric artery and the aorta. This impingement once again causes left renal venous hypertension, with resulting late stage left gonadal vein valvular incompetence and reflux.[10]

During conventional venograms, diagnosis of pelvic congestion includes a tortuous pelvic vein with a diameter greater than 4 mm, poor blood flow (less than 3 cm/s), and distended communicating veins.[5]

In 1993, Edwards et al described the first case of bilateral embolization of the ovarian vein to treat PCS.[11] Since then, innumerable case reports and nonrandomized studies have been reported, with a mean success rate of 75%.[12] Based on this, embolization is typically performed with coils, plugs, and sclerosant to occlude the gonadal vein once the venographic diagnosis is made.[13]

References

[1] APGO Educational Series on Women's Health Issues. Chronic pelvic pain: An Integrated approach. Crofton, MD: APGO; January 2000

[2] Taylor HC, Jr. Vascular congestion and hyperemia; their effect on function and structure in the female reproductive organs; the clinical aspects of the congestion-fibrosis syndrome. Am J Obstet Gynecol. 1949; 57(4):637–653

[3] Topolanski-Sierra R. Pelvic phlebography. Am J Obstet Gynecol. 1958; 76 (1):44–52

[4] Tu FF, Hahn D, Steege JF. Pelvic congestion syndrome-associated pelvic pain: a systematic review of diagnosis and management. Obstet Gynecol Surv. 2010; 65(5):332–340

[5] Beard RW, Highman JH, Pearce S, Reginald PW. Diagnosis of pelvic varicosities in women with chronic pelvic pain. Lancet. 1984; 2(8409):946–949

[6] Freedman J, Ganeshan A, Crowe PM. Pelvic congestion syndrome: the role of interventional radiology in the treatment of chronic pelvic pain. Postgrad Med J. 2010; 86(1022):704–710

[7] Liddle AD, Davies AH. Pelvic congestion syndrome: chronic pelvic pain caused by ovarian and internal iliac varices. Phlebology. 2007; 22(3):100–104

[8] Ahlberg NE, Bartley O, Chidekel N. Circumference of the left gonadal vein. An anatomical and statistical study. Acta Radiol Diagn (Stockh). 1965; 3(6): 503–512

[9] Ahlberg NE, Bartley O, Chidekel N. Right and left gonadal veins. An anatomical and statistical study. Acta Radiol Diagn (Stockh). 1966; 4(6): 593–601

[10] Scultetus AH, Villavicencio JL, Gillespie DL. The nutcracker syndrome: its role in the pelvic venous disorders. J Vasc Surg. 2001; 34(5):812–819

[11] Edwards RD, Robertson IR, MacLean AB, Hemingway AP. Case report: pelvic pain syndrome—successful treatment of a case by ovarian vein embolization. Clin Radiol. 1993; 47(6):429–431

[12] Daniels JP, Champaneria R, Shah L, Gupta JK, Birch J, Moss JG. Effectiveness of embolization or sclerotherapy of pelvic veins for reducing chronic pelvic pain: a systematic review. J Vasc Interv Radiol. 2016; 27(10):1478–1486.e8

[13] Capasso P, Simons C, Trotteur G, Dondelinger RF, Henroteaux D, Gaspard U. Treatment of symptomatic pelvic varices by ovarian vein embolization. Cardiovasc Intervent Radiol. 1997; 20(2):107–111

44 Caudal Block

Roger Williams and Thomas Murphy

44.1 Case Presentation

A 49-year-old man with a history of metastatic prostate cancer presented with left knee pain. He was currently being treated with Lupron, Abiraterone/Prednisone, and monthly Zometa. He stated that his prostate specific antigen (PSA) was over 100 ng/dL at diagnosis, and that he underwent left femoral rodding followed by postoperative radiation therapy. He was unclear about specifics of his radiation therapy other than that he underwent simulation, temporary tattoo placement, and approximately 2 weeks of treatments. He reported pelvic pain since radiation. He was currently admitted to the hospital for severe left-sided sciatic-type pain radiating down the left lower extremity. He underwent magnetic resonance imaging (MRI) of the lumbar spine demonstrating some extra-osseous metastatic disease with impingement of the S2 nerve root (▶ Fig. 44.1). He was admitted for pain control and radiation oncology consultation. Palliative medicine requested a consult from interventional radiology (IR) after radiation oncology stated that there was no role for treatment and persistent pain with analgesics.

History and physical examination demonstrated 9/10 pain with tenderness over the lower lumbar spine and sacrum. He had a normal range of motion and severe left radicular pain with 5+ strength bilaterally. All of these findings occurred alongside chronic pelvic pain for about 6 months.

Because of his diffuse axial disease and pelvic pain with radiculopathy, the decision at multidisciplinary tumor board was to perform a nerve block. Given the diffuse sclerotic osseous disease involving the lumbar spine and sacrum (▶ Fig. 44.2) with multilevel foraminal narrowing including at S2 cause, the decision was made to perform a caudal block. The plan was to obtain access via a trans-sacral hiatus (sacrococcygeal access) approach, with infusion to at least the L3 level.

The procedure was performed in standard fashion under computed tomography (CT) guidance via a trans-sacral approach (▶ Fig. 44.3, ▶ Fig. 44.4, ▶ Fig. 44.5, ▶ Fig. 44.6, and ▶ Fig. 44.7). The procedure was uneventful. After 1 hour of the caudal block, the patient reported partial pain relief in his pelvis and lower extremity, relating the pain to be 4/10. At 24 hours post-procedure, he was transitioned to oral analgesics, was able to ambulate without gait dysfunction, and reported significant improvement in his deep pelvic pain. Given the drastic decreased pain at 36 hours, particularly in the region of the pathologic neuropathy at S2, the patient was discharged that day.

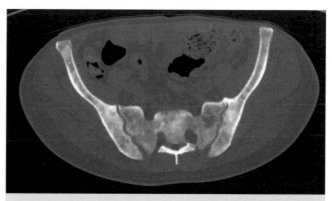

Fig. 44.2 Axial computed tomography (CT) of the pelvis demonstrating diffuse osteoblastic metastatic disease involving all osseous structures.

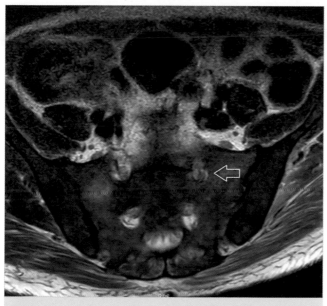

Fig. 44.1 T1 W axial magnetic resonance imaging (MRI) of the pelvis demonstrating extra-osseous disease impinging on the left of midline involving the left S2 foramen (arrow).

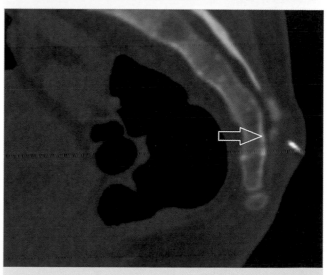

Fig. 44.3 Intraprocedural sagittally reconstructed computed tomography (CT) scan demonstrating the needle directed toward the sacral hiatus (arrow).

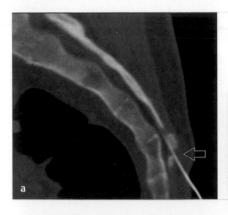

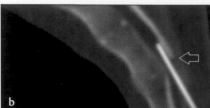

Fig. 44.4 (a, b) Following a trajectory change, the needle (arrows) is noted to be in line with the ventral sacrum.

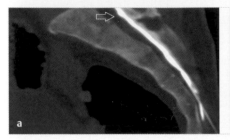

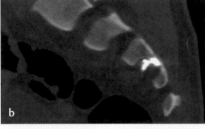

Fig. 44.5 (a, b) The needle was advanced toward S3 and remained extradural. Contrast is noted extending cephalad into the epidural space (arrow).

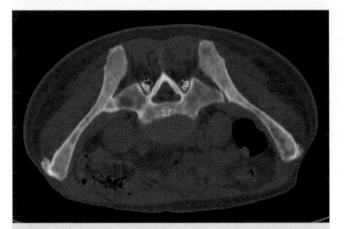

Fig. 44.6 Axial computed tomography (CT) scan following injection confirmed epidural placement with contrast noted diffusely in the epidural space (arrows).

44.2 Discussion

Radiologists were the first to perform caudal injections in the early 1900s, describing infusing a dilute solution of cocaine caudally through the sacral hiatus in a patient with an intractable sciatic pain.[1] The first use of corticosteroids into the epidural space via a caudal approach was performed in 1957 by Cappio.[2] He reported good results of approximately 67% of the 80 patients treated. Since that seminal report, there have been several prospective, retrospective, and meta-analyses studies demonstrating the efficacy of caudal blocks in palliating chronic back pain. The results, however, have been less favorable in controlling pelvic pain.

Fig. 44.7 Final sagittally reconstructed computed tomography (CT) image following analgesic and nonparticulate steroid injection. Note the epidural contrast (arrow) that is less dense than noted previously (compare to ▶ Fig. 44.5a) due to dilution following the therapeutic injection.

Indications of caudal epidural injection are chronic low back pain and failure of conservative therapy including bracing, and oral and/or intravenous analgesics. Additionally, caudal injections can be utilized in patients with sacral involvement (as in the case presented).

Anecdotally, given the high local concentration of corticosteroids over the inflamed sacral nerve roots (particularly S2–S4), deep pelvic pain has been successfully treated with caudal injection (▶ Fig. 44.6).[3] Given the pudendal supply from these nerves and extrapolating the experience with pudendal blockade, the relief seen with epidural caudal steroid injection can be presumed.

References

[1] Sicard JA. Les injections medica-menteuse extraduraqles per voie saracoccygiene. Comptes Renues des Senances de la Societe de Biolgie et de ses Filliales. 1901; 53:396–398

[2] Cappio M. Il trattamento Idrocortisonico per via epidurale sacrale delle lombosciatalgie. Reumatismo. 1957; 9(1):60–70

[3] Abdi S, Datta S, Trescot AM, et al. Epidural steroids in the management of chronic spinal pain: a systematic review. Pain Physician. 2007; 10(1):185–212

45 Superior Hypogastric Nerve Block I

Roger Williams and Thomas Murphy

45.1 Case Presentation

A 45-year-old Black/African-American woman presented with symptomatic fibroids. On prior imaging, the fibroids avidly enhanced on contrast magnetic resonance imaging (MRI). Pertinent history included heavy menses requiring multiple pads during the day and night, with her menstrual cycle lasting from 9 to 14 days monthly; her cycles, however, were highly variable. The patient also reported some dyspareunia and new-onset back pain. She declined myomectomy/hysterectomy, and was referred to interventional radiology for uterine artery embolization.

Prior to the clinic visit, the patient underwent a complete gynecologic evaluation including Pap smear and endometrial biopsy. Physical examination demonstrated a palpable uterus of about 12 to 16 weeks size compared to the gravid state. The patient stated that at that time she had increased dysmenorrhea over the previous few months, which was not palliated with over-the-counter nonsteroidal anti-inflammatory drugs (NSAIDs).

A superior hypogastric nerve block with local anesthetic and steroids was injected under fluoroscopic guidance during the fibroid embolization procedure (▶ Fig. 45.1). The patient experienced no significant cramping or pain 3 hours following the procedure. She reported her pain to be 2/10. The patient was discharged as an outpatient having received no oral or intravenous (IV) narcotics. She was counseled to take NSAIDs as directed and oral narcotics as needed. At 1-week follow-up call, the patient had no issues with pain and minimal cramping, which did not require narcotics.

45.2 Discussion

Superior hypogastric nerve block is a recognized therapy for chronic oncologic-based pelvic pain.[1,2] As in the case presented here, superior hypogastric neurolysis can also be performed in a woman with severe pelvic pain with cyclical hemorrhage thought to be secondary to large fibroids.

Initial postembolization pain usually peaks 6 to 8 hours after fibroid embolization, and lasts up to 24 hours. This initial pain is usually severe and caused primarily by tissue ischemia.[3,4] The more manageable outpatient pain occurs between 2 and 7 days post procedure, and is likely secondary to release of inflammatory cells triggered by cell death and may present with flu-like symptoms referred to as postembolization syndrome.[5,6] Postembolization syndrome has been noted to improve with preprocedural Superior Hypogastric Block (SHB).[7,8]

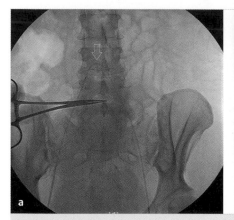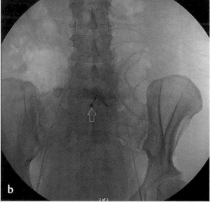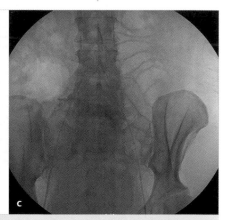

Fig. 45.1 (a) Following embolization of the left uterine artery and prior to relocating the catheter to the right uterine artery, the angiographic catheter (Roberts uterine artery catheter [RUC]; Cook Medical, Inc., Bloomington, IN) was used as a localizer for the aortic bifurcation (arrow). The L4–L5 interdisc space is identified with a hemostat. (b) A 22-G Chiba needle (arrow) was advanced to the cortex of L5, and contrast was injected to confirm extravascular location. (c) Following administration of the analgesic mixture of steroid and bupivacaine, the 22-G needle was removed. The final image demonstrates the dilute contrast tracing appropriately along the descending nerve roots.

References

[1] Abd-Elsayed A, ed. Pain: A Review Guide. Cham: Springer Nature Switzerland; 2019

[2] Plancarte R, Amescua C, Patt RB, Aldrete JA. Superior hypogastric plexus block for pelvic cancer pain. Anesthesiology. 1990; 73(2):236–239

[3] Ruuskanen A, Sipola P, Hippeläinen M, Wüstefeld M, Manninen H. Pain after uterine fibroid embolisation is associated with the severity of myometrial ischaemia on magnetic resonance imaging. Eur Radiol. 2009; 19(12):2977–2985

[4] Scheurig-Muenkler C, Wagner M, Franiel T, Hamm B, Kroencke TJ. Effect of uterine artery embolization on uterine and leiomyoma perfusion: evidence of transient myometrial ischemia on magnetic resonance imaging. J Vasc Interv Radiol. 2010; 21(9):1347–1353

[5] Spencer EB, Stratil P, Mizones H. Clinical and periprocedural pain management for uterine artery embolization. Semin Intervent Radiol. 2013; 30(4):354–363

[6] Worthington-Kirsch RL, Koller NE. Time course of pain after uterine artery embolization for fibroid disease. Medscape Womens Health. 2002; 7(2):4

[7] Pereira K, Morel-Ovalle LM, Taghipour M, et al. Superior hypogastric nerve block (SHNB) for pain control after uterine fibroid embolization (UFE): technique and troubleshooting. CVIR Endovasc. 2020; 3(1):50

[8] Pereira K, Morel-Ovalle LM, Wiemken TL, et al. Intraprocedural superior hypogastric nerve block allows same-day discharge following uterine artery embolization. J Vasc Interv Radiol. 2020; 31(3):388–392

46 Hypogastric Nerve Block II

Shenise Gilyard, Nariman Nezami, and Nima Kokabi

46.1 Case Presentation

A 52-year-old woman with locally advanced unresectable cervical cancer presented to the emergency department with uncontrolled vaginal bleeding and unremitting abdominal pain. She was being managed with vaginal packing and intravenous (IV) opiates. Throughout her hospital course, her pain continued to be a barrier to discharge despite treatment with local radiation and chemotherapy. Interventional radiology (IR) was consulted for pain management, and the patient was deemed to be an appropriate candidate for superior hypogastric plexus block (SHPB). The patient reported 10/10 pain prior to the procedure and 0/10 pain post-treatment. No immediate side effects were reported. ▶ Fig. 46.1 demonstrates the procedure performed for the patient (superior hypogastric nerve block [SHNB]).

46.2 Discussion

46.2.1 Superior Hypogastric Plexus Anatomy

The superior hypogastric plexus (SHP) provides sympathetic visceral innervation to the pelvic viscera including the uterus, descending colon, and rectum, except the ovaries and fallopian tubes.[1,2] The SHP receives nerve fibers from the celiac and inferior mesenteric plexuses, arising from L4 to S1.[2] The plexus is retroperitoneal and resides at the bifurcation of the common iliac arteries, at L5–S1. The ureters lie just lateral to the nervous plexus.[3]

Given the extent of visceral innervation of the SHP, nerve blockade has been used as a means to treat a wide range of pelvic pain etiologies. SHP block was first introduced in 1990 by Plancarte et al as a means of managing neurolyisis in patients with locally advanced cancer pain.[4] In this original study, 28 oncology patients were successfully managed using a posterior/Transdiscal approach to treat the SHP. The authors followed this study up with a 227-patient study validating SHPB as an effective means of achieving pain control in patients with advanced pelvic cancer.[5] Since then, SHPB has been adopted to manage a number of pelvic visceral pain etiologies including malignancy, chronic pelvic pain, and surgical pain.[6] SHP blockade has been widely employed in alleviating visceral pain from ovarian, cervical, bladder, rectal, and prostate malignancies.[7] A recent study demonstrated that SHPB in abdominal hysterectomy reduced the need for opiate analgesia.[1] One retrospective study found SHPB in uterine fibroid embolization results in significantly lower opiate usage than epidural anesthesia.[8] A recent study by Park et al found that SHPB significantly reduced required opiate analgesia in patients undergoing uterine fibroid embolization (Park, 2020).

The inferior hypogastric nerve conversely is not a purely sympathetic plexus. It contains sympathetic fibers from the hypogastric plexus, and visceral afferent fibers from pelvic viscera.[9] Nerve supply to the urinary bladder, corpora cavernosa, and urethra primarily arises from the inferior hypogastric plexus.[10] A case series described transscacral blockade of the inferior hypogastric plexus as a means of managing chronic pelvic pain.[9]

46.2.2 Indications

The American Society of Anesthesiology recommends considering sympathetic nerve blockade for short-term visceral pain management.[11]

46.2.3 Relative Contraindications

SHP anesthesia should not be performed in cases of local or systemic infection, coagulopathy, or anatomic aberrancies which

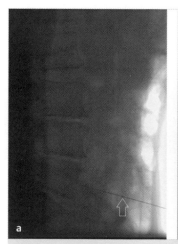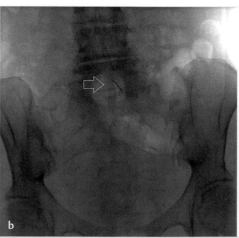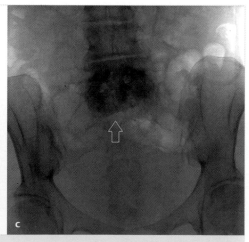

Fig. 46.1 Technical approach of superior hypogastric nerve block. (**a**) Cross-table lateral view of 22-gauge Chiba needle in the infraumbilical position angled toward the L5 vertebral body (arrow). (**b**) Posteroanterior view of the properly positioned needle before contrast administration (arrow). (**c**) Contrast pooling (arrow) along the anterior surface of the vertebral bodies in the location of the hypogastric plexus post contrast administration.

would preclude safe needle placement. Additionally, allergies to phenol are an additional contraindication.

46.2.4 Techniques

There are three methodologies which are in common practice, namely, posterior paravertebral, trans-diskal, and trans-abdominal approaches.

For diagnostic or temporary blockade, 6 to 8 mL of 25% bupivacaine is administered. For neurolysis, 6 to 10 mL of 10% phenol or 50% ethanol is injected.[12]

Posterior Paravertebral Approach

The trans-diskal approach evolved from the initial posterior paravertebral approach, in which two Chiba needles positioned at 45-degree angles are advanced lateral to the midline at the L4–L5 interspace and advanced so that the needle tip lies anterolateral to the L5–S1 disk space[12,13] (▶ Fig. 46.2). Bupivacaine is administered once retroperitoneal location was confirmed.

Trans-diskal Approach

A modified trans-diskal approach has been validated as a safe and effective method of performing hypogastric nerve blockade in multiple case series.[14] In a randomized control trial of trans-diskal approach versus classic blockade, Gamal et al demonstrated superior efficacy of the trans-diskal approach. Patients undergoing the trans-diskal approach had lower procedure time, no intravascular puncture, no urinary injury, and the ability to use a single needle.[15]

Under fluoroscopic guidance, the patient is positioned prone with a pillow placed under the iliac crest. The pillow placement is essential as this allows for opening of the intradiskal space at L5–S1.[14] A 22- to 25-gauge needle attached to a 5-mL syringe is advanced through the disk space under lateral fluoroscopic

positioning until resistance is lost. The needle is aspirated to confirm position (the absence of blood). Water-soluble contrast is then injected, and positioning is confirmed. Then 5 mL of neurolytic agent is administered. When withdrawing the needle, cephazolin 50 mg should be administered to prevent infection of the disk.[14]

In an effort to improve precision of needle targeting, computed tomography (CT)-guided posterior approach can be considered. Yang et al evaluated the efficacy of CT-guided hypogastric block for refractory menstrual pain due to adenomyosis or endometriosis.[16] The patient is positioned prone with a pillow placed under the pelvis. A CT scan with slice thickness of 3 mm is obtained through the pelvis to confirm the L5–S1 disk space. Puncture path is planned based upon the images. A paravertebral puncture is made anterolateral to the margin of the L5 vertebral body. The position is confirmed, and the needle is advanced to the depth as measured on cross-sectional imaging. A second puncture is made through the disk space. A solution of 2% lidocaine and iohexol (lipophilic contrast) is injected and distribution assessed on subsequent CT. If the solution distributed along the anterior margin of the psoas major muscle and the anterior margin of the disk space, the injection site is deemed appropriate (▶ Fig. 46.3).

Risks

Infection: Given the interruption of the disk space, there is an increased risk of diskitis. To reduce this risk, Erdine et al suggest administering 50 mg intradiskal cephazolin.[14]

Hemorrhage and off-target drug administration: Anatomically, there is a risk of interrupting vasculature. Once the disk is traversed, aspirate to ensure no blood flow. Inject contrast to ensure retroperitoneal placement in the extra-vascular space.

Anterior/Trans-abdominal Approach

The anterior approach has been increasingly employed as it is considered less technically challenging than the trans-diskal approach.[2] A randomized control trial of conventional medical analgesia versus anterior approach SHNB for uterine fibroid embolization demonstrated significant reduction in pain score among the SHNB group.[17] Using the method described by Kanazi et al[2], the patient is positioned prone in Trendelenburg at 15 degrees. The periumbilical region is prepped in usual sterile

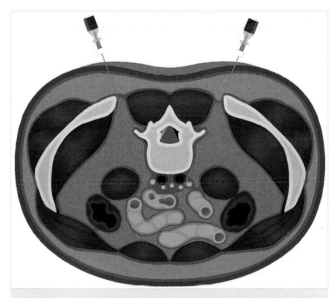

Fig. 46.2 Posterior paravertebral approach demonstrating two Chiba needles positioned at 45-degree angles with the bevel posterior to the superior hypogastric plexus.

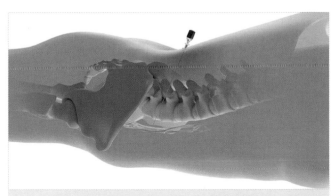

Fig. 46.3 Transdiscal approach at the L5–S1 interspace with the bevel angled toward the superior hypogastric plexus.

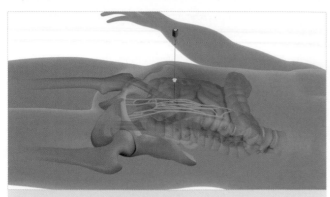

Fig. 46.4 Three-dimensional rendering of anterior transabdominal approach showing positioning of a Chiba needle relative to the superior hypogastric plexus.

fashion. Lidocaine is infiltrated 2 to 3 cm below the umbilicus and the region is prepped. From this position, a 22-gauge, 6-inch needle is advanced perpendicular to L5 vertebral body.[2] Once the needle contacts the inferior two-thirds of the vertebral body, the needle is aspirated to evaluate for vascular puncture. Radiopaque solution is injected and then assessed for spread over the anterior L5 vertebral body. After confirmation, 20 to 30 mL of bupivacaine is administered (▶ Fig. 46.4).

CT can be employed in an anterior approach as demonstrated by Cariati et al in a case series of 10 patients treated with SHPB for cancer pain.[18] This group completed a series of contiguous scans from the L3–L4 disk space to S1 to locate the aortic bifurcation. A 10-cm, 20-guage needle was introduced, and the needle tip was positioned anterior to the left iliac vein below the aortic bifurcation. The needle was aspirated to ensure extravascular position. To confirm position 1 mL of contrast was administered. An alcoholic solution was administered with 4 mL of bupivacaine HCL and 2 mL of contrast medium. This study found cessation of opioid therapy in 70% of the patients.[18]

Risks

Compared with the trans-diskal approach, there is a theoretical risk of damage to the overlying bowel and mesenteric plexus. Kanzi et al[2] recommend using a 22-guage needle to minimize consequential perforation risk. Additionally, bowel preparation should be performed prior to the procedure, as collapsed bowel tends to move away from the needle.[19] As with any intra-abdominal procedure there is a risk of intra-abdominal infection. With the numerous overlying vascular plexuses which accompany the hypogastric plexus, there is a risk of injecting into a vascular plexus.[18] Aspirating and injecting contrast prior to administration of the bupivacaine are essential to ensure targeted therapy.

Ultrasound-Guided Approach

Although less commonly used, an ultrasound-guided SHPB can be accomplished in areas with limited access to IR. Mishra et al positioned the patients supine and used an abdominal probe to identify the abdominal aorta and common iliac arteries to find L5.[19] The transducer was placed transversely once the L5 vertebrae was identified, and the skin was infiltrated with lidocaine 3 cm below the umbilicus.[19] A 22-guage Chiba needle was advanced anterior to the L5 vertebral body. After aspiration to confirm extra-vascular placement, bupivacaine was administered.[19]

References

[1] Aytuluk HG, Kale A, Astepe BS, Basol G, Balci C, Colak T. Superior hypogastric plexus blocks for postoperative pain management in abdominal hysterectomies. Clin J Pain. 2020; 36(1):41–46

[2] Kanazi GE, Perkins FM, Thakur R, Dotson E. New technique for superior hypogastric plexus block. Reg Anesth Pain Med. 1999; 24(5):473–476

[3] Bosscher H. Blockade of the superior hypogastric plexus block for visceral pelvic pain. Pain Pract. 2001; 1(2):162–170

[4] Plancarte R, Amescua C, Patt RB, Aldrete JA. Superior hypogastric plexus block for pelvic cancer pain. Anesthesiology. 1990; 73(2):236–239

[5] Plancarte R, de Leon-Casasola OA, El-Helaly M, Allende S, Lema MJ. Neurolytic superior hypogastric plexus block for chronic pelvic pain associated with cancer. Reg Anesth. 1997; 22(6):562–568

[6] Choi JW, Kim WH, Lee CJ, Sim WS, Park S, Chae HB. The optimal approach for a superior hypogastric plexus block. Pain Pract. 2018; 18(3):314–321

[7] Sindt JE, Brogan SE. Interventional treatments of cancer pain. Anesthesiol Clin. 2016; 34(2):317–339

[8] Binkert CA, Hirzel FC, Gutzeit A, Zollikofer CL, Hess T. Superior hypogastric nerve block to reduce pain after uterine artery embolization: advanced technique and comparison to epidural anesthesia. Cardiovasc Intervent Radiol. 2015; 38(5):1157–1161

[9] Schultz DM. Inferior hypogastric plexus blockade: a transsacral approach. Pain Physician. 2007; 10(6):757–763

[10] Röthlisberger R, Aurore V, Boemke S, et al. The anatomy of the male inferior hypogastric plexus: what should we know for nerve sparing surgery. Clin Anat. 2018; 31(6):788–796

[11] American Society of Anesthesiologists Task Force on Chronic Pain Management, American Society of Regional Anesthesia and Pain Medicine. Practice guidelines for chronic pain management: an updated report by the American Society of Anesthesiologists Task Force on Chronic Pain Management and the American Society of Regional Anesthesia and Pain Medicine. Anesthesiology. 2010; 112(4):810–833

[12] Gundavarpu S, Lema MJ. Superior hypogastric nerve block for pelvic pain. Tech Reg Anesth Pain Manage. 2001; 5(3):116–119

[13] de Leon-Casasola OA, Kent E, Lema MJ. Neurolytic superior hypogastric plexus block for chronic pelvic pain associated with cancer. Pain. 1993; 54(2):145–151

[14] Erdine S, Yucel A, Celik M, Talu GK. Transdiscal approach for hypogastric plexus block. Reg Anesth Pain Med. 2003; 28(4):304–308

[15] Gamal G, Helaly M, Labib YM. Superior hypogastric block: transdiscal versus classic posterior approach in pelvic cancer pain. Clin J Pain. 2006; 22(6):544–547

[16] Yang X, You J, Tao S, Zheng X, Xie K, Huang B. Computed tomography-guided superior hypogastric plexus block for secondary dysmenorrhea in perimenopausal women. Med Sci Monit. 2018; 24:5132–5138

[17] Rasuli P, Jolly EE, Hammond I, et al. Superior hypogastric nerve block for pain control in outpatient uterine artery embolization. J Vasc Interv Radiol. 2004; 15(12):1423–1429

[18] Cariati M, De Martini G, Pretolesi F, Roy MT. CT-guided superior hypogastric plexus block. J Comput Assist Tomogr. 2002; 26(3):428–431

[19] Mishra S, Bhatnagar S, Rana SP, Khurana D, Thulkar S. Efficacy of the anterior ultrasound-guided superior hypogastric plexus neurolysis in pelvic cancer pain in advanced gynecological cancer patients. Pain Med. 2013; 14(6):837–842

47 Coccydynia

Anthony Brown

47.1 Case Presentation

A 52-year-old man with a long history of back pain and depression presented to clinic for coccygeal pain. He had a history of two lumbar spine surgeries including a microdiskectomy and laminectomy for right lower extremity radiculopathy. He also had a history of several falls onto his tail bone. His pain was centered on the very low sacrum and tail bone, preventing him from sitting without an offloading cushion. The pain was reproduced by palpation of the coccyx and did not radiate. He did not have hyper- or hypomobility of the coccyx on examination. Interventions for his pain included epidural steroid injections at L4 and L5 as well as daily tramadol, acetaminophen, and naproxen. With medication his pain was 7/10; without medication his pain was unbearable.

Cross-sectional imaging of his pelvis and sacrum was negative for fracture, bone spur, or other visible pain generator. With this constellation of findings, he was diagnosed with idiopathic coccydynia refractory to conservative management.

47.2 Procedural Details

A ganglion impar nerve block (GIB) was performed (▶ Fig. 47.1). The patient was positioned prone on a fluoroscopy table. The sacrococcygeal junction was localized in anteroposterior and lateral projections. A 22-gauge spinal needle was advanced through the sacrococcygeal junction to just beyond the ventral border of the bone. Contrast injection within the presacral space demonstrated a comma-shaped appearance. At this point a mixture of local anesthetic and steroid was injected.

The patient had immediate improvement in his coccygeal pain (from 7/10 to 2/10). This effect lasted for 6 weeks, after which the patient returned for a repeat block which resulted in significant pain relief.

47.3 Discussion

Coccydynia is a rare and often vague sacrococcygeal pain syndrome that occurs in 1% of patients who complain of spinal pain. Coccygeal pain is five times more common in women than men and is most commonly noted after childbirth.[1,2] The etiologies of coccydynia are varied; however, in most patients it is post-traumatic or idiopathic. Nontraumatic coccydynia can result from spinal degenerative disease, hypermobility or hypomobility of the sacrococcygeal joint, obesity, infection, and cancers of the pelvis and anorectal region. Importantly, cases of chronic therapy recalcitrant idiopathic coccydynia can reflect somatization disorder and other psychological disturbances.[2,3,4]

Numerous treatment options are available for coccydynia ranging from conservative therapy to interventional procedures. Conservative treatment includes nonsteroidal anti-inflammatory drugs (NSAIDs), analgesic suppositories, hot or cold application, transcutaneous electrical nerve stimulation, coccygeal offloading cushions, and pelvic floor relaxation exercises. A percentage of patients do not respond, and interventional methods of pain relief are employed, including direct injection around the coccyx, caudal epidural block, ganglion impar block, neurolysis, and coccygectomy.

The ganglion impar is the most caudal sympathetic ganglion, located in the retroperitoneum behind the rectum at the level of the sacrococcygeal joint. Ganglion impar blockade was first described by Plancarte et al, but it is currently performed as image-guided procedure.[5] It can be used as a treatment option for chronic refractory coccydynia and pelvic pain. The injection is safe and most effective when anesthetic is combined with corticosteroid. The block can be repeated when the benefit wanes or if only partial pain relief is achieved. A statistically significant decrease in coccygeal pain and improvement in depressed mood has been shown to persist for up to 6 months after administration of GIB.[6]

47.4 Companion Case

A 60-year-old woman with history of stage III anal cancer was referred to the interventional pain clinic for tailbone pain. She was unable to sit due to pain, had pain when rising from a seated position, and had pain with ambulation. She had undergone multi-fraction radiation treatments to her pelvis for her anal cancer, resulting in cure of her cancer. However, due to these treatments she subsequently suffered a radiation-related,

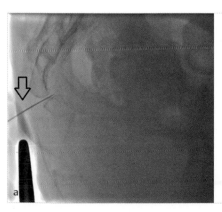
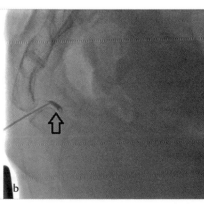

Fig. 47.1 (a, b) Intraprocedural images demonstrate 22-gauge needle access through the sacrococcygeal junction (arrow) in the lateral projection (a). Contrast injection demonstrates the typical comma-shaped appearance of the presacral retroperitoneum (arrow) at the anatomic location of the ganglion impar.

H-shaped sacral fracture with bilateral ala and S2 vertebral body involvement. She had no history of steroid use or vertebral compression fractures, and had a normal dual-energy X-ray absorptiometry (DEXA) from 1 year previously. She underwent sacral vertebral augmentation and had resolution of pain.

The patient presented 3 months post sacral augmentation, complaining of acute and different pain that was centered lower in her tailbone area. On physical examination, the patient reported 9/10 pain that was exacerbated by movement. Palpation of the low sacrum and coccyx revealed focal tenderness. Her pain was minimal in lying position. She had no bowel or bladder dysfunction, and had 5 + strength in her lower extremities. Her gait was steady but hesitant due to pain. Imaging revealed new fractures at the S4 vertebral body with soft tissue edema extending to the sacrococcygeal junction (▶ Fig. 47.2).

Given the magnetic resonance imaging (MRI) findings and significant mechanical pain associated with the fracture, cement augmentation of the fracture was considered the best choice for treatment of her pain. The patient was positioned prone and underwent monitored anesthesia care. A 13-gauge bone trocar was advanced in the midline from a caudal approach through S4 and S5 vertebral bodies (▶ Fig. 47.3). Sacral vertebral augmentation was performed with a total of 3 mL polymethylmethacrylate (PMMA). Given the coccygeal pain was associated with the S4 fracture, a ganglion impar block was performed to maximize pain relief and treat local inflammation (▶ Fig. 47.4).

47.5 Discussion

Patients who have a distal sacral or coccygeal fracture as a cause of pain can have the fracture stabilized with PMMA. There is scant literature regarding the efficacy of cement augmentation as a treatment for fractures near the sacrococcygeal junction. These fractures can be equally debilitating as fracture of the more proximal sacral elements. Dean et al initially reported a case of injection of PMMA in a patient with coccygeal fracture resulting in immediate relief of pain.[6] Augmentation for sacral fractures is a well-established treatment that results in marked reduction of pain after cement is injected into one or both affected ala, typically at the S1/2 levels.[7] Treatment of midline vertebral body fractures in the proximal sacrum is not typical as access is more technically difficult compared to the ala, and must often be performed from a lateral trans-iliac approach. The approach for augmentation in the distal sacrum and coccyx is opposite, as the ala are quite small and difficult to access. For this reason, PMMA injection directly into the midline vertebral body is performed, and has been shown to be efficacious for pain relief and stability. Distal sacral vertebral bodies are accessed from a direct caudal approach, and only a small volume of cement is required for stability. The addition of a ganglion impar block in patients with distal sacral fractures who undergo augmentation may add additional relief for local sacrococcygeal and sympathetic nervous inflammation.[5]

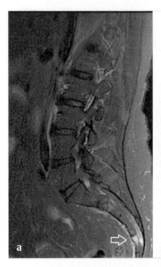
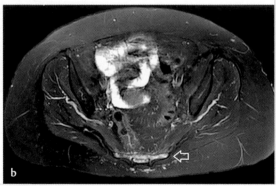

Fig. 47.2 (a, b) Sagittal and axial magnetic resonance images demonstrating localized edema (arrows) within the S4 vertebral body as well as the adjacent soft tissue near the sacrococcygeal junction.

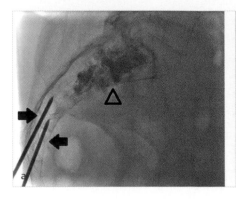
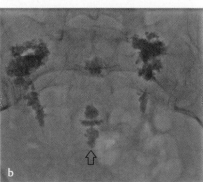

Fig. 47.3 Intraprocedural images demonstrating previous sacral augmentation change in the higher sacral elements (arrowhead) proximally. (a) A bone trocar is placed through S4 and S5 vertebral bodies in the midline as well as caudal ala (closed arrows). (b) Postaugmentation image demonstrating new polymethylmethacrylate (PMMA) in the midline at S4 (open arrow).

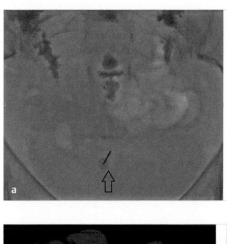

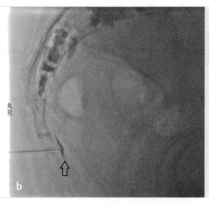

Fig. 47.4 (a) Intraprocedural images demonstrating a 22-gauge spinal needle placed in the midline at the sacrococcygeal junction (arrow). (b) The needle was advanced into the ventral presacral space, with placement confirmed by contrast injection (arrow). Then 4 mL of 0.5% bupivacaine with 40 mg methylprednisolone was injected for ganglion impar nerve block (GIB).

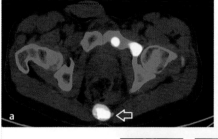

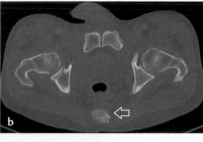

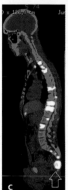

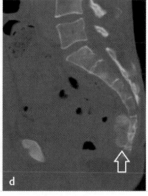

Fig. 47.5 Axial (a, b) and sagittal (c, d) positron emission tomography–computed tomography (PET/CT) images demonstrating extensive metastatic disease involving multiple bones. A focus of intense uptake with an expansile mass in the low sacrum at the sacrococcygeal junction (arrows) corresponded to the area of pain and tenderness.

47.6 Companion Case

A 38-year-old man with metastatic neuroendocrine cancer presented with intractable pain of the tailbone for more than 10 years, resulting in general loss of function and clinical depression. The patient had undergone two courses of radiation therapy to the affected area, and was taking regular narcotic medications with minimal relief. The patient reported pain with direct pressure to the coccyx including with sitting and with transition from sitting to standing. His insurance company had denied authorization for peptide receptor radionuclide therapy.

Positron emission tomography (PET) images demonstrated intense radionuclide uptake in the low sacrum at the sacrococcygeal junction secondary to an expansile metastatic lesion (▶ Fig. 47.5). Physical examination revealed pain with palpation of the coccyx that was both in the midline and to the right of midline, corresponding to the location of the metastasis. Focused cryoablation for palliation of pain was offered with sparing of his two S4 nerve roots, given his young age and desire to retain full sexual function (▶ Fig. 47.6).

After the procedure the patient experienced a gradual decrease in his pain over 2 weeks. He had no loss of bowel, bladder, or sexual function. His follow-up PET imaging demonstrated persistent uptake at the periphery of the lesion (▶ Fig. 47.7), but he rated his pain as 3/10 at that point and was satisfied with his relief.

47.7 Discussion

Tumors of the sacrococcygeal junction may result in severe pain and debility due to displacement of adjacent structures and de stabilization of the involved bone. The most common tumors involving the coccyx include chordoma, giant cell tumor, and metastatic disease. Treatment for tumors at the sacrococcygeal junction includes surgery, radiation, embolization, and ablation. Cryoablation has been shown to be effective for palliation of painful tumors of bone, including those at the sacrococcygeal junction. The level of aggressiveness of the ablation should be tailored to the goals of the patient as well as the potential complications in patients with preserved neurologic function. Cryoablation has excellent safety profile when performed using CT with the advantage of allowing for intraprocedural visualization of the

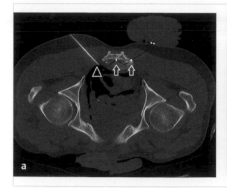
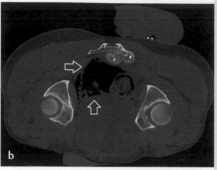

Fig. 47.6 **(a)** Images from an intraprocedural ablation procedure demonstrating cryoablation probe tips (arrows) directed from a caudal approach within the midline and right aspect of the expansile mass at the sacrococcygeal junction. A separate needle (arrowhead) was advanced to the presacral space, and protective CO_2 dissection of the rectum was performed during ablation. **(b)** An axial image obtained more cranially demonstrating the probes to be well positioned in the expansile mass with good dissection of soft tissue in the presacral space (arrows = CO_2 gas).

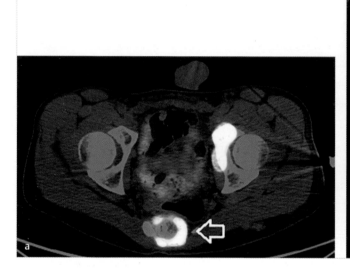
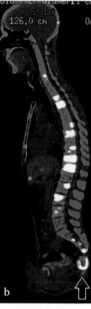

Fig. 47.7 **(a, b)** Positron emission tomography (PET) images demonstrating postablation reduction in avidity (compare with ▶ Fig. 47.5) of the mass at the sacrococcygeal junction (arrow). This reduction in avidity corresponded to significant improvement in the patient's pain.

ablation margin. However, unlike in the soft tissue visualizing the ice-ball may be difficult in bone. Therefore, cryoablation in the sacrum requires preprocedural planning with an understanding of which nerve roots are at risk during ablation and how injury to those nerves may manifest clinically. If there is potential for encroachment on the sciatic or pudendal nerves, precise needle positioning, use of gas or hydrodissection, and neurologic monitoring during ablation are all useful for protection.[8,9]

The nerve roots most likely to sustain damage during ablation at the sacrococcygeal junction are the S3–S5 nerve roots and may result in bowel, bladder, or sexual dysfunction. Motor function is unlikely to be affected. Sparing of at least one S3 nerve root is essential for preservation of erectile function and will also result in preserved bowel and bladder function in the majority of patients.[10] When both S4 nerve roots are spared, the patient's sexual, bowel, and bladder function should be completely preserved.[11]

References

[1] Dampc B, Słowiński K. Coccygodynia—pathogenesis, diagnostics and therapy. Review of the writing. Pol Przegl Chir. 2017; 89(4):33–40

[2] Gonnade N, Mehta N, Khera PS, Kumar D, Rajagopal R, Sharma PK. Ganglion impar block in patients with chronic coccydynia. Indian J Radiol Imaging. 2017; 27(3):324–328

[3] Kodumuri P, Raghuvanshi S, Bommireddy R, Klezl Z. Coccydynia—could age, trauma and body mass index be independent prognostic factors for outcomes of intervention? Ann R Coll Surg Engl. 2018; 100(1):12–15

[4] Sencan S, Cuce I, Karabiyik O, Demir FU, Ercalik T, Gunduz OH. The influence of coccygeal dynamic patterns on ganglion impar block treatment results in chronic coccygodynia. Interv Neuroradiol. 2018; 24 (5):580–585

[5] Plancarte R, Amescua C, Patt RB, Allende S. Presacral blockade of the ganglion of Walther (ganglion impar). Anesthesiology. 1990; 73:A751

[6] Dean LM, Syed MI, Jan SA, et al. Coccygeoplasty: treatment for fractures of the coccyx. J Vasc Interv Radiol. 2006; 17(5):909–912

[7] Chandra V, Wajswol E, Shukla P, Contractor S, Kumar A. Safety and efficacy of sacroplasty for sacral fractures: a systematic review and meta-analysis. J Vasc Interv Radiol. 2019; 30(11):1845–1854

[8] Kurup AN, Woodrum DA, Morris JM, et al. Cryoablation of recurrent sacrococcygeal tumors. J Vasc Interv Radiol. 2012; 23(8):1070–1075

[9] Kurup AN, Morris JM, Schmit GD, et al. Neuroanatomic considerations in percutaneous tumor ablation. Radiographics. 2013; 33(4):1195–1215

[10] Li CJ, Liu XZ, Zhou GX, et al. [Impact of sacral nerve root resection on the erectile and ejaculatory function of the sacral tumor patient] [in Chinese]. Zhonghua Nan Ke Xue. 2015; 21(3):251–255

[11] Zoccali C, Skoch J, Patel AS, Walter CM, Maykowski P, Baaj AA. Residual neurological function after sacral root resection during en-bloc sacrectomy: a systematic review. Eur Spine J. 2016; 25(12):3925–3931

48 Regenerative Medicine—Mesenchymal Stromal Cells

R. Amadeus Mason and Kenneth Mautner

48.1 Introduction

An appropriateness criterion should be utilized when considering a patient for lumbar intradiskal treatment because of the likelihood of postprocedure diskitis and significant postprocedure pain that commonly occurs after the procedure. The ideal patient will be between the age of 18 and 60 years of age with axial lower back pain that is worse with sitting, flexion, and twisting at the waist. A recent lumbar magnetic resonance imaging (MRI) scan should demonstrate disk degeneration with or without disk herniation, with preservation of at least 50% of the disk height. There may be an annular tear as well (i.e., high intensity zone [HIZ]) present at the level(s) of interest. Radicular symptoms from either a chemical or mechanical radiculitis may be absent or present. Conservative measures will have failed in most patients including: physical therapy, chiropractic care, massage, acupuncture, and epidural steroid injections (with no lasting long-term benefit).

48.2 Case Presentation

A 40-year-old woman presented with axial lower back pain (left greater than right) after falling off a porch 3 years previously. She consulted an orthopedist who ordered a lumbar MRI, after which the orthopedist recommended a transforaminal epidural steroid injection. The patient underwent two such procedures in 2017, and two in 2018. She also completed physical therapy, acupuncture, and chiropractic care. With no significant improvement after those measures, she presented to a neurosurgeon who recommended a repeat epidural injection at L5–S1, which was completed in January of 2019, and a left hip corticosteroid infection to determine if the hip was contributing to her low back pain. She reported no significant improvement from either of those procedures.

At this point, she had a sitting tolerance of approximately 30 minutes, with pain occasionally radiating to the lateral thighs. Her pain improved with rest and walking, but was worse with bowel movements. A visual analog scale assessment at its worse was 7 to 8 out of 10, and on average was 5 to 6 out of 10. She was taking some ibuprofen as needed for pain, and

had previously been taking meloxicam. An MRI in February 2019 demonstrated lumbar degenerative disk disease most notable at L5–S1, with a small leftward herniation and annular tearing, but no significant stenosis. Some mild multifidus atrophy and facet arthropathy were also noted. After an at length discussion with the patient, she decided to proceed with an intradiskal injection of bone marrow concentrate (BMC) with Platelet-rich plasma (PRP) at L5–S1. The procedure was performed in standard fashion without complication.

At 14 weeks post treatment she reported 50 to 60% improvement in her lower back pain and sitting intolerance. She reported waxing and waning clinical course after the procedure, but described steady improvement overall. In comparison to the preprocedure MRI, a repeat MRI demonstrated improved disk hydration at L5–S1 (▶ Fig. 48.1). It was expected that she would continue to have additional improvement and postprocedural rehabilitation with a focus on weight loss, multifidus and transversus abdominus muscle activation, and strengthening.

48.3 Discussion

48.3.1 Brief History of Regenerative Medicine and MSCs

Mesenchymal stromal cells (MSCs) can be isolated from a variety of tissues, including bone marrow, adipose tissue, umbilical cord blood tissue, and synovial tissue.[1] These cells are of interest within the field of regenerative orthopedics due to their potential for pluripotent differentiation into multiple tissue types, including bone, cartilage muscle, tendon, ligament, and adipose.[2] The first application of MSCs in orthopedics occurred in the 1970s when bone marrow allografts demonstrated efficacy in reversing osteonecrosis and osteopetrosis in murine models.[3,4,5,6] Hernigou et al first published a similar application in humans in 1997 with the reconstruction of an osteonecrotic humeral head following human leukocyte antigen compatible bone marrow transplantation.[7] This was later expanded to autologous bone marrow grafting in conjunction with core decompression (CD) as a therapy for hip osteonecrosis,[8] and the addition of bone

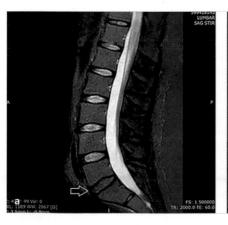
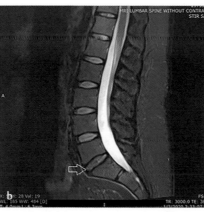

Fig. 48.1 Pre- and postprocedure magnetic resonance imaging (MRI) demonstrating improved disk hydration at L5–S1 (arrows).

marrow plus CD was demonstrated to confer superior outcomes than CD alone.[9] Centeno et al were the first to publish a nonsurgical orthopedic application of MSCs with a case study reporting pain and functional improvements following percutaneous intra-articular injection of bone marrow–derived, culture-expanded MSCs for the treatment of hip osteoarthritis (OA).[10] Since then, several other studies have been published on the topic of MSCs for treating musculoskeletal pathology.

48.3.2 Rationale for Use and Mechanisms of Action

Regenerative medicine is an emerging industry in health care and is expected to reach 8 billion US dollars by 2020.[11] Regenerative medicine uses cellular mechanisms to regain normal tissue function. MSCs produce and secrete a variety of growth factors, chemokines, and cytokines, which play a role in arteriogenesis, protection of renal and limb from tissue injury, promoting neovascularization, and increasing angiogenesis. MSC secretion is derived from endosomes; however, its function is not completely understood. MSCs likely carry cellular materials, including nucleic acids, protein, and lipids, from secreting cells to receiving cells. Cellular material is secreted to the extracellular environment via exosomes, which have abundant enzymes to maintain homeostasis in the tissue and respond to the surrounding environment, particularly if the environment is affected by injury or damage.[12] Multiple mechanisms have been theorized that may contribute to the therapeutic potential of MSCs in orthopedic use including BMC and adipose tissue derived stem cells.

BMC preparations are centrifuged to concentrate the product to obtain MSCs, hematopoietic stem cells, platelets, and cytokines, including platelet-derived growth factor, transforming growth factor-b, interleukin (IL)-1 receptor antagonist, and bone morphogenetic proteins 2 and 7. The various cytokines in BMC are known to promote stem cell differentiation and proliferation.[13]

Bone marrow derived stem cells can be derived in two ways: cultured and noncultured. Cultured cells undergo an in-vitro process to increase cell count by several hundred to thousandfold. Noncultured cells are used directly after concentrating the cells from the initial aspirate by centrifugation.[13] MSCs derived from bone marrow have the potential to differentiate into bone, cartilage, muscle, and tendon. They also promote the secretion of transforming growth factor-b, vascular epidermal growth factor, basic fibroblast growth factor, and other factors to recruit neighboring cells to stimulate tissue repair.[13]

Adipose tissue derived stromal cells (ASCs) have a very rich blood supply and can help with tissue repair. ASCs can be harvested in one of two ways. The first involves washing the adipose tissue, digesting the extracellular matrix, neutralizing, and rewashing the suspension. The second is via micro-fragmentation which involves lipo-aspiration.[13] One method for the micro-fragmentation of adipose tissue is processing utilizing a device containing saline which is washed and filtered and then broken up by steel beads to release components including oils, connective tissue, and blood components. There are several mechanisms by which ASCs may contribute to tissue repair and regeneration. ASCs can secrete cytokines and growth factors in a paracrine manner similar to bone marrow derived MSCs.

Additionally, ASCs can recruit endogenous stem cells at the site of tissue damage to promote differentiation. Lastly, ASCs are believed to release antioxidants and free radicals to remove toxic substances.[13] As previously mentioned, there are many sources of MSCs. In the United States, currently, the Food and Drug Administration (FDA) regulations restrict the use of MSCs to BMC or micro-fragmented adipose tissue (MFAT) for orthopedic use. Other sources of MSCs include stromal vascular fraction (SVF) derived from enzymatically processed adipose tissue and culture-expanded bone marrow or adipose-derived MSCs, among others.

48.3.3 Evidence in Other Joints and Tissues

Numerous studies have now been published on the efficacy of MSCs for treatment of orthopedic conditions using a variety of sources, from adipose tissue to synovium and culture-expanded as well as same-day grafting. Since it is the most ubiquitous FDA-approved MSC source documented in the literature, evidence for use of BMC will be summarized here. As previously discussed, many studies have evaluated the efficacy of autologous BMC for the treatment of Osteonecrosis (ON) of the hip.[7,8,14] Although a handful of studies showed equivocal results,[15,16,17] the majority of publications do support the use of BMC for treatment of femoral head ON, particularly in stage I or II disease.[18,19,20,21,22,23,24,25,26] The literature also supports the use of BMC for treatment of Avascular necrosis (AVN) of the talus[24,27,28] although, as of this writing, it has not shown clear efficacy for humeral head AVN.[29] Percutaneous subchondral BMC injection for knee osteonecrosis with advanced OA has been shown to be equally as effective as total knee arthroplasty with fewer complications.[30]

In addition to applications for AVN, much of the literature on BMC is on the topic of OA. Although two studies showed similar outcomes in BMC-treated patients versus placebo group treated with intra-articular saline,[31,32] the majority of case series and randomized controlled trials have shown improvements in pain and functional outcomes in patients treated with BMC for knee OA.[33,34,35,36] Additionally, it is important to keep in mind that dosage has been shown to affect results. Patients receiving a minimum of $>4 \times 10^8$ total nucleated cells (TNCs) for intra-articular knee injection demonstrated superior outcomes compared with those who received a smaller number.[37] BMC has also been shown to be effective in a limited number of studies for shoulder OA[38] and hip OA,[39] although there does appear to be a higher likelihood of success in patients under the age of 55 when treating hips.[39] For the treatment of ankle pathology, studies support the use of BMC for augmentation of surgical treatment of osteochondral lesions of the talus.[40,41,42,43]

Regarding tendons, one recent study showed promising results for treatment of lateral epicondylitis with BMC injection in a case series of 30 patients with significant improvements in outcomes at 6 weeks post-procedure.[44] BMC augmentation of surgical rotator cuff repair demonstrated superior outcomes to surgical repair alone at 10-year follow-up, and those patients with higher cell counts at the time of augmentation showed greater tendon integrity at long-term follow-up.[45] Nonsurgical treatment of rotator cuff pathology with percutaneous BMC injection has also shown significant improvements in pain and function at up to 2-year follow-up in a large case series[38] and at 3-month follow-up in a smaller case control study compared with physical therapy alone.[46] Successful treatments of anterior cruciate ligament tears with < 1 cm retraction via percutaneous, fluoroscopically guided BMC injection have been evaluated in two published case series, with improvements seen in ligament integrity, pain, and functional scores.[47,48]

For applications in the spine, the majority of studies investigate the use of cultured MSCs for intradiskal treatment. Pettine et al showed improvements in the Owestry Disability Index, visual analog scale, and, in some cases, improvements in Pfirrmann grading in a case series of patients with diskogenic low back pain treated with percutaneous intradiskal injection of BMC with follow-up data reports at 12, 24, and 36 months.[49,50,51] At the final follow-up, data was consistent with studies in other regions showing a positive dose–response correlation with the number of cells injected.[51]

Although the evidence for the use of MSCs for several musculoskeletal tissue types of various pathogenic etiology is very promising, there remains the need for continued investigation via multicenter, well-powered randomized controlled trials.[52]

48.3.4 Postprocedure Course

Rehabilitation is an integral part of the treatment process for many musculoskeletal disorders.[53] Development of effective rehabilitation protocols is an important objective in order to elicit maximum efficacy following regenerative therapies.

Current understanding of the tissue healing process comes mostly from animal studies, from which three phases of the healing cascade are commonly described: inflammatory, proliferative, and remodeling.[54,55,56] The inflammatory phase lasts from 4 to 7 days, during which inflammatory cells such as monocytes and macrophages enter the site of injury and clean up cellular debris.[57] In the proliferative phase, there is neovascularization with subsequent formation of granulation tissue and upregulation of fibroblasts.[57] Around week 6, the maturation phase begins, with functional tissue being formed.[57] This process can continue for up to 1 year after the initial injury.

Understanding of this basic framework has guided clinicians in developing rehabilitation protocols after orthobiologic cellular injections with phases to mirror those of the healing process.[58,59] For postinjection days 0 to 3, the inflammatory cascade is allowed to proceed with relative rest of the affected structures. Pain control is a priority, with nonsteroidal anti-inflammatory drugs (NSAIDs) and icing often avoided due to their anti-inflammatory nature.[60,61] For postinjection days 3 to 14, there is a gradual transition to weight bearing as tolerated and full range of motion exercises. Mechanical stress on healing tendons during the proliferative phase has been shown to improve regeneration.[62]

For postinjection weeks 2 to 4, as the proliferative phase proceeds, strength and endurance training will be added in addition to full range of motion exercises. A progressive strengthening program starting with isometric to concentric then to eccentric exercises is recommended.[58] Proprioceptive training can be initiated as well, although it is not a common component of existing rehabilitation protocols.[58,63]

For postinjection weeks 5 and beyond, there is a gradual return to full activity. However, there is not yet a consensus regarding the exact timing of returning to full sports and/or daily functional activities.[58]

There is currently heterogeneity among existing protocols. Further research is needed to determine the specific timing and types of stretching and strengthening exercises, duration of rest, timing of resumption of normal activity, and necessity of therapist supervision.[58]

Close postprocedure follow-up is critical to ensure no significant prolonged or worsening pain, which can be indicative of diskitis. Also, appropriate postprocedure pain control is necessary. A 5 to 7 days prescription of oxycodone with 1 to 2 days of 2 mg hydromorphone tablets is reasonable for severe pain. A prescription for a muscle relaxant should also be considered to help deal with the significant paraspinal muscle spasms that commonly occur post-procedure.

References

[1] Sensebé L, Bourin P. Mesenchymal stem cells for therapeutic purposes. Transplantation. 2009; 87(9) Suppl:S49–S53

[2] Caplan AI. Mesenchymal stem cells. J Orthop Res. 1991; 9(5):641–650

[3] Walker DG. Control of bone resorption by hematopoietic tissue. The induction and reversal of congenital osteopetrosis in mice through use of bone marrow and splenic transplants. J Exp Med. 1975; 142(3):651–663

[4] Walker DG. Spleen cells transmit osteopetrosis in mice. Science. 1975; 190 (4216):785–787

[5] Walker DG. Bone resorption restored in osteopetrotic mice by transplants of normal bone marrow and spleen cells. Science. 1975; 190(4216):784–785

[6] Walker DG. Experimental osteopetrosis. Clin Orthop Relat Res. 1975(97): 785–787

[7] Hernigou P, Bernaudin F, Reinert P, Kuentz M, Vernant JP. Bone-marrow transplantation in sickle-cell disease. Effect on osteonecrosis: a case report with a four-year follow-up. J Bone Joint Surg Am. 1997; 79(11):1726–1730

[8] Hernigou P, Beaujean F. Treatment of osteonecrosis with autologous bone marrow grafting. Clin Orthop Relat Res. 2002(405):14–23

[9] Gangji V, Hauzeur J-P, Matos C, De Maertelaer V, Toungouz M, Lambermont M.. Treatment of osteonecrosis of the femoral head with implantation of autologous bone-marrow cells. A pilot study. J Bone Joint Surg Am. 2004; 86 (6):1153–1160

[10] Centeno CJ, Kisiday J, Freeman M, Schultz JR. Partial regeneration of the human hip via autologous bone marrow nucleated cell transfer: A case study. Pain Physician. 2006; 9(3):253–256

[11] Andia I, Maffulli N. Biological therapies in regenerative sports medicine. Sports Med. 2017; 47(5):807–828

[12] Lai RC, Yeo RW, Lim SK. Mesenchymal stem cell exosomes. Semin Cell Dev Biol. 2015; 40:82–88

[13] Borg-Stein J, Osoria HL, Hayano T. Regenerative sports medicine: past, present, and future (adapted from the PASSOR Legacy Award Presentation; AAPMR; October 2016). PM R. 2018; 10(10):1083–1105

[14] Gangji V, Hauzeur JP. Treatment of osteonecrosis of the femoral head with implantation of autologous bone-marrow cells. Surgical technique. J Bone Joint Surg Am. 2005; 87(Pt 1) Suppl 1:106–112

[15] Cruz-Pardos A, Garcia-Rey E, Ortega-Chamarro JA, Duran-Manrique D, Gomez-Barrena E. Mid-term comparative outcomes of autologous bone-marrow concentration to treat osteonecrosis of the femoral head in standard practice. Hip Int. 2016; 26(5):432–437

[16] Hauzeur JP, De Maertelaer V, Baudoux E, Malaise M, Beguin Y, Gangji V. Inefficacy of autologous bone marrow concentrate in stage three osteonecrosis: a randomized controlled double-blind trial. Int Orthop. 2018; 42(7):1429–1435

[17] Nally FJ, Zanotti G, Buttaro MA, et al. THA conversion rate comparing decompression alone, with autologous bone graft or stem cells in osteonecrosis. Hip Int. 2018; 28(2):189–193

[18] Daltro GC, Fortuna V, de Souza ES, et al. Efficacy of autologous stem cell-based therapy for osteonecrosis of the femoral head in sickle cell disease: a five-year follow-up study. Stem Cell Res Ther. 2015; 6(1):110

[19] Persiani P, De Cristo C, Graci J, Noia G, Gurzì M, Villani C. Stage-related results in treatment of hip osteonecrosis with core-decompression and autologous mesenchymal stem cells. Acta Orthop Belg. 2015; 81(3):406–412

[20] Zhao D, Liu B, Wang B, et al. Autologous bone marrow mesenchymal stem cells associated with tantalum rod implantation and vascularized iliac

grafting for the treatment of end-stage osteonecrosis of the femoral head. BioMed Res Int. 2015; 2015:240506

[21] Mishima H, Sugaya H, Yoshioka T, et al. The safety and efficacy of combined autologous concentrated bone marrow grafting and low-intensity pulsed ultrasound in the treatment of osteonecrosis of the femoral head. Eur J Orthop Surg Traumatol. 2016; 26(3):293–298

[22] Pepke W, Kasten P, Beckmann NA, Janicki P, Egermann M. Core decompression and autologous bone marrow concentrate for treatment of femoral head osteonecrosis: a randomized prospective study. Orthop Rev (Pavia). 2016; 8(1):6162

[23] Pilge H, Bittersohl B, Schneppendahl J, et al. Bone marrow aspirate concentrate in combination with intravenous Iloprost increases bone healing in patients with avascular necrosis of the femoral head: a matched pair analysis. Orthop Rev (Pavia). 2017; 8(4):6902

[24] Hernigou P, Dubory A, Homma Y, et al. Cell therapy versus simultaneous contralateral decompression in symptomatic corticosteroid osteonecrosis: a thirty year follow-up prospective randomized study of one hundred and twenty five adult patients. Int Orthop. 2018; 42(7):1639–1649

[25] Hernigou P, Thiebaut B, Housset V, et al. Stem cell therapy in bilateral osteonecrosis: computer-assisted surgery versus conventional fluoroscopic technique on the contralateral side. Int Orthop. 2018; 42(7):1593–1598

[26] Houdek MT, Wyles CC, Collins MS, et al. Stem cells combined with platelet-rich plasma effectively treat corticosteroid-induced osteonecrosis of the hip: a prospective study. Clin Orthop Relat Res. 2018; 476(2):388–397

[27] Hernigou P, Dubory A, Flouzat Lachaniette CH, Khaled I, Chevallier N, Rouard H. Stem cell therapy in early post-traumatic talus osteonecrosis. Int Orthop. 2018; 42(12):2949–2956

[28] Hernigou P, Guissou I, Homma Y, et al. Percutaneous injection of bone marrow mesenchymal stem cells for ankle non-unions decreases complications in patients with diabetes. Int Orthop. 2015; 39(8):1639–1643

[29] Makihara T, Yoshioka T, Sugaya H, Yamazaki M, Mishima H. Autologous concentrated bone marrow grafting for the treatment of osteonecrosis of the humeral head: a report of five shoulders in four cases. Case Rep Orthop. 2017; 2017:4898057

[30] Hernigou P, Auregan JC, Dubory A, Flouzat-Lachaniette CH, Chevallier N, Rouard H. Subchondral stem cell therapy versus contralateral total knee arthroplasty for osteoarthritis following secondary osteonecrosis of the knee. Int Orthop. 2018; 42(11):2563–2571

[31] Shapiro SA, Kazmerchak SE, Heckman MG, Zubair AC, O'Connor MI. A prospective, single-blind, placebo-controlled trial of bone marrow aspirate concentrate for knee osteoarthritis. Am J Sports Med. 2017; 45(1):82–90

[32] Shapiro SA, Arthurs JR, Heckman MG, et al. Quantitative T2 MRI mapping and 12-month follow-up in a randomized, blinded, placebo controlled trial of bone marrow aspiration and concentration for osteoarthritis of the knees. Cartilage. 2019; 10(4):432–443

[33] Centeno C, Pitts J, Al-Sayegh H, Freeman M. Efficacy of autologous bone marrow concentrate for knee osteoarthritis with and without adipose graft. BioMed Res Int. 2014; 2014:370621

[34] Centeno C, Sheinkop M, Dodson E, et al. A specific protocol of autologous bone marrow concentrate and platelet products versus exercise therapy for symptomatic knee osteoarthritis: a randomized controlled trial with 2 year follow-up. J Transl Med. 2018; 16(1):355

[35] Goncars V, Kalnberzs K, Jakobsons E, et al. Treatment of knee osteoarthritis with bone marrow-derived mononuclear cell injection: 12-month follow-up. Cartilage. 2019; 10(1):26–35

[36] Di Matteo B, Vandenbulcke F, Vitale ND, et al. Minimally manipulated mesenchymal stem cells for the treatment of knee osteoarthritis: a systematic review of clinical evidence. Stem Cells Int. 2019; 2019:1735242

[37] Centeno CJ, Al-Sayegh H, Bashir J, Goodyear S, Freeman MD. A dose response analysis of a specific bone marrow concentrate treatment protocol for knee osteoarthritis. BMC Musculoskelet Disord. 2015; 16:258

[38] Centeno CJ, Al-Sayegh H, Bashir J, Goodyear S, Freeman MD. A prospective multi-site registry study of a specific protocol of autologous bone marrow concentrate for the treatment of shoulder rotator cuff tears and osteoarthritis. J Pain Res. 2015; 8:269–276

[39] Centeno CJ, Pitts. JA, Al-Sayegh H, Freeman MD. Efficacy and safety of bone marrow concentrate for osteoarthritis of the hip; treatment registry results for 196 patients. J Stem Cell Res Ther. 2014; 4(10):1–7

[40] Giannini S, Buda R, Vannini F, Cavallo M, Grigolo B. One-step bone marrow-derived cell transplantation in talar osteochondral lesions. Clin Orthop Relat Res. 2009; 467(12):3307–3320

[41] Shimozono Y, Yasui Y, Hurley ET, Paugh RA, Deyer TW, Kennedy JG. Concentrated bone marrow aspirate may decrease postoperative cyst occurrence rate in autologous osteochondral transplantation for osteochondral lesions of the talus. Arthroscopy. 2019; 35(1):99–105

[42] Murphy EP, Fenelon C, Egan C, Kearns SR. Matrix-associated stem cell transplantation is successful in treating talar osteochondral lesions. Knee Surg Sports Traumatol Arthrosc. 2019; 27(9):2737–2743

[43] Murphy EP, McGoldrick NP, Curtin M, Kearns SR. A prospective evaluation of bone marrow aspirate concentrate and microfracture in the treatment of osteochondral lesions of the talus. Foot Ankle Surg. 2019; 25(4):441–448

[44] Singh A, Gangwar DS, Singh S. Bone marrow injection: a novel treatment for tennis elbow. J Nat Sci Biol Med. 2014; 5(2):389–391

[45] Hernigou P, Flouzat Lachaniette CH, Delambre J, et al. Biologic augmentation of rotator cuff repair with mesenchymal stem cells during arthroscopy improves healing and prevents further tears: a case-controlled study. Int Orthop. 2014; 38(9):1811–1818

[46] Kim SJ, Kim EK, Kim SJ, Song DH. Effects of bone marrow aspirate concentrate and platelet-rich plasma on patients with partial tear of the rotator cuff tendon. J Orthop Surg Res. 2018; 13(1):1

[47] Centeno CJ, Pitts J, Al-Sayegh H, Freeman MD. Anterior cruciate ligament tears treated with percutaneous injection of autologous bone marrow nucleated cells: a case series. J Pain Res. 2015; 8:437–447

[48] Centeno C, Markle J, Dodson E, et al. Symptomatic anterior cruciate ligament tears treated with percutaneous injection of autologous bone marrow concentrate and platelet products: a non-controlled registry study. J Transl Med. 2018; 16(1):246

[49] Pettine K, Suzuki R, Sand T, Murphy M. Treatment of discogenic back pain with autologous bone marrow concentrate injection with minimum two year follow-up. Int Orthop. 2016; 40(1):135–140

[50] Pettine KA, Murphy MB, Suzuki RK, Sand TT. Percutaneous injection of autologous bone marrow concentrate cells significantly reduces lumbar discogenic pain through 12 months. Stem Cells. 2015; 33(1):146–156

[51] Pettine KA, Suzuki RK, Sand TT, Murphy MB. Autologous bone marrow concentrate intradiscal injection for the treatment of degenerative disc disease with three-year follow-up. Int Orthop. 2017; 41(10):2097–2103

[52] Navani A, Manchikanti L, Albers SL, et al. Responsible, safe, and effective use of biologics in the management of low back pain: American Society of Interventional Pain Physicians (ASIPP) Guidelines. Pain Physician. 2019; 22 (1S) 1s:S1–S74

[53] Ilieva EM, Oral A, Küçükdeveci AA, et al. Osteoarthritis. The role of physical and rehabilitation medicine physicians. The European perspective based on the best evidence. A paper by the UEMS-PRM Section Professional Practice Committee. Eur J Phys Rehabil Med. 2013; 49(4):579–593

[54] Carpenter JE, Thomopoulos S, Flanagan CL, DeBano CM, Soslowsky LJ. Rotator cuff defect healing: a biomechanical and histologic analysis in an animal model. J Shoulder Elbow Surg. 1998; 7(6):599–605

[55] Fortier LA, Smith RK. Regenerative medicine for tendinous and ligamentous injuries of sport horses. Vet Clin North Am Equine Pract. 2008; 24(1):191–201

[56] Ortved KF. Regenerative medicine and rehabilitation for tendinous and ligamentous injuries in sport horses. Vet Clin North Am Equine Pract. 2018; 34(2):359–373

[57] Broughton G , 2nd, Janis JE, Attinger CE.. Wound healing: an overview. Plast Reconstr Surg. 2006;; 117(7 Suppl):1e-S–32e-S

[58] Sussman WI, Mautner K, Malanga G. The role of rehabilitation after regenerative and orthobiologic procedures for the treatment of tendinopathy: a systematic review. Regen Med. 2018; 13(2):249–263

[59] Wu PI, Diaz R, Borg-Stein J. Platelet-rich plasma. Phys Med Rehabil Clin N Am. 2016; 27(4):825–853

[60] Reynolds JF, Noakes TD, Schwellnus MP, Windt A, Bowerbank P. Non-steroidal anti-inflammatory drugs fail to enhance healing of acute hamstring injuries treated with physiotherapy. S Afr Med J. 1995; 85(6):517–522

[61] Mautner K, Malanga G, Colberg R. Optimization of ingredients, procedures and rehabilitation for platelet-rich plasma injections for chronic tendinopathy. Pain Manag (Lond). 2011; 1(6):523–532

[62] Virchenko O, Aspenberg P. How can one platelet injection after tendon injury lead to a stronger tendon after 4 weeks? Interplay between early regeneration and mechanical stimulation. Acta Orthop. 2006; 77(5):806–812

[63] McKay J, Frantzen K, Vercruyssen N, et al. Rehabilitation following regenerative medicine treatment for knee osteoarthritis—current concept review. J Clin Orthop Trauma. 2019; 10(1):59–66

49 Biologics II: Platelet-Rich Plasma

Robert L. Bowers, Walter I. Sussman, Oluseun A. Olufade, David J. Park, and John R. Hermansen

49.1 Case Presentation

A 33-year-old man with chronic right lateral shoulder pain presented to an outpatient orthopedic clinic. There was no inciting event or trauma. He had a previous orthopedic evaluation and had completed over 8 months of physical therapy and a landmark-guided subacromial cortisone injection. A magnetic resonance imaging (MRI) scan (▶ Fig. 49.1) demonstrated an interstitial tear of the supraspinatus tendon, and mild long head bicep brachii tendinopathy.

On physical examination, the patient's range of motion and strength were within normal limits. There was tenderness over the lateral shoulder adjacent to the acromion and anterior shoulder. The patient had positive provocative impingement and biceps testing, but there were no signs of instability. An ultrasound-guided diagnostic injection into the interstitial tear resolved 60% of the patient's pain, and a subsequent lidocaine injection into the biceps brachii tendon resolved the residual pain.

Treatment options were discussed with the patient and the decision was made to proceed with a platelet-rich plasma (PRP) injection. The patient was prepped for a blood draw, and 60 mL of whole blood was collected from the antecubital fossa vein and processed using the Emcyte PurePRP II system (Emcyte, Fort Myers, FL, USA). A two-spin cycle, 1.5 minutes (min) and 5 min at 3,800 revolutions/min, was used, producing 6 mL of leukocyte-poor and red blood cell–poor PRP. The supraspinatus and long head biceps brachii tendon were anesthetized with a mixture of 1% lidocaine (4 mL) and 0.2% ropivacaine (4 mL). The

PRP was then injected using ultrasound guidance into the supraspinatus tear (▶ Fig. 49.2) and long head of the biceps brachii.

The postprocedure protocol involved 2 weeks of rest, and then an isometric strengthening program progressing to a concentric and eccentric program over the next 6 weeks. At the 2-month follow-up visit, the patient reported his pain was 65% improved compared to preprocedure. At the 4-month follow-up visit, the symptoms had completely resolved with the patient having returned to all gym activities. The patient presented 1 year later after reinjuring the arm and examination was concerning for a labral injury. An MR arthrogram (▶ Fig. 49.2) at that time demonstrated resolution of the rotator cuff tear with mild insertional supraspinatus tendinopathy and a new anterior labral tear.

49.2 Discussion

49.2.1 Basics of PRP Therapy

PRP is defined as any sample of autologous blood that is processed in order to obtain a plasma sample with a platelet concentration greater than baseline blood values.[1] PRP is a concentration of platelets and their growth factors, which is then isolated with the goal of facilitating healing and/or pain relief in injured tissue. There are multiple methods of preparing PRP, with various laboratory protocols or commercial kits available. In general, PRP is prepared from autologous whole blood utilizing a centrifuge to separate the blood components. Red blood cells precipitate to the bottom, white blood cells and platelets

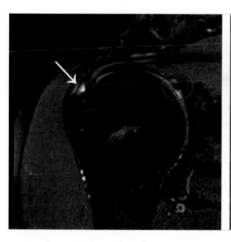 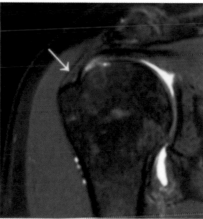

Fig. 49.1 (a, b) Representative coronal images obtained during magnetic resonance (MR) arthrography demonstrating inflammation of the supraspinatous tendon insertion (solid white arrows) and an anterior labral tear (red circle, better seen on axial images).

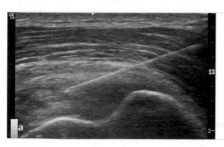 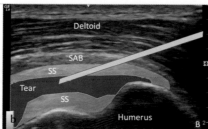

Fig. 49.2 Injection of platelet-rich plasma (PRP) into the supraspinatous muscle. (a) Ultrasound image obtained during injection. (b) The same image as a with superimposed anatomic annotations. Abbreviations: SAB, subacromial bursa; SS, supraspinatous muscle.

("buffy coat" or PRP layer) collect in the middle, and the remaining plasma (platelet-poor plasma) collects on the top. Depending on the PRP kit used and the centrifugation process, different concentrations of cellular components are obtained from the middle buffy coat layer (PRP layer).[2] The normal human platelet count in whole blood ranges from 150,000 to 450,000 µL. Commercial PRP kits vary widely, and after centrifugation, platelet concentrations can range from 0.52 to 9 times baseline depending on the kit used.[3,4] PRP preparations are further categorized into leukocyte-rich PRP (LR-PRP), defined as a leukocyte concentration above baseline, and leukocyte-poor PRP (LP-PRP), defined as a leukocyte concentration below baseline.[5] The presence of erythrocytes (RBCs) in PRP preparations should also be noted, as the iron in heme molecules may contribute to the induction of apoptosis in nearby cells and reduce the efficacy of tissue healing.[6] Furthermore, after preparation of the PRP, the platelets can either be directly injected into the patient or be "activated" via the addition of calcium chloride or thrombin, causing the platelets to degranulate and release growth factors. Overall, multiple variables relating to the PRP product, including platelet concentration, the presence or absence of leukocytes and erythrocytes, as well as the activation status of the platelets are suspected to play a role in the success of the procedure.[7] The clinical ramifications and cellular effects of these different PRP preparations are yet to be fully determined.[5]

In addition to their role in hemostasis, platelets are known to contain a milieu of essential growth factors and cytokines in their alpha granules. Alpha granules are the predominating organelles of the platelet intracellular body and have been shown to contain more than 300 different proteins. The proteins found in the alpha granules are believed to play a fundamental role in normal tissue repair.[8] Notable growth factors released from platelets that are involved in the healing process include platelet-derived growth factor (PDGF), tissue growth factor-β1 (TGF-β1), vascular endothelial growth factor (VEGF), epidermal growth factor (EGF), basic fibroblast growth factor (bFGF), and insulin-like growth factor (IGF-1).[9] These cytokines contribute to a host of functions, including stimulation of cell proliferation and differentiation, chemotaxis and angiogenesis, as well as secondary effects such as increased matrix secretions from osteoblasts and increased production of collagen and other proteins. It is theorized that by introducing PRP into damaged tissue, especially musculoskeletal tissue, the elevated levels of growth and repair factors may augment healing potential and improve pain. However, although therapeutic effects of PRP are often attributed to these bioactive factors, the true biological response to PRP is poorly understood since there is no clear *in vivo* mechanism accounting for the therapeutic effects of PRP.

49.2.2 Limitations to the PRP Literature

Basic science studies have consistently shown the beneficial effects of PRP, but the efficacy of PRP in clinical trials has been mixed. Interpreting the clinical literature is challenging, particularly as many studies have a small sample size.[10,11] The specific composition of PRP can vary from person to person and can also be influenced by patient-specific factors (e.g., gender, medications taken) and the commercial system used to prepare the PRP.[12,13,14,15,16,17,18] The correct dose of PRP is not definitively known and likely varies depending on the target tissue. *In vitro*

experiments have demonstrated a dose-dependent increase in stem cell proliferation up to a certain concentration, but in many studies the commercial system, actual dose of platelets delivered, and/or the specific composition of the PRP is not reported.[19,20] By definition, PRP has a platelet concentration of at least 1,000,000 platelets/µL in 5 mL of plasma which is a three- to eight-fold increase in platelet concentration.[21] Autologous conditioned plasma (ACP) is a platelet concentration that has 1.5 to 3 times the normal platelet, and although it does not meet the threshold of PRP, it is often confused with PRP in the literature. Several attempts have been made to create a standardized classification system for future biologic research; however, no system has been validated and no consensus has been reached regarding such a classification scheme.[7,22,23]

Studies also vary in the type of tear or pathology involved, the method of injecting the PRP, the follow-up period, and the rehabilitation protocols. Outcomes vary according to the tendon treated and severity of the arthritis.[24,25] Accuracy of joint and tendon injections is higher with image guidance, and the efficacy of PRP is likely dependent on accurate placement of the injectate.[26,27,28,29] This makes image guidance preferable during the procedures. Yet, in one review of regenerative and orthobiologic procedures for tendinopathy, only 24 of the 60 articles (40%) reviewed used image guidance.[30] The length of follow-up can also influence how a study is interpreted, and in studies with truncated follow-up it is difficult to know if the PRP had reached maximum efficacy. PRP has been shown to have continued positive benefits at 2-year follow-up in some studies and it is difficult to interpret outcomes in studies with follow-up periods as short as 4 weeks.[25,31,32] Significant variability in the postprocedure protocols also exists and there is a lack of research on how immobilization and rehabilitation impacts outcomes.

49.2.3 Evidence for the Use of PRP

Evidence for Use of PRP in Joints

The majority of the literature on PRP injections for joint pathology is for knee osteoarthritis (OA), with fewer published studies describing the technique for hip OA. There is a paucity of literature on PRP injections for shoulder OA, and only case reports or case series for other joints (i.e., first carpometacarpal, ankle, etc.). Although the basic science is still in its early stages, when used with an appropriate scaffold for osteochondral defects, PRP is thought to promote cartilage regeneration.[33,34] In osteoarthritic joints, PRP has been shown to induce chondrocyte proliferation, synoviocyte production of hyaluronic acid (HA), and decreased apoptosis.[35,36] The reduction in pain experienced by patients may be explained by downregulation of the inflammatory cascade.[35,37]

The majority of randomized controlled trials (RCTs) in knee OA have directly compared PRP to HA. A systematic review by Delanois et al of 11 RCTs on biologic therapies in the management of knee OA found that the majority of studies reported improved pain and/or function in the PRP groups when compared to controls.[37] However, there are limitations to the current literature, including small sample sizes, short-term follow-up, variations in controls and outcome measures, inconsistent dose or number of PRP injections, and differences in the severity of knee OA. These differences make interpreting the literature challenging; however, at a minimum the literature suggests that patients with mild to moderate OA generally have better outcomes compared to those with more advanced disease, and LP-PRP injections have better outcomes that LR-PRP.[38,39,40,41,42,43]

Only four RCTS of PRP injections for hip OA have been reported, and results have been conflicting. All of the studies compared PRP to HA injections.[44,45,46,47] Although Dallari et al found significant short-term improvement in pain with PRP compared to HA at 2 and 6 months, there was no difference when compared to HA at 12 months.[45] The other three studies failed to demonstrate differences between the PRP and HA groups.[44,46,47] Although PRP may have different effects depending on the joint injected, further research is needed to determine if outcomes are truly more favorable in knee OA compared to hip OA.

Evidence for Use of PRP in Tendons/Ligaments

PRP and ACP have been used to treat tendon and ligament pathology throughout the body. Several *in vivo* studies have demonstrated the effects of PRP on tendons, including tendon cell proliferation, increased tenocyte growth factors, and total collagen synthesis.[48,49,50] Despite promising results in basic science and clinical research, lack of standardization and heterogeneity of PRP used in clinical studies make it difficult to come to definitive conclusions.

Advances in the understanding of the pathophysiology of degenerative chronic tendon injuries have increased the interest in using PRP for these disease processes. There have been a growing number of RCTs studying PRP in tendinopathy, but analyzing the clinical efficacy of PRP in patients with tendinopathy remains challenging. For example, six systematic reviews published between 2010 and 2014 evaluating the same data reported conflicting conclusions on the effectiveness of PRP in tendinopathy.[51,52,53,54,55,56] A systematic review by Fitzpatrick et al reported that the outcome of studies is likely dependent on the method of preparation of PRP. This study also found strong evidence for LR-PRP performed under ultrasound guidance.[57]

The majority of RCTs have looked at the role of PRP for lateral epicondylitis and rotator cuff pathology, comprising nearly three-quarters of the 37 RCTs in the literature.[58] Treatment of lateral epicondylitis with PRP has been compared to operative and nonoperative interventions, including dry needling, corticosteroid injections, and arthroscopic debridement.[59,60,61,62] A systematic review and network meta-analysis of 10 RCTs by Arirachakaran et al found that PRP was superior at reducing pain with lower rates of complications to autologous blood and corticosteroid injections.[63] A separate meta-analysis by Chen et al concluded that PRP may provide symptomatic relief for lateral epicondylitis in the short (< 6.5 months) and long term (> 1 year), but not all trials have demonstrated a positive benefit.[58] When comparing PRP to arthroscopic debridement, both treatments have been reported to be safe and effective. The results of a retrospective cohort study comparing PRP to surgical release of the extensor tendon origin suggested that PRP is a suitable alternative to surgical intervention, with comparable rates of pain resolution and return to work.[64] Karaduman et al suggested in their retrospective study that

PRP reduced pain to a greater degree than surgery in the short term and mid-term. However, a prospective study by Merolla et al that compared arthroscopic debridement and PRP found similar pain reductions at 1 year, but better pain relief in the arthroscopy group at 2-year follow-up.[62,65]

Most studies published exclusively on PRP for rotator cuff tendinopathy and tears are under powered, limiting their clinical utility. To further cloud the issue, recent systematic reviews have come to different conclusions on the efficacy of PRP in managing pain with rotator cuff pathology.[58,66] Care should be taken when reviewing the literature to distinguish between the use of PRP injections for rotator cuff pathology and those used to augment arthroscopic rotator cuff repair. Results with PRP used as augmentation of rotator cuff repairs are inconsistent,[67,68] and PRP injections for rotator cuff tendinopathy and tears have likewise shown controversial results. The nature of the rotator cuff disease, use of landmark or ultrasound guidance, number of PRP injections (single versus multiple), and PRP preparation varies across the studies making data interpretation difficult. In addition, some studies targeted the tendon tear with the PRP injection, while some intentionally injected the subacromial space or glenohumeral joint.[69,70,71,72,73,74] Further clinical investigations are needed to better define the role of PRP in rotator cuff pathology.

There are also promising high level data supporting the use of PRP for greater trochanteric pain syndrome/gluteal tendinopathy. An RCT by Fitzpatrick et al compared PRP to corticosteroid injection in patients with chronic gluteal tendinopathy and reported significantly better improvements in pain and function with a single intratendinous LR-PRP injection versus corticosteroid injection. These improvements were sustained at 2-year follow-up.[75] Furthermore, a recent systematic review by Walker-Santiago et al determined PRP to be a safe and effective alternative to surgery in patients with recalcitrant greater trochanteric pain syndrome.[76]

As noted earlier, although the majority of the clinical research has focused on lateral epicondylitis and rotator cuff pathology, PRP has also been reported for the treatment of other tendon and ligament pathology, including medial epicondylitis, gluteal tendinopathy, hamstring tendinopathy, patella tendinopathy, Achilles tendinopathy, plantar fasciopathy, chronic ankle and syndesmotic sprains, and ulnar collateral ligament tears.[77,78,79,80,81,82]

Evidence for Use of PRP in the Spine

In the spine, PRP has been used in the treatment zygapophyseal (facet joint), nerve root, sacroiliac joint, and intervertebral disk pathology, but the majority of published studies address PRP injections for intervertebral disk disease. The results of *in vitro* and *in vivo* studies assessing the effects of PRP on intervertebral disk degeneration are promising. PRP has been shown to stimulate cell proliferation and extracellular matrix metabolism, and the anti-inflammatory and anti-apoptotic effects of PRP may facilitate disk repair and symptomatic relief.[83,84,85,86,87] Disk height and disk hydration also improved with PRP in an *in vivo* animal model.[88]

The clinical literature on PRP for diskogenic pain at the time of this study is limited to six studies, including three case reports or case series, two prospective trials, and one double-blinded RCT.[87,89,90,91,92,93] The RCT demonstrated improvement in pain scores at 2 years, but in this study at 2 months 83% of the control group crossed over, resulting in a single group cohort that could no longer be compared to the control group.[91] In addition, in this study there was a high risk for attrition bias with 23 out of 47 patients lost to follow-up at 1 year.[94]

Recently, the effects of PRP on zygapophyseal joint pain have been evaluated in one case series, one prospective study, and one randomized controlled study.[95,96,97] After confirming the short-term benefits of PRP on lumbar facet joint injections in their prospective cohort study, Wu et al performed an RCT comparing PRP to steroids.[85,86] Both PRP and steroids relieved pain in the short term, but the therapeutic effects of PRP were more prolonged.[97] The literature on the treatment of sacroiliac joint pathology with PRP is likewise limited.[98] One RCT by Singla et al reported that PRP injections for sacroiliac joint pathology were superior to steroid injections at 3 months post injection, albeit with a mild increase in complications such as postinjection pain and stiffness.[99,100] PRP has scarcely been evaluated as an epidural treatment of back pain, with only one pilot study reporting positive results.[101]

49.2.4 Rehabilitation

The literature on rehabilitation protocols after PRP injections for tendon/ligament, joint, and spine pathology is limited, resulting in a paucity of evidence to help guide postprocedure caregivers. Attempts have been made to catalogue variables in the rehabilitation period, but most guidelines are based on expert recommendation rather than stronger evidence.[30,102] Common features of PRP rehabilitation protocols for tendinopathy include a short period of weight-bearing restriction, nonspecific activity restrictions for 1 to 2 weeks, range of motion exercises within 1 to 2 weeks following the injection, a strengthening program beginning 2 weeks after injection, and initiation of dynamic loading/plyometrics at 6 to 8 weeks post injection.

Rehabilitation protocols after PRP injections are often overlooked, despite evidence that mechanical stress on the tendon is needed to optimize outcomes. In one study using a rat tendon model, calf muscles that were unloaded by injecting botulinum toxin after an Achilles PRP injection demonstrated no effect from the PRP injection.[103] Rats that were not treated with botulinum toxin showed neo-tendon development, suggesting mechanical stimulation as a driver in the early phases of tendon regeneration. In a pilot study of PRP for chronic patellar tendinopathy, Kon et al found that subjects who did not follow postprocedure stretching and strengthening programs had poorer results than those subjects who did follow such programs.[104]

McCarrel et al reported that 70% of growth factors from PRP are released within the first 10 min following injection[105]; therefore, a very short period of immobilization (approximately 10–15 min) is often recommended after PRP injections. Some operators believe that there is little diffusion of injectate; in a cadaveric study, PRP with dye injected into the Achilles tendon did not show any significant difference in dye spread after movement of the limbs compared to those without movement.[106] Longer periods of immobilization are not recommended since it is believed that mechanical stimulus, such as early active range of motion, will aid the necessary cellular response for tissue healing.[107] Active range of motion can begin 2 to 5 days after the injection, allowing for the inflammatory

stage of healing to subside. After several weeks, the rehabilitation process should progress from active range of motion and light resistive range of motion to concentric and eccentric strengthening exercises. An eccentric loading rehabilitation protocol has previously been described by Alfredson for Achilles and patellar tendinopathy, and is the most commonly prescribed exercise regimen for tendinopathy.[108] Strengthening exercises should continue during the proliferative phase of healing for up to 6 to 8 weeks post injection. The remodeling phase of healing begins at 6 to 8 weeks after injection; during this phase, the rehabilitation protocol can progress to dynamic functional activity, plyometrics, and return to sport programs.[109,110,111,112,113]

Rehabilitation is vital to the success of PRP injections. However, there is much to be learned in this area since rehabilitative protocols after PRP injections lack strong evidence. Knowing that significant variability in the literature exists, at the very least it is imperative that both physicians and physical therapists understand the phases of healing in order to best outline the rehabilitative process following PRP procedures.

References

[1] Mazzocca AD, McCarthy MB, Chowaniec DM, et al. The positive effects of different platelet-rich plasma methods on human muscle, bone, and tendon cells. Am J Sports Med. 2012; 40(8):1742–1749

[2] Araki J, Jona M, Eto H, et al. Optimized preparation method of platelet-concentrated plasma and noncoagulating platelet-derived factor concentrates: maximization of platelet concentration and removal of fibrinogen. Tissue Eng Part C Methods. 2012; 18(3):176–185

[3] Fadadu PP, Mazzola AJ, Hunter CW, Davis TT. Review of concentration yields in commercially available platelet-rich plasma (PRP) systems: a call for PRP standardization. Reg Anesth Pain Med. 2019:rapm-2018–100356 [Online ahead of print]

[4] Oudelaar BW, Peerbooms JC, Huis In 't Veld R, Vochteloo AJH. Concentrations of blood components in commercial platelet-rich plasma separation systems: a review of the literature. Am J Sports Med. 2019; 47(2):479–487

[5] Le ADK, Enweze L, DeBaun MR, Dragoo JL. Current clinical recommendations for use of platelet-rich plasma. Curr Rev Musculoskelet Med. 2018; 11(4): 624–634

[6] Braun HJ, Kim HJ, Chu CR, Dragoo JL. The effect of platelet-rich plasma formulations and blood products on human synoviocytes: implications for intra-articular injury and therapy. Am J Sports Med. 2014; 42(5): 1204–1210

[7] Mautner K, Malanga GA, Smith J, et al. A call for a standard classification system for future biologic research: the rationale for new PRP nomenclature. PM R. 2015; 7(4) Suppl:S53–S59

[8] Rainys D, Samulėnas G, Kievišas M, Samulėnienė E, Pilipaitytė L, Rimdeika R. Platelet biology and the rationale of PRP therapy in chronic wounds. Eur J Plast Surg. 2017; 40(2):87–96

[9] Boswell SG, Cole BJ, Sundman EA, Karas V, Fortier LA. Platelet-rich plasma: a milieu of bioactive factors. Arthroscopy. 2012; 28(3):429–439

[10] Zhu Y, Yuan M, Meng HY, et al. Basic science and clinical application of platelet-rich plasma for cartilage defects and osteoarthritis: a review. Osteoarthritis Cartilage. 2013; 21(11):1627–1637

[11] Zhou Y, Wang JH. PRP treatment efficacy for tendinopathy: a review of basic science studies. BioMed Res Int. 2016; 2016:9103792

[12] Xiong G, Lingampalli N, Koltsov JCB, et al. Men and women differ in the biochemical composition of platelet-rich plasma. Am J Sports Med. 2018; 46 (2):409–419

[13] Schippinger G, Prüller F, Divjak M, et al. Autologous platelet-rich plasma preparations: influence of nonsteroidal anti-inflammatory drugs on platelet function. Orthop J Sports Med. 2015; 3(6):2325967115588896

[14] Jayaram P, Yeh P, Patel SJ, et al. Effects of aspirin on growth factor release from freshly isolated leukocyte-rich platelet-rich plasma in healthy men: a prospective fixed-sequence controlled laboratory study. Am J Sports Med. 2019; 47(5):1223–1229

[15] Magalon J, Bausset O, Serratrice N, et al. Characterization and comparison of 5 platelet-rich plasma preparations in a single-donor model. Arthroscopy. 2014; 30(5):629–638

[16] Castillo TN, Pouliot MA, Kim HJ, Dragoo JL. Comparison of growth factor and platelet concentration from commercial platelet-rich plasma separation systems. Am J Sports Med. 2011; 39(2):266–271

[17] Kushida S, Kakudo N, Morimoto N, et al. Platelet and growth factor concentrations in activated platelet-rich plasma: a comparison of seven commercial separation systems. J Artif Organs. 2014; 17(2):186–192

[18] Kaux JF, Le Goff C, Renouf J, et al. Comparison of the platelet concentrations obtained in platelet-rich plasma (PRP) between the GPS™ II and GPS™ III systems. Pathol Biol (Paris). 2011; 59(5):275–277

[19] Lucarelli E, Beccheroni A, Donati D, et al. Platelet-derived growth factors enhance proliferation of human stromal stem cells. Biomaterials. 2003; 24 (18):3095–3100

[20] Zhou Y, Zhang J, Wu H, Hogan MV, Wang JH. The differential effects of leukocyte-containing and pure platelet-rich plasma (PRP) on tendon stem/progenitor cells—implications of PRP application for the clinical treatment of tendon injuries. Stem Cell Res Ther. 2015; 6:173

[21] Foster TE, Puskas BL, Mandelbaum BR, Gerhardt MB, Rodeo SA. Platelet-rich plasma: from basic science to clinical applications. Am J Sports Med. 2009; 37(11):2259–2272

[22] Magalon J, Chateau AL, Bertrand B, et al. DEPA classification: a proposal for standardising PRP use and a retrospective application of available devices. BMJ Open Sport Exerc Med. 2016; 2(1):e000060

[23] DeLong JM, Russell RP, Mazzocca AD. Platelet-rich plasma: the PAW classification system. Arthroscopy. 2012; 28(7):998–1009

[24] Jang SJ, Kim JD, Cha SS. Platelet-rich plasma (PRP) injections as an effective treatment for early osteoarthritis. Eur J Orthop Surg Traumatol. 2013; 23(5):573–580

[25] Mautner K, Colberg RE, Malanga G, et al. Outcomes after ultrasound-guided platelet-rich plasma injections for chronic tendinopathy: a multicenter, retrospective review. PM R. 2013; 5(3):169–175

[26] Daniels EW, Cole D, Jacobs B, Phillips SF. Existing evidence on ultrasound-guided injections in sports medicine. Orthop J Sports Med. 2018; 6(2):2325967118756576

[27] Sussman WI, Williams CJ, Mautner K. Ultrasound-guided elbow procedures. Phys Med Rehabil Clin N Am. 2016; 27(3):573–587

[28] Aly AR, Rajasekaran S, Ashworth N. Ultrasound-guided shoulder girdle injections are more accurate and more effective than landmark-guided injections: a systematic review and meta-analysis. Br J Sports Med. 2015; 49 (16):1042–1049

[29] Finnoff JT, Hall MM, Adams E, et al. American Medical Society for Sports Medicine. American Medical Society for Sports Medicine position statement: interventional musculoskeletal ultrasound in sports medicine. Clin J Sport Med. 2015; 25(1):6–22

[30] Sussman WI, Mautner K, Malanga G. The role of rehabilitation after regenerative and orthobiologic procedures for the treatment of tendinopathy: a systematic review. Regen Med. 2018; 13(2):249–263

[31] Gosens T, Peerbooms JC, van Laar W, den Oudsten BL. Ongoing positive effect of platelet-rich plasma versus corticosteroid injection in lateral epicondylitis: a double-blind randomized controlled trial with 2-year follow-up. Am J Sports Med. 2011; 39(6):1200–1208

[32] Park PYS, Cai C, Bawa P, Kumaravel M. Platelet-rich plasma vs. steroid injections for hamstring injury—is there really a choice? Skeletal Radiol. 2019; 48(4):577–582

[33] Marx RE. Platelet-rich plasma (PRP): what is PRP and what is not PRP? Implant Dent. 2001; 10(4):225–228

[34] Kon E, Filardo G, Di Matteo B, Perdisa F, Marcacci M. Matrix assisted autologous chondrocyte transplantation for cartilage treatment: a systematic review. Bone Joint Res. 2013; 2(2):18–25

[35] Mifune Y, Matsumoto T, Takayama K, et al. The effect of platelet-rich plasma on the regenerative therapy of muscle derived stem cells for articular cartilage repair. Osteoarthritis Cartilage. 2013; 21(1):175–185

[36] Dhillon MS, Patel S, John R. PRP in OA knee—update, current confusions and future options. SICOT J. 2017; 3:27

[37] Delanois RE, Etcheson JI, Sodhi N, et al. Biologic therapies for the treatment of knee osteoarthritis. J Arthroplasty. 2019; 34(4):801–813

[38] Duymus TM, Mutlu S, Dernek B, Komur B, Aydogmus S, Kesiktas FN. Choice of intra-articular injection in treatment of knee osteoarthritis: platelet-rich plasma, hyaluronic acid or ozone options. Knee Surg Sports Traumatol Arthrosc. 2017; 25(2):485–492

[39] Görmeli G, Görmeli CA, Ataoglu B, Çolak C, Aslantürk O, Ertem K. Multiple PRP injections are more effective than single injections and hyaluronic acid in knees with early osteoarthritis: a randomized, double-blind, placebo-controlled trial. Knee Surg Sports Traumatol Arthrosc. 2017; 25(3):958–965

[40] Lana JF, Weglein A, Sampson SE, et al. Randomized controlled trial comparing hyaluronic acid, platelet-rich plasma and the combination of both in the treatment of mild and moderate osteoarthritis of the knee. J Stem Cells Regen Med. 2016; 12(2):69–78

[41] Montañez-Heredia E, Irízar S, Huertas PJ, et al. Intra-articular injections of platelet-rich plasma versus hyaluronic acid in the treatment of osteoarthritic knee pain: a randomized clinical trial in the context of the Spanish national health care system. Int J Mol Sci. 2016; 17(7):E1064

[42] Paterson KL, Nicholls M, Bennell KL, Bates D. Intra-articular injection of photo-activated platelet-rich plasma in patients with knee osteoarthritis: a double-blind, randomized controlled pilot study. BMC Musculoskelet Disord. 2016; 17:67

[43] Riboh JC, Saltzman BM, Yanke AB, Fortier L, Cole BJ. Effect of leukocyte concentration on the efficacy of platelet-rich plasma in the treatment of knee osteoarthritis. Am J Sports Med. 2016; 44(3):792–800

[44] Battaglia M, Guaraldi F, Vannini F, et al. Efficacy of ultrasound-guided intra-articular injections of platelet-rich plasma versus hyaluronic acid for hip osteoarthritis. Orthopedics. 2013; 36(12):e1501–e1508

[45] Dallari D, Stagni C, Rani N, et al. Ultrasound-guided injection of platelet-rich plasma and hyaluronic acid, separately and in combination, for hip osteoarthritis: a randomized controlled study. Am J Sports Med. 2016; 44 (3):664–671

[46] Doria C, Mosele GR, Caggiari G, Puddu L, Ciurlia E. Treatment of early hip osteoarthritis: ultrasound-guided platelet rich plasma versus hyaluronic acid injections in a randomized clinical trial. Joints. 2017; 5(3):152–155

[47] Di Sante L, Villani C, Santilli V, et al. Intra-articular hyaluronic acid vs platelet-rich plasma in the treatment of hip osteoarthritis. Med Ultrason. 2016; 18(4):463–468

[48] Anitua E, Andía I, Sanchez M, et al. Autologous preparations rich in growth factors promote proliferation and induce VEGF and HGF production by human tendon cells in culture. J Orthop Res. 2005; 23(2):281–286

[49] McCarrel T, Fortier L. Temporal growth factor release from platelet-rich plasma, trehalose lyophilized platelets, and bone marrow aspirate and their effect on tendon and ligament gene expression. J Orthop Res. 2009; 27(8):1033–1042

[50] Zhang J, Wang JH. Platelet-rich plasma releasate promotes differentiation of tendon stem cells into active tenocytes. Am J Sports Med. 2010; 38(12):2477–2486

[51] Ahmad Z, Brooks R, Kang SN, et al. The effect of platelet-rich plasma on clinical outcomes in lateral epicondylitis. Arthroscopy. 2013; 29(11):1851–1862

[52] Baksh N, Hannon CP, Murawski CD, Smyth NA, Kennedy JG. Platelet-rich plasma in tendon models: a systematic review of basic science literature. Arthroscopy. 2013; 29(3):596–607

[53] de Vos RJ, van Veldhoven PL, Moen MH, Weir A, Tol JL, Maffulli N. Autologous growth factor injections in chronic tendinopathy: a systematic review. Br Med Bull. 2010; 95:63–77

[54] de Vos RJ, Windt J, Weir A. Strong evidence against platelet rich plasma injections for chronic lateral epicondylar tendinopathy: a systematic review. Br J Sports Med. 2014; 48(12):952–956

[55] Krogh TP, Bartels EM, Ellingsen T, et al. Comparative effectiveness of injection therapies in lateral epicondylitis: a systematic review and network meta-analysis of randomized controlled trials. Am J Sports Med. 2013; 41 (6):1435–1446

[56] Moraes VY, Lenza M, Tamaoki MJ, Faloppa F, Belloti JC. Platelet-rich therapies for musculoskeletal soft tissue injuries. Cochrane Database Syst Rev. 2014(4):CD010071

[57] Fitzpatrick J, Bulsara M, Zheng MH. The effectiveness of platelet-rich plasma in the treatment of tendinopathy: a meta-analysis of randomized controlled clinical trials. Am J Sports Med. 2017; 45(1):226–233

[58] Chen X, Jones IA, Park C, Vangsness CT , Jr. The efficacy of platelet-rich plasma on tendon and ligament healing: a systematic review and meta-analysis with bias assessment. Am J Sports Med. 2018; 46(8):2020–2032

[59] Mi B, Liu G, Zhou W, et al. Platelet rich plasma versus steroid on lateral epicondylitis: meta-analysis of randomized clinical trials. Phys Sportsmed. 2017; 45(2):97–104

[60] Ben-Nafa W, Munro W. The effect of corticosteroid versus platelet-rich plasma injection therapies for the management of lateral epicondylitis: a systematic review. SICOT J. 2018; 4:11

[61] Mishra AK, Skrepnik NV, Edwards SG, et al. Efficacy of platelet-rich plasma for chronic tennis elbow: a double-blind, prospective, multicenter, randomized controlled trial of 230 patients. Am J Sports Med. 2014; 42(2): 463–471

[62] Merolla G, Dellabiancia F, Ricci A, et al. Arthroscopic debridement versus platelet-rich plasma injection: a prospective, randomized, comparative study of chronic lateral epicondylitis with a nearly 2-year follow-up. Arthroscopy. 2017; 33(7):1320–1329

[63] Arirachakaran A, Sukthuayat A, Sisayanarane T, Laoratanavoraphong S, Kanchanatawan W, Kongtharvonskul J. Platelet-rich plasma versus autologous blood versus steroid injection in lateral epicondylitis: systematic review and network meta-analysis. J Orthop Traumatol. 2016; 17(2):101–112

[64] Ford RD, Schmitt WP, Lineberry K, Luce P. A retrospective comparison of the management of recalcitrant lateral elbow tendinosis: platelet-rich plasma injections versus surgery. Hand (N Y). 2015; 10(2):285–291

[65] Karaduman M, Okkaoglu MC, Sesen H, Taskesen A, Ozdemir M, Altay M. Platelet-rich plasma versus open surgical release in chronic tennis elbow: a retrospective comparative study. J Orthop. 2016; 13(1):10–14

[66] Warth RJ, Dornan GJ, James EW, Horan MP, Millett PJ. Clinical and structural outcomes after arthroscopic repair of full-thickness rotator cuff tears with and without platelet-rich product supplementation: a meta-analysis and meta-regression. Arthroscopy. 2015; 31(2):306–320

[67] Hak A, Rajaratnam K, Ayeni OR, et al. A double-blinded placebo randomized controlled trial evaluating short-term efficacy of platelet-rich plasma in reducing postoperative pain after arthroscopic rotator cuff repair: a pilot study. Sports Health. 2015; 7(1):58–66

[68] Zhao JG, Zhao L, Jiang YX, Wang ZL, Wang J, Zhang P. Platelet-rich plasma in arthroscopic rotator cuff repair: a meta-analysis of randomized controlled trials. Arthroscopy. 2015; 31(1):125–135

[69] Jo CH, Lee SY, Yoon KS, Oh S, Shin S. Allogenic pure platelet-rich plasma therapy for rotator cuff disease: a bench and bed study. Am J Sports Med. 2018; 46(13):3142–3154

[70] Tahririan MA, Moezi M, Motififard M, Nemati M, Nemati A. Ultrasound guided platelet-rich plasma injection for the treatment of rotator cuff tendinopathy. Adv Biomed Res. 2016; 5:200

[71] Shams A, El-Sayed M, Gamal O, Ewes W. Subacromial injection of autologous platelet-rich plasma versus corticosteroid for the treatment of symptomatic partial rotator cuff tears. Eur J Orthop Surg Traumatol. 2016; 26(8):837–842

[72] Ilhanli I, Guder N, Gul M. Platelet-rich plasma treatment with physical therapy in chronic partial supraspinatus tears. Iran Red Crescent Med J. 2015; 17(9):e23732

[73] von Wehren L, Blanke F, Todorov A, Heisterbach P, Sailer J, Majewski M. The effect of subacromial injections of autologous conditioned plasma versus cortisone for the treatment of symptomatic partial rotator cuff tears. Knee Surg Sports Traumatol Arthrosc. 2016; 24(12):3787–3792

[74] Ibrahim DH, El-Gazzar NM, El-Saadany HM, El-Khouly RM. Ultrasound-guided injection of platelet rich plasma versus corticosteroid for treatment of rotator cuff tendinopathy: effect on shoulder pain, disability, range of motion and ultrasonographic findings. Egypt Rheumatol. 2019; 41(2):157–161

[75] Fitzpatrick J, Bulsara MK, O'Donnell J, Zheng MH. Leucocyte-rich platelet-rich plasma treatment of gluteus medius and minimus tendinopathy: a double-blind randomized controlled trial with 2-year follow-up. Am J Sports Med. 2019; 47(5):1130–1137

[76] Walker-Santiago R, Wojnowski NM, Lall AC, Maldonado DR, Rabe SM, Domb BG. Platelet-rich plasma versus surgery for the management of recalcitrant greater trochanteric pain syndrome: a systematic review. Arthroscopy. 2020; 36(3):875–888

[77] Kia C, Baldino J, Bell R, Ramji A, Uyeki C, Mazzocca A. Platelet-rich plasma: review of current literature on its use for tendon and ligament pathology. Curr Rev Musculoskelet Med. 2018; 11(4):566–572

[78] Akşahin E, Doğruyol D, Yüksel HY, et al. The comparison of the effect of corticosteroids and platelet-rich plasma (PRP) for the treatment of plantar fasciitis. Arch Orthop Trauma Surg. 2012; 132(6):781–785

[79] Fitzpatrick J, Bulsara MK, O'Donnell J, McCrory PR, Zheng MH. The effectiveness of platelet-rich plasma injections in gluteal tendinopathy: a randomized, double-blind controlled trial comparing a single platelet-rich plasma injection with a single corticosteroid injection. Am J Sports Med. 2018; 46(4):933–939

[80] Laver L, Carmont MR, McConkey MO, et al. Plasma rich in growth factors (PRGF) as a treatment for high ankle sprain in elite athletes: a randomized control trial. Knee Surg Sports Traumatol Arthrosc. 2015; 23(11):3383–3392

[81] Davenport KL, Campos JS, Nguyen J, Saboeiro G, Adler RS, Moley PJ. Ultrasound-guided intratendinous injections with platelet-rich plasma or autologous whole blood for treatment of proximal hamstring tendinopathy: a double-blind randomized controlled trial. J Ultrasound Med. 2015; 34(8): 1455–1463

[82] Le ADK, Enweze L, DeBaun MR, Dragoo JL. Platelet-rich plasma. Clin Sports Med. 2019; 38(1):17–44

[83] Masuda K, An HS. Prevention of disc degeneration with growth factors. Eur Spine J. 2006; 15 Suppl 3:S422–S432

[84] Kim HJ, Yeom JS, Koh YG, et al. Anti-inflammatory effect of platelet-rich plasma on nucleus pulposus cells with response of TNF-α and IL-1. J Orthop Res. 2014; 32(4):551–556

[85] Liu MC, Chen WH, Wu LC, et al. Establishment of a promising human nucleus pulposus cell line for intervertebral disc tissue engineering. Tissue Eng Part C Methods. 2014; 20(1):1–10

[86] Cho H, Holt DC , III, Smith R, Kim SJ, Gardocki RJ, Hasty KA. The effects of platelet-rich plasma on halting the progression in porcine intervertebral disc degeneration. Artif Organs. 2016; 40(2):190–195

[87] Akeda K, Ohishi K, Masuda K, et al. Intradiscal injection of autologous platelet-rich plasma releasate to treat discogenic low back pain: a preliminary clinical trial. Asian Spine J. 2017; 11(3):380–389

[88] Moriguchi Y, Alimi M, Khair T, et al. Biological treatment approaches for degenerative disk disease: a literature review of in vivo animal and clinical data. Global Spine J. 2016; 6(5):497–518

[89] Bodor MTA, Aufiero D. Disc regeneration with platelets and growth factors. In: Lana JFSD ASM, Dias Belangero W, Malheiros Luzo AC, eds. Platelet-Rich Plasma: Regenerative Medicine: Sports Medicine, Orthopedic, and Recovery of Musculoskeletal Injuries. Berlin: Springer Berlin Heidelberg; 2014:265–279

[90] Navani A, Hames A. Platelet-rich plasma injections for lumbar discogenic pain: a preliminary assessment of structural and functional changes. Tech Reg Anesth Pain Manage. 2015; 19(1–2):38–44

[91] Tuakli-Wosornu YA, Terry A, Boachie-Adjei K, et al. Lumbar intradiskal platelet-rich plasma (PRP) injections: a prospective, double-blind, randomized controlled study. PM R. 2016; 8(1):1–10, quiz 10

[92] Lutz GE. Increased nuclear T2 signal intensity and improved function and pain in a patient one year after an intradiscal platelet-rich plasma injection. Pain Med. 2017; 18(6):1197–1199

[93] Levi D, Horn S, Tyszko S, Levin J, Hecht-Leavitt C, Walko E. Intradiscal platelet-rich plasma injection for chronic discogenic low back pain: preliminary results from a prospective trial. Pain Med. 2016; 17(6):1010–1022

[94] Burnham T, Conger A, Tate Q, et al. The effectiveness and safety of percutaneous platelet-rich plasma and bone marrow aspirate concentrate for the treatment of suspected discogenic low back pain: a comprehensive review. Curr Phys Med Rehabil Rep. 2019; 7(4):372–384

[95] Aufiero D, Vincent H, Sampson S, Bodor M. Regenerative injection treatment in the spine: review and case series with platelet rich plasma. J Stem Cells Res Rev Rep. 2015; 2(1):1–9

[96] Wu J, Du Z, Lv Y, et al. A new technique for the treatment of lumbar facet joint syndrome using intra-articular injection with autologous platelet rich plasma. Pain Physician. 2016; 19(8):617–625

[97] Wu J, Zhou J, Liu C, et al. A prospective study comparing platelet-rich plasma and local anesthetic (LA)/corticosteroid in intra-articular injection for the treatment of lumbar facet joint syndrome. Pain Pract. 2017; 17(7):914–924

[98] Urits I, Viswanath O, Galasso AC, et al. Platelet-rich plasma for the treatment of low back pain: a comprehensive review. Curr Pain Headache Rep. 2019; 23(7):52

[99] Singla V, Batra YK, Bharti N, Goni VG, Marwaha N. Steroid vs. platelet-rich plasma in ultrasound-guided sacroiliac joint injection for chronic low back pain. Pain Pract. 2017; 17(6):782–791

[100] Wallace P, Bezjian Wallace L, Tamura S, Prochnio K, Morgan K, Hemler D. Effectiveness of ultrasound-guided platelet-rich plasma injections in relieving sacroiliac joint dysfunction. Am J Phys Med Rehabil. 2020; 99(8): 689–693

[101] Bhatia R, Chopra G. Efficacy of platelet rich plasma via lumbar epidural route in chronic prolapsed intervertebral disc patients—a pilot study. J Clin Diagn Res. 2016; 10(9):UC05–UC07

[102] Mautner K, Malanga G, Colberg R. Optimization of ingredients, procedures and rehabilitation for platelet-rich plasma injections for chronic tendinopathy. Pain Manag. 2011; 1(6):523–532

[103] Virchenko O, Aspenberg P. How can one platelet injection after tendon injury lead to a stronger tendon after 4 weeks? Interplay between early regeneration and mechanical stimulation. Acta Orthop. 2006; 77(5):806–812

[104] Kon E, Filardo G, Delcogliano M, et al. Platelet-rich plasma: new clinical application: a pilot study for treatment of jumper's knee. Injury. 2009; 40 (6):598–603

[105] McCarrel TM, Mall NA, Lee AS, Cole BJ, Butty DC, Fortier LA. Considerations for the use of platelet-rich plasma in orthopedics. Sports Med. 2014; 44(8): 1025–1036

[106] Wiegerinck JI, de Jonge S, de Jonge MC, Kerkhoffs GM, Verhaar J, van Dijk CN. Comparison of postinjection protocols after intratendinous Achilles platelet-rich plasma injections: a cadaveric study. J Foot Ankle Surg. 2014; 53(6): 712–715

[107] Dunn SL, Olmedo ML. Mechanotransduction: relevance to physical therapist practice—understanding our ability to affect genetic expression through mechanical forces. Phys Ther. 2016; 96(5):712–721

[108] Alfredson H. The chronic painful Achilles and patellar tendon: research on basic biology and treatment. Scand J Med Sci Sports. 2005; 15(4): 252–259

[109] Yuan T, Zhang CQ, Wang JH. Augmenting tendon and ligament repair with platelet-rich plasma (PRP). Muscles Ligaments Tendons J. 2013; 3 (3):139–149

[110] Sharma P, Maffulli N. Tendon injury and tendinopathy: healing and repair. J Bone Joint Surg Am. 2005; 87(1):187–202

[111] Murtaugh B, Ihm JM. Eccentric training for the treatment of tendinopathies. Curr Sports Med Rep. 2013; 12(3):175–182

[112] O'Neill S, Watson PJ, Barry S. Why are eccentric exercises effective for Achilles tendinopathy? Int J Sports Phys Ther. 2015; 10(4):552–562

[113] Khan KM, Scott A. Mechanotherapy: how physical therapists' prescription of exercise promotes tissue repair. Br J Sports Med. 2009; 43(4):247–252

50 Nerve Ablations (Peripheral Neuropathy)

Ross Bittman

50.1 Case Presentation

A 51-year-old man presented with a 2-year history of constant aching, tingling pain, and hypersensitivity along the left medial calf. He worked as a carpenter, and stated that his symptoms started after he was hit in the leg by a swinging board. His primary care physician and a pain specialist physician attempted to treat these symptoms with trials of amitriptyline, duloxetine, and gabapentin that did not provide significant relief. Topical lidocaine provided only minor, temporary relief. Physical examination revealed constant tingling pain, allodynia, and hyperalgesia along the cutaneous territory of the left saphenous nerve, and no other abnormality. There were no skin changes, and strength was preserved throughout the left lower extremity. There was no abnormality of the right lower extremity.

History and physical examination were most consistent with neuropathy of the left saphenous nerve. Since conservative management failed to provide relief, further intervention was warranted. After consultation with an interventional radiologist, the patient scheduled a diagnostic nerve block in preparation for percutaneous cryoneurolysis. Under ultrasound guidance, the left saphenous nerve was infiltrated with a mixture of bupivacaine and triamcinolone, at a site proximal to the area of pain. The patient reported relief of symptoms within 10 minutes, lasting for 8 hours. After injection, there were no motor deficits, the left medial calf was numb, and there were no other sensory deficits.

After the successful diagnostic nerve block, the patient was scheduled for ultrasound-guided percutaneous cryoneurolysis at the same site. Like the diagnostic nerve block, this procedure was performed on an outpatient basis. After infiltration of the site with lidocaine, a cryoprobe was advanced to the target nerve. Ultrasound guidance was used to ensure that the target nerve was immediately adjacent to but not transected by the probe tip. Two 8-minute freeze cycles are performed, separated by a 3-minute passive thaw. Immediately following the procedure, the patient reported relief of symptoms and had no complications, other than numbness of the left medial calf, which was expected based on the results of the diagnostic nerve block. The patient experienced complete relief of symptoms for about 6 months, at which point some constant pain returned, but to a lesser degree than before. Repeat cryoneurolysis will be pursued.

50.2 Discussion

Peripheral neuropathy is caused by aberrant signaling from injured or diseased nervous tissue. Symptoms vary by the type of nerve affected (motor or sensory) and can include neuropathic pain, numbness, weakness, paralysis, and/or spasticity. Neuropathic pain is often described as prickling, burning, tingling, or shooting. Additional features may include increased sensitivity to pain (hyperalgesia) and painful response to normally nonpainful stimuli (allodynia) in the distribution of the affected nerve.[1]

Chronic/repetitive nerve compression, leading to demyelination and, in severe cases, Wallerian degeneration, is a common cause of lower extremity nerve injury. Unifocal peripheral neuropathies may also be caused by traumatic or surgical transection.[2,3] Other causes include ischemia, radiation injury, and inflammatory processes such as those caused by herpes zoster virus. When considering intervention, it is important to establish that symptoms are not secondary to a systemic process such as diabetic neuropathy, vasculitis, or medication side effect (e.g., chemotherapy).[4] The differential diagnosis of peripheral neuropathy is broad and may warrant pain specialist consultation. Typically, involvement of more than one nerve, especially in a symmetric pattern, indicates a systemic process, although bilateral focal nerve injury secondary to trauma or overuse is possible. Radiculopathy must also be identified, as peripheral nerve interventions may not adequately treat pain secondary to more central pathology.

Potentially useful diagnostic tests include electromyography (EMG), nerve conduction studies (NCS), ultrasound, and magnetic resonance imaging (MRI). EMG and NCS are useful to identify areas of slowed impulse conduction representing peripheral nerve injury. Ultrasound can identify areas of nerve trauma, compression, inflammation, or neoplasm. MRI may be the most appropriate initial study if there is a high suspicion for lumbosacral/nerve root disease.

Initial treatment includes treating the source of nerve injury whenever possible, including removal of any suspected external source of compression and/or physical therapy for physiologic compression, as well as treatment of any systemic illness (e.g., diabetes mellitus, herpes zoster). First-line pharmacologic options for symptomatic relief of neuropathic pain include tricyclic antidepressants and α2δ ligands (gabapentin and pregabalin). Topical lidocaine or capsaicin may provide additional relief. Opioids or tramadol may be considered as second-line treatment options, although they have significant side effects and the added risk of dependence.

For cases of peripheral neuropathy refractory to conservative management, further intervention should be pursued. Certain peripheral neuropathies may be amenable to surgical decompression of the nerve. Other treatment options include analgesic injections, chemical neurolysis, and surgical neurectomy. Relatively recently, percutaneous nerve ablation has emerged as a safe and effective method of interrupting peripheral nerve conduction in order to treat neuropathic pain. Both cryoablation (often referred to as cryoneurolysis) and radiofrequency ablation have been successfully used to treat peripheral neuropathies. Cryoneurolysis has been demonstrated to be effective in treating peripheral neuropathy at many anatomic sites.[5,6,7] Symptomatic relief can last for a period of months to years, and in some cases may allow for permanent relief. Retreatment after the return of symptoms is safe and effective. Radiofrequency ablation of nerves has been studied most in the setting of knee pain (genicular nerve) and lumbar pain (rhizotomy). Superficial nerves can often be targeted percutaneously via nerve stimulator or surface landmark guidance.[8] Deeper nerves, or nerves adjacent to delicate structures, are better targeted with image guidance—ultrasound, fluoroscopy, computed tomography, and MRI have been used successfully.[9]

Complications of image-guided percutaneous cryoneurolysis are rare and most commonly include minor bleeding, pain, or swelling at the treatment site. However, there are risks of nontarget tissue ablation, especially when targeting nerves adjacent to blood vessels or other delicate structures. With consistent use of a diagnostic nerve block at the planned treatment site prior to treatment, unexpected post-treatment nerve deficits are rare.

50.3 Conclusion

Peripheral neuropathy refractory to conservative treatment is often amenable to image-guided percutaneous nerve ablation, which may provide months or years of relief. Cryoneurolysis is the preferred method of nerve ablation for most peripheral neuropathies. A variety of imaging modalities can be employed, and ultrasound is especially useful in the extremities. Complications are rare, and patients are often able to decrease the use of medications that may have significant side effects and/or risks of dependence.

References

[1] Gilron I, Baron R, Jensen T. Neuropathic pain: principles of diagnosis and treatment. Mayo Clin Proc. 2015; 90(4):532–545

[2] Dales JG, Meals R. Peripheral neuropathy of the upper extremity: medical comorbidity that confounds common orthopedic pathology. Orthopedics. 2009; 32(10):758

[3] Bowley MP, Doughty CT. Entrapment neuropathies of the lower extremity. Med Clin North Am. 2019; 103(2):371–382

[4] Katona I, Weis J. Diseases of the peripheral nerves. Handb Clin Neurol. 2017; 145:453–474

[5] Bittman RW, Peters GL, Newsome JM, et al. Percutaneous image-guided cryoneurolysis. AJR Am J Roentgenol. 2018; 210(2):454–465

[6] Yoon JH, Grechushkin V, Chaudhry A, Bhattacharji P, Durkin B, Moore W. Cryoneurolysis in patients with refractory chronic peripheral neuropathic pain. J Vasc Interv Radiol. 2016; 27(2):239–243

[7] Bonham LW, Phelps A, Rosson GD, Fritz J. MR imaging-guided cryoneurolysis of the sural nerve. J Vasc Interv Radiol. 2018; 29(11):1622–1624

[8] Trescot AM. Cryoanalgesia in interventional pain management. Pain Physician. 2003; 6(3):345–360

[9] Connelly NR, Malik A, Madabushi L, Gibson C. Use of ultrasound-guided cryotherapy for the management of chronic pain states. J Clin Anesth. 2013; 25(8):634–636

Index

Note: Page numbers set **bold** or *italic* indicate headings or figures, respectively.